Defibrillation of the Heart
ICDs, AEDs, and Manual

Defibrillation of the Heart
ICDs, AEDs, and Manual

EDITED BY

W. A. Tacker, Jr., M.D., Ph.D.

Professor,
Executive Director,
William A. Hillenbrand
Biomedical Engineering Center
Purdue University
West Lafayette, Indiana

with 110 *illustrations and 8 color illustrations in 2 plates*

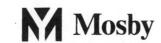

St. Louis Baltimore Boston Chicago London
Madrid Philadelphia Sydney Toronto

Executive Editor: Stephanie Manning
Managing Editor: Laura DeYoung
Project Manager: Barbara Bowes Merritt
Editing and Production: University Graphics, Inc.
Book and Cover Design: Suzanne Bennett
Manufacturing Supervisor: Theresa Fuchs

Printed in the United States of America
Composition by University Graphics, Inc.
Printing/binding by Maple Vail—York

Mosby–Year Book, Inc.
11830 Westline Industrial Drive
St. Louis, Missouri 63146

International Standard Book Number: 0-8016-7292-9

93 94 95 96 97 / 9 8 7 6 5 4 3 2 1

Contributors

Dianne L. Atkins, M.D.
Associate Professor of Pediatrics
Department of Pediatric Cardiology
University of Iowa Hospital and
   Clinics
Iowa City, Iowa

Charles F. Babbs, M.D., Ph.D.
Associate Research Scholar
Hillenbrand Biomedical
   Engineering Center
Purdue University
West Lafayette, Indiana

Francis M. Charbonnier, Ph.D.
Professional Relations Manager
McMinnville Division
Hewlett-Packard Company
McMinnville, Oregon

Nathan Every, M.D.
Acting Clinical Instructor
Department of Medicine
Division of Cardiology
University of Washington Medical
   Center
Senior Research Fellow
Department of Medicine
Division of Cardiology
University of Washington, School of
   Medicine
Seattle, Washington

Gordon A. Ewy, M.D.
Professor of Medicine
Associate Head, Department of
   Medicine
Chief, Section of Cardiology
Director, University Heart
   Center
Department of Internal
   Medicine
University of Arizona College of
   Medicine
Tucson, Arizona

Leslie A. Geddes, Ph.D.
Showalter Distinguished
   Professor Emeritus of
   Bioengineering
Hillenbrand Biomedical
   Engineering Center
Purdue University
West Lafayette, Indiana

Gerard M. Guiraudon, M.D.
Professor
Department of Surgery
University of Western Ontario
London, Ontario,
Canada

Raymond E. Ideker, M.D., Ph.D.
Professor of Pathology
Associate Professor of Medicine
Associate Professor of Biomedical
    Engineering
Department of Pathology/Medicine
Duke University Medical Center
Durham, North Carolina

Janice L. Jones, Ph.D.
Associate Professor
Department of Physiology and
    Biophysics
Georgetown University
Chief, Cardiac Research
V.A. Medical Center
Washington, D.C.

Richard E. Kerber, M.D.
Professor of Medicine
Associate Director
Cardiovascular Division
Department of Internal Medicine
University of Iowa Hospital
Iowa City, Iowa

Karl B. Kern, M.D.
Associate Professor of Medicine
University of Arizona College of
    Medicine
Department of Internal Medicine
Section of Cardiology
University Medical Center
Associate Director
Cardiac Catheterization Laboratory
Department of Internal Medicine
Section of Cardiology
University of Arizona
Tucson, Arizona

George J. Klein, M.D.
Professor
Department of Medicine
University of Western Ontario
London, Ontario
Canada

W. A. Tacker, Jr., M.D., Ph.D.
Executive Director
William A. Hillenbrand Biomedical
    Engineering Center
Purdue University
West Lafayette, Indiana

Anthony S. L. Tang, M.D.
Assistant Professor
University of Ottawa
Ottawa, Ontario
Canada

R. K. Thakur, M.D.
Assistant Professor
Department of Medicine (Service
    Cardiology)
University of Western Ontario
London, Ontario
Canada

John F. Van Fleet, D.V.M., Ph.D.
Professor of Pathology
Associate Dean of Academic
    Affairs
Department of Veterinary
    Pathobiology
School of Veterinary Medicine
Purdue University
West Lafayette, Indiana

W. Douglas Weaver, M.D.
Director, Cardiovascular Critical
    Care
Department of Medicine
Division of Cardiology
University of Washington Medical
    Center
Professor of Medicine
Department of Medicine
Division of Cardiology
University of Washington School of
    Medicine
Seattle, Washington

Patrick D. Wolf, Ph.D.
Assistant Professor
Department of Biochemical
  Engineering
Duke University
Durham, North Carolina

Raymond Yee, M.D.
Associate Professor
Department of Medicine
University of Western Ontario
London, Ontario
Canada

To my family,
Martha, Sarah, Betsy, and Katherine;
and to my scientific colleagues,
whose quest for improved medical
care makes this book possible

Preface

This book is for use as a resource for practicing physicians and medical scientists who have professional interest in the prevention of sudden cardiac death and who use ICDs or external defibrillators in any of the various applications for which they are intended. Two new devices, ICDs and AEDs, comprise the most dynamic and promising new technology for prevention of sudden death. Indeed, technology and clinical application improve the applications almost daily.

Cardiologists, who are the physicians primarily responsible for defibrillation in the hospital, and who select patients for ICDs, will find the book valuable. The book is also for physicians in the emergency room, or those responsible for out-of-hospital use of defibrillators—in ambulances, for example. The book is also written for internists who have a practice with a significant cardiology component or whose practice leads them to refer patients to cardiologists for evaluation of arrhythmic disease and possible implantation of devices to control tachyarrhythmias. It is also for surgeons with an interest in implanting these devices.

Other medical scientists who will find the book valuable are the faculty of medical schools or of biomedical engineering training programs who train the research and development personnel who conduct research and improve, design, and manufacture defibrillators. The students in such programs should find the book to be an up-to-date source of information about defibrillators and defibrillation. The book will also be a resource for the medical device engineers who work for companies that manufacture defibrillators and the companies that provide supplies and accessories for defibrillators. Finally, the clinical engineer or biomedical engineer responsible for equipment and devices in the hospital, emergency room, or ambulance service will find the book valuable.

The book is truly an interdisciplinary one, with chapters of interest to anyone interested in defibrillation, but also with chapters focused on areas of infrequently addressed but critical interest to developers of defibrillators. An example is standards for defibrillators.

This book is not a competitor to the publications, guidelines, or training materials of the American Heart Association. Instead, it is complementary and supplementary to those publications. Likewise, it is not intended as a handbook for the use of defibrillators but as a text for use by those who are seeking a thorough understanding of the many aspects of defibrillation.

In order to make the book easy to read, the authors do not attempt to make it exhaustive. The intent is to include material relevant to the practicing physician, medical scientist, or engineer who is currently active in his or her profession.

Contents

Color Plates 1 and 2 are between pp. 146 and 147.

Defibrillation of the Heart
ICDs, AEDs, and Manual

Chapter 1
Fibrillation Causes and Criteria for Defibrillation

W. A. Tacker

MECHANISM OF FIBRILLATION

Fibrillation is the manifestation of chaotic electrical excitation of the heart chambers, and its consequence is loss of coordinated contraction of myocytes around the chambers. The common element that predisposes the myocardium to this relative chaos is conduction block (either transient or permanent) of cardiac excitation. The block increases heterogeneity of conduction and recovery to produce conditions necessary for initiation and continuation of fibrillation. In combination with other factors and conditions, fibrillation may ensue. The mechanisms by which block can cause fibrillation and the other contributing factors are as follows.

The reentrant, or circus motion, theory of fibrillation is based on findings of Mines[14] and Garrey[7] in rings cut from excitable tissue, and their work demonstrates the phenomenon of reentry. As shown in Fig. 1-1, *A*, if a ring of excitable tissue is stimulated at a single point, the wave of depolarization will travel around the ring in both directions Fig. 1-1, *B*, until the two waves meet each other on the other side of the ring Fig. 1-1, *C*. At that point the waves will extinguish each other, because each waveform will encounter the cells that have been depolarized by the other wave. The already depolarized cells are not excitable, and as a consequence both waves of excitation will be extinguished.

Figs. 1-1, *D*, to 1-1, *G*, depict how transient block due to a prolonged refractory period in one area can lead to reentrant electrical activity. If there is an area of transient block as shown by the crosshatched area in Fig. 1-1, *D*, the wavefront will be conducted only in the lower part of the ring, as shown in Fig. 1-1, *E*. However, since the block is transient, as shown in Fig. 1-1, *F*

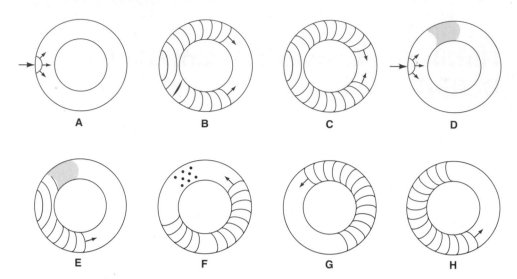

Fig. 1-1, A to **H.** Events leading to established reentry.

(where stippling shows almost complete recovery), the wavefront going counterclockwise will reach the area of transient block after the area has recovered and will be propagated onward, as seen in Fig. 1-1, *G.* Thus the counterclockwise wave can proceed around the ring indefinitely, as shown in Fig. 1-1, *H,* given that the ring is sufficiently large, the wave is advancing at a sufficiently slow velocity, and the recovery time of the cells is sufficiently brief. These conditions assure that the "head" will never catch the "tail" of the advancing dipole.

Recovery times of the cells of the heart vary somewhat and are dependent on many factors. It is apparent that a critical factor in the model depicted by the ring is the recovery time (refractory period) of the cells in the area of transient block, the propagation velocity of the advancing wavefront, and the size of the ring. Conditions that favor continuation of reentrant electrical activity are slow conduction, a short refractory period, or a large ring.[23] It follows that enlarged heart chambers and conditions that block or slow conduction, or change the refractory period of cardiac cells, might reasonably be expected to predispose the heart to fibrillation. Many factors alter these critical variables. In fact, even in the normal heart there is some heterogeniety of recovery time in adjacent cells, which at rapid stimulation rates may cause fibrillation. Therefore the situation in Fig. 1-1 may produce reentry even in normal myocardium, because even slight differences in recovery time of cells in the two sides of the ring can cause fibrillation at rapid rates of stimulation.

Lewis[12] proposed a theory of "reentrant excitation" of the myocardium using the principle of circus motion, stating that a propagated impulse spreading through the heart tissue must always encounter excitable tissue if it is to be sustained. If the wave encounters temporary or permanent areas (islands) of block, it will be divided into two, or even more, daughter waves, which may then be further divided into more daughter waves as more areas of block are encountered. This condition may create complex, ever-changing pathways for the daughter waves to follow as the myocardium is converted to islands of cells repeatedly exposed to rapidly recurring depolarization waves from different directions. In addition to encountering permanent block areas, transient block areas may be constantly appearing and moving in location. In fact, when an island of transient block recovers and is stimulated from one side, the island becomes a source of excitation for all other cells in contact with it. The pathways for reentrant excitation as proposed by Lewis are constantly changing and it is in this respect that his concept is more detailed than Mines's or Garry's.

In chambers of the heart the situation is more complex, because the heart is a three-dimensional structure, but it is easy to visualize that if the atrial or ventricular chambers are completely depolarized before any repolarization occurs, there can be no reentry. However, if there are areas that recover (repolarize) before the entire chamber has been depolarized, there is some chance that the repolarized cells will be depolarized by an advancing wavefront. This requires, of course, that the depolarizing wavefront come into immediate contact with the repolarized cells, and this is a condition that does not normally happen, because the time intervals between normal pacemaker impulses are long enough that all cells repolarize before the chamber is restimulated.

An alternative mechanism was proposed by Scherf and Teranova[19] to be simultaneous activation of multiple latent pacemakers in a chamber. In fact, it may also be correct that multiple pacemakers initiate circus motion and that the latter sustains the fibrillation.

From the examples cited above where rapid stimulation predisposes the myocardium to reentry and fibrillation (Fig. 1-1, *D*), it is easy to understand that conditions that activate latent pacemakers to cause tachycardia will also increase the heart's propensity to fibrillate. Conditions such as myocardial ischemia that may cause conduction block and also activate latent pacemaker sites are especially dangerous.

SUDDEN CARDIAC DEATH

Sudden cardiac death is the sudden and unexpected loss of cardiac function, that is, loss of the heart's ability to pump blood. It is usually due to electrical asystole of the ventricles, commonly referred to as an Adams-Stokes attack, or is due to ventricular tachycardia progressing to ventricular fibrillation.[21] The loss of mechanical function due to these abnormalities of electrophysiology causes death in a very short period of time, which is generally thought to be a few minutes.

CPR

The proximate cause of death is the loss of blood flow and oxygen supply to the vital organs of the body. The definitive treatment for sudden cardiac death is correction of the electrical abnormality, but in many instances the temporary measure is the administration of CPR, or cardiopulmonary resuscitation.[21] CPR is effective in some patients to prevent irreversible damage to tissues and organs, because some oxygenation of blood is achieved and some of the oxygenated blood flows to the tissues. This keeps the vital organs viable during the time needed to prepare for and apply the electrical shocks to restore effective cardiac function. Of course, mechanical failure of the heart due to weakened myocytes will not be effectively treated by electrical shocks, since that disorder is not due to failure of periodic pacing by cardiac autostimulation.

Details of CPR, which is comprised of basic life support (BLS) and advanced life support (ALS), are beyond the scope of this book. The reader is referred to the standards of the American Heart Association for these procedures,[21] but a few points should be made about BLS and ALS. First, Adams-Stokes attacks should be treated by pacing; atrial tachyrhythmia and ventricular tachycardia should be treated by relatively low-energy synchronized shocks from a defibrillator (cardioversion); and ventricular fibrillation must be treated with higher energy unsynchronized defibrillator shocks. Second, the effectiveness of CPR is very limited and will prolong viability for only a short period of time. Therefore, the most effective means for treating cardiac arrest is rapid correction of the underlying disorder, either by pacing, cardioversion, or defibrillation. Third, BLS and ALS are very important methods for prolonging by a few minutes the time during which a patient may be successfully treated for sudden cardiac death. Fourth, it is now generally held that CPR applied by persons having only moderate skills may improve the outcome of resuscitation efforts. CPR has been widely publicized and taught in the U.S. during the past decade, with large numbers of patients having their lives prolonged as a consequence.

The problem of sudden cardiac death is enormous in the U.S., with an estimated several hundred thousand deaths per year occurring, many of which would be preventable with improved use of available medical knowledge and treatment. Of course, not all cases are amenable to correction of the rhythm disorders, since they are complicated by heart failure due to loss of strength in individual myocytes. The approach to reducing the incidence of sudden cardiac death is wide-ranging and includes better education of people about ways to reduce their risk of heart disease, medical and surgical treatment of patients with heart disease, training of professional and lay persons in CPR, and widespread deployment of defibrillators.

PREDISPOSING FACTORS FOR VENTRICULAR FIBRILLATION

Although sudden cardiac death is characteristic of several disorders, by far the major cause is ventricular fibrillation due to ischemic heart disease (IHD); hence the greatest numbers of patients at risk are those at risk of IHD, with the risk factors of increased age, male sex, and so forth. Of course, other causes account for a large number of cases of sudden cardiac death, including other heart diseases, drug side effects, hypothermia, electrolyte disorders, hypoxia and other metabolic disorders, and electric shock. These predisposing factors will be discussed briefly.

The most common predisposing factor is myocardial ischemia and infarction. The insufficient supply of blood, with associated hypoxia, localized metabolic changes, and changes in autonomic nervous system output of neurohormones are conducive to arrhythmiagenesis. This includes the appearance of areas of transient and/or permanent block combined with increased excitability and increased sinoatrial or latent pacemaker activity. Often the chambers will be enlarged due to cardiac failure, and the enlarged cardiac mass provides a more favorable size for onset and sustainment of fibrillation.

Likewise, severe congestive failure from any cause may combine with increased sympathetic nervous system activity and perhaps other factors to lead to fibrillation. Cardiomyopathies may lead to death by either gradual pump failure or sudden cardiac death due to a fatal arrhythmia.

Many of the drugs used to treat cardiac abnormalities, drugs used for other purposes, toxic chemicals, or naturally occurring chemicals or ions cause cardiac arrhythmias as a side effect, and this toxicity may lead to fibrillation. Commonly cited examples are digitalis, epinephrine, and potassium.

Hypothermia is another well-documented cause of ventricular fibrillation, probably due to the effects of cooling to alter myocyte refractoriness. The greatest danger occurs at a temperature of about 28°C, and risk is as great during rewarming as during cooling. Either intentionally induced hypothermia (such as during cardioplegia for surgery) or accidental hypothermia from cold exposure carries the risk, but of course the latter is much more likely to result in death, since it is unanticipated and the means for defibrillation may not be readily available, or even used if the subject is not discovered and treated. It is important to note that the electrical dose for ventricular defibrillation of the hypothermic subject is not higher than for the normothermic patient.[24]

Electric shock is another cause of fibrillation and appears to produce fibrillation by as many as three mechanisms. The first mechanism is the well-known effect of rapidly repeated electrical stimulation of myocardium. These stimuli need not be excessively strong, and they probably fibrillate the heart by stimulation at such a rapid rate that the inherent inhomogeneity of repolarization rates of the different cardiac cells produces transient block and fibrillation via the mechanism depicted in Fig. 1-1. The second is the fibrillation reported by Peleska,[15] caused by the application of extremely strong electrical currents. This ventricular fibrillation is unresponsive to treatment with subsequent shocks, and it is likely that these shocks damage the heart cells directly and cause long-term or permanent changes in both refractoriness and excitability. The third mechanism, called vulnerable period stimulation, is exemplified by single pulse stimulation with a stronger than physiologic voltage during the repolarization phase of the chamber (that is, the T-wave).[25]

Such single stimuli, if they are not excessively strong, do not cause the irreversible fibrillation described by Peleska and must therefore have some differentiating features.

STRENGTH-DURATION CURVES FOR DEFIBRILLATION

Defibrillation with electric shocks, first reported in 1889,[17] requires stimulation of cells by passing an adequate current intensity through the cells for an adequate period of time. The strength-duration curve is the classic way to describe the shock intensity and duration relationships for stimulation by unipolar pulses and has been used for many decades to describe both pacing requirements for electronic pacemakers and defibrillation requirements. A strength-duration curve can be determined by testing shocks of known duration and strength and plotting them as a success (+) or failure (−). Fig. 1-2 shows such a hypothetical plot for multiple test shocks. A line connecting the lowest intensity points that were successful for each duration describes the minimum shock strength required for success as a strength-duration curve; that is the solid line in Fig. 1-2.

The electronic pacemaker is required to stimulate only a small myocardial tissue mass, since the depolarization will spread throughout the myocardium in a normal heart. Hence, the shock intensity required is small compared to a defibrillation shock that must affect a large proportion of the chambers being

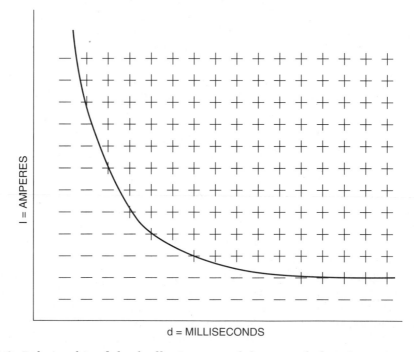

Fig. 1-2. Relationship of shock effectiveness and the strength-duration curve.
    I = current; d = duration

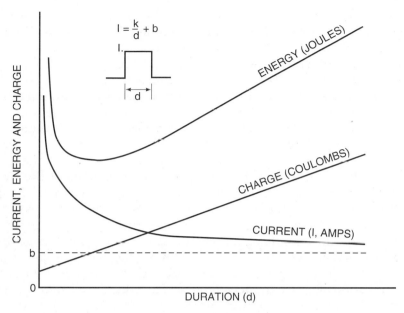

Fig. 1-3. Strength-duration curves for current, energy, and charge. (From Tacker WA, Geddes LA: *Electrical defibrillation*, Boca Raton, FL, 1980, CRC Press.)

treated. In either pacing or defibrillation the strength-duration curve for a pulse of prescribed configuration describes the shock intensity required for a given pulse duration.[23] Fig. 1-3 shows a strength-duration curve for a rectangular pulse, that is, one with constant current amplitude throughout the full duration of the pulse. The relationship between current intensity and pulse durations is described as a hyperbolic curve, and it shows that as the pulse duration increases the current required to defibrillate decreases until a minimum current capable of stimulation is reached. This value is labeled *B* in Fig. 1-3 and is known as the rheobase. The reason the curve does not continue to decrease is that the cell membrane is able to resist depolarization indefinitely at such low current intensity.

DEFIBRILLATION THRESHOLD

From the strength-duration curve we can illustrate the concept of "threshold," which is defined as the shock intensity at a given duration that is just high enough to stimulate or defibrillate. In Fig. 1-2 each of the connected +'s is a defibrillation threshold (DFT) value for a rectangular pulse at the specified duration. The concept of threshold is very useful because it is possible to use only a few shocks to determine the parameters for a successful shock.[2]

Strength-duration curves for energy or charge can also be measured, or they can be calculated from the strength-duration curve for current; energy is the time integral of the current squared, multiplied by the resistance of the discharge circuit, and charge is obtained by integration of the current-time curve. Fig. 1-3 shows strength-duration curves calculated for charge and energy using the current curve shown. Due to the basic laws of electronics, the forms of the three curves are very different. The energy curve has a minimum, which for the rectangular wave and ventricular cells is about 5 milliseconds in duration. The charge curve is linear and increases with pulse duration. Thus for defibrillation with minimum current long-duration pulses (near rheobase) are best; for defibrillation with minimum charge short-duration pulses are best; for minimum energy an intermediate duration is best, as shown by the nadir of the energy curve.

Strength-duration curves for waveforms other than the rectangular wave have been determined, and they follow the general shape of the rectangular wave curve in most cases.[23] The clinically used waveforms (damped sine wave and truncated exponential decay waveforms) have similar curves at the durations used. The behavior of strength-duration curves for monotonic pulses of relatively short duration (which are used for clinical transchest defibrillation) has been found by Bourland et al.[2,3] to follow the "average current law" for these pulses. The average current law states that comparison of pulse effectiveness is equivalent when the two pulses have the same average current.

However, not all strength-duration curves for damped sine wave and monophasic truncated waveforms have this shape. The exceptions are waveforms with durations greater than about 20 msec or waveforms that terminate with a gradually decreasing slope rather than an abrupt ending.[20] It is generally thought that the long pulse or the pulse that gradually decreases can refibrillate the heart after it has been defibrillated.

DEFIBRILLATION PROBABILITY

Threshold is a very useful but not perfect criterion for defibrillation. An alternative to the "threshold for defibrillation" approach is to determine the "probability of defibrillation" for a particular defibrillation shock. Due to the biologic variability of the defibrillation process, a shock with identical electrical parameters may or may not defibrillate. Fig. 1-4 demonstrates the practical effect of biologic variability. The dashed line in the figure shows how defibrillation behavior would appear if there were no variability in defibrillation of a subject, the impedance of the discharge circuit, etc. In that case a shock below threshold (to the left of the line) would never defibrillate, but a shock above threshold (to the right) would always defibrillate. In practice any factor that changes the shock waveform changes the current distribution through the heart, or changes in the myocytes' response to a shock will change the intensity of shock strength required to defibrillate. That is to say it will change the threshold intensity depending on the existing conditions. Considering that the dashed vertical line may move to the left or right as successive shocks are applied in attempts to defibrillate, the threshold will become "smeared" or "blurred." Actually, this will also produce a sigmoid-shaped curve, shown as a solid line in Fig. 1-4, due to the probabilistic nature of defibrillation at progressively lower or higher intensity.

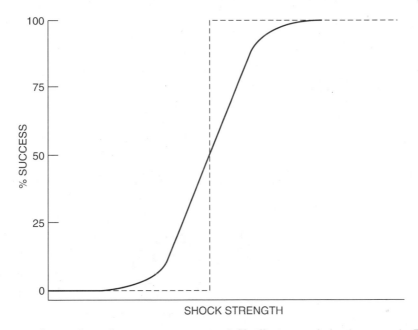

Fig. 1-4. Relationship of percent success in defibrillation and shock strength. Dashed line is theoretical, solid line is empirical.

The sigmoid curve shows the effect produced because of changes in the shock strength required to defibrillate. As shock intensities are reduced to progressively lower intensity, the probability of success will decrease, and within limits the opposite is also true. That is, as shock intensity increases the probability of success will increase, assuming that some other phenomenon does not confound the results. In fact, of course, there are confounding factors, such as the intractable fibrillation of Peleska,[15] for which the heart is probably temporarily defibrillated, but immediately refibrillates, thus masking the defibrillation; or the descending ramp effect of Schuder et al.[20] In these instances, from a practical standpoint, the ultrashort period of defibrillation (assuming it exists) is not of clinical significance.

The effect of strong shocks to obscure or prevent defibrillation has an effect on the strength-duration curve of such waveforms, which is depicted in Fig. 1-5. Success above and to the right of the solid curves will occur only if the shocks are not too long, too short, or too strong. If they are too strong, short, or long, then the dashed curve depicted in Fig. 1-5 will form a "ceiling" for the area of effectiveness, which will then make the curve close in an approximate "ellipse" of success. This "bullseye" pattern was first described by Gold et al.,[10] as shown in Fig. 1-6. In theory it is a very valuable descriptor of defibrillation success, because it describes closed boundaries for defibrillation, and it can be used to describe either 100% success or lesser degrees of success. However, one disadvantage of this method is that it requires many more shocks than threshold measurements do, and therein has practical limi-

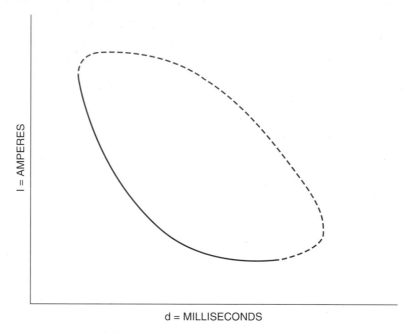

Fig. 1-5. Composite effect to achieve defibrillation with combinations of shock duration and intensity. Area in "ellipse" shows successful combinations.

tations, especially for clinical use or for human studies. It must be remembered also that since passage of time is associated with changes in the shock strength that will defibrillate the long times required to generate the probability curves and "bullseyes" will compromise accuracy of defibrillation criteria. Exact reproduction of a set of concentric ellipses using a subject as its own control has never been reported and may be impractical due to the large number of shocks required. Admittedly, there is no evidence to support the hypothesis that the probability or "bullseye" technique would be more reproduceable in the same subject than the threshold technique.

There are advantages to each of the methods for determining defibrillation success. The probability method takes into account the fact that attempts to apply perfectly identical shocks under identical conditions is impossible, and it emphasizes variability in defibrillation success. This is to say that a shock may be successful at one time but not at another. The threshold method has the advantage of being more practical, because fewer shocks are required to evaluate a waveform's performance. This is true since the S-D curve is known to be hyperbolic and therefore only a few points on the curve have to be measured to characterize the curve. The two are related, of course, and in fact the threshold method does correspond in most cases to a success probability of slightly above 50%, as one would expect. Several investigators have attempted to develop other means (such as unique shock protocols) to measure effectiveness in a way to achieve the advantages of both the threshold and proba-

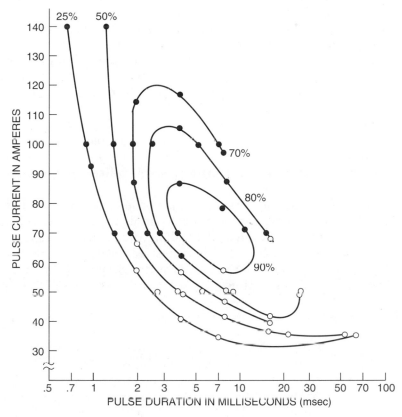

Fig. 1-6. Contour graph for defibrillation success rates. (From Gold JH, Schuder JC, Stoeckle H: Contour graph for relating percent success in achieving ventricular defibrillation to duration, current, and energy content of shock, *Am Heart J* 98:207, 1979.)

bility methods,* but to date no method shows a substantial advantage over other methods.

In conclusion and summary, the various methods are based on the concept that defibrillation success can be determined with reasonable reliability, that the biologic variability makes all methods somewhat limited, and that the trade-offs for choosing a method are practical ones related to the time required and the objectives of the study or treatment being undertaken.

DEFIBRILLATION DOSE

The concept of the defibrillation dose has been that the strength of electrical shock required to defibrillate can be considered analogous to the dose of a drug given to treat a medical disorder.[23] This requires consideration of the

*References 1, 2, 5, 6, 16, 18, 26.

best way to relate the dose to the subject's characteristics, such as the specific medical problem being treated, the side effects or toxicity of the shock, the presence or absence of proportionality of the shock strength to side effects and toxicity, the patient's size, sex, or other factors that would be important in selecting the best shock strength for treatment. The issue of whether divided doses of shock are cumulative either in effectiveness or toxicity must also be included.

Some of these factors have been worked out fairly well in experimental animals, and general principles can be applied clinically, but exact relationships are unknown, and some of the issues involved in the past have been controversial.[4] However, it is possible to identify some principles that are widely agreed upon.

Subject size is one variable for which it has been clearly shown that over a wide range of body sizes, for experimental animals without severe heart disease the shock intensity required to defibrillate the ventricles increases with subject size, both for transchest or open-chest defibrillation with electrodes applied to the heart surface.[8,9] Also, small pediatric patients require lower energy than adult patients.[11] However, it has not been possible to predict with certainty the appropriate doses for adults of varying weights. Many factors probably affect this, but some are of special note. First, there is considerable variability (also in the animal studies) of threshold for a specific body size.[8,9] Another is the altered condition of the diseased heart (for example, metabolic derangement or cardiomegaly) in humans who are shocked in defibrillation attempts. Disease is considered by most investigators to account for some of the variability. Also the effects of some drugs on defibrillation success have been documented. These will be covered in detail in Chapter 11.

Other effects of body size are also important. For example, addition of body mass in the form of fat on the abdomen and hips should have little or no effect on current density in the heart. The added tissue on the chest wall, which puts added impedance between the electrodes and the heart, might have considerable effect. The type of tissue may be important also, since impedance of tissues varies widely. An example of the possible importance of this is the very high impedance of lung tissue (due to the presence of air, which insulates against electric current), which in the barrel-chested, emphysematous patient could make defibrillation difficult due to interference with passage of current through the lungs to the heart.

It has been shown in experimental animal subjects that larger hearts require stronger shocks for ventricular defibrillation.[8,9] This is not surprising in view of the effect of a larger heart in reducing the current density of the shock through each cell. Again, however, application of the principle to humans has been confounded by the effects of disease, drugs, etc.

The effect of species differences is important in determination of the importance of animal studies with respect to human clinical application.

Indirect evidence strongly suggests that humans are easier to defibrillate than animals.[23] Defibrillation threshold for 70 kg animals is higher than the energy for defibrillation of human subjects. Also, with electrodes applied directly to the heart only about half as much energy is required to defibrillate human hearts directly following cardiovascular surgery than is required to defibrillate animals during direct defibrillation experiments without cardiovascular surgery. Some difference may be due to differences in anatomy of the chest and tissue impedance encountered with different animal species.

In summary, it has been shown that important determinants in the defibrillation dose for animals are size, chest impedance, electrode size and location, and species. Other variables that are important are disease, drugs, metabolic state of the subject, and the type of current waveform used.

CRITICAL MASS

If there is a critical mass of heart size required to sustain fibrillation, there may be a volume of myocardium or "critical mass" for defibrillation. This would mean enough cells (that is, a critical mass) must be stimulated to extinguish fibrillation.

The concept of depolarizing a critical mass of myocardium for defibrillation is related to the theory that it is necessary to depolarize enough of the heart cells to prevent spread of wavefronts of depolarization through reentrant pathways. That is to say that advancing wavefronts of depolarization do not encounter enough excitable tissue to be propagated further. There is strong empirical support for this in the observation that smaller hearts do not support fibrillation and that spontaneous defibrillation is common in small hearts.[13] Also, large hearts are very difficult to defibrillate. Finally, Zipes et al.[27] reported that depolarization of about three fourths of the heart with KCl was effective to defibrillate, which supports the critical mass hypothesis.

One theory about the difficulty of defibrillation of large hearts is that some area is not depolarized and hence at least one of the daughter waves of depolarization survives by being propagated through this volume of excitable myocardium that has a mass "critically" large enough to propagate the wave while cells depolarized by the shock are recovering. After recovery, these cells can perpetuate the fibrillatory chaos. It is tempting to suppose that this would be some area far from the current-carrying electrodes, such as the septum of the heart, since maldistribution of current and uneven current density, with low density areas, would be more likely in that part of the heart. Technical difficulties of measuring an adequate number of sample sites in the heart to test this hypothesis have so far prevented obtaining a definitive answer to this question. Nevertheless, achieving even distribution of current is, at present, a major research issue.

REFERENCES

1. Babbs CF et al: Therapeutic indices for transchest defibrillator shocks: effective, damaging and lethal electrical doses, *Am Heart J* 99:734, 1980.
2. Bourland JD, Tacker WA, Geddes LA: Strength-duration curves for trapezoidal waveforms of various tilts for transchest defibrillation in animals, *Med Instrum* 12:38, 1978.
3. Bourland JD et al: Comparative efficacy of damped sine wave and square wave current for transchest ventricular defibrillation in animals, *Med Instrum* 12:42, 1978.
4. Crampton R: Accepted, controversial and speculative aspects of ventricular defibrillation, *Prog Cardiovasc Dis* 23:167, 1980.
5. Davy JM et al: The relationship between successful defibrillation and delivered energy in open-chest dogs: reappraisal of the "defibrillation threshold" concept, *Am Heart J* 113:77, 1987.
6. Fujimura O, Jones DL, Klein GJ: The defibrillation threshold: how many measurements are enough? *Am Heart J* 117:977, 1989.
7. Garrey WE: The nature of fibrillary contraction of the heart. Its relation to tissue mass and form, *Am J Physiol* 33:297, 1914.
8. Geddes LA et al: The electrical dose for ventricular defibrillation with electrodes applied directly to the heart, *J Thorac Cardiovasc Surg* 68:593, 1974.
9. Geddes LA et al: Electrical dose for ventricular defibrillation of large and small animals using precordial electrodes, *J Clin Invest* 53:10, 1974.
10. Gold JH, Schuder JC, Stoeckle H: Contour graph for relating percent success in achieving ventricular defibrillation to duration, current and energy content of shock, *Am Heart J* 98:207, 1979.
11. Gutgesell HP et al: Energy dose for ventricular defibrillation of children, *Pediatrics* 58:898, 1976.
12. Lewis T: Observations upon flutter and fibrillation, *Heart* 7:127, 1920.
13. McWilliam JA: Fibrillary contraction of the heart, *J Physiol* 8:296, 1887.
14. Mines GR: On dynamic equilibrium in the heart, *J Physiol* 46:349, 1913.
15. Peleska C: Cardiac arrhythmias following condenser discharges and their dependence upon strength of current and phase of cardiac cycle, *Circ Res* 13:21, 1963.
16. Peng-Wie H, Rehan M: Genesis of sigmoidal dose-response curve during defibrillation by random shock: a theoretical model based on experimental evidence for a vulnerable window during ventricular fibrillation, *PACE* 13:1326, 1990.
17. Prevost JL, Batelli F: Some effects of electric discharge on the hearts of mammals, *C.R. Academy of Science* 129:1267, 1899
18. Rattes MF et al: Defibrillation threshold: a simple and quantitative estimate of the ability to defibrillate, *PACE* 10:70, 1987.
19. Scherf D, Teranova R: Mechanisms of auricular flutter and fibrillation, *Am J Cardiol* 15:137, 1949.
20. Schuder J, Rahmoeller G, Stoeckle H: Transthoracic ventricular defibrillation with triangular and trapezoidal waveforms, *Circ Res* 19:689, 1966
21. Guidelines for cardiopulmonary resuscitation and emergency cardiac care, *JAMA* 268:2171, 1992.
22. Tacker WA et al: The electrical dose for direct ventricular defibrillation in man, *J Thorac Cardiovasc Surg* 75:224, 1978.
23. Tacker WA, Geddes LA: *Electrical defibrillation*, Chapter 1, Boca Raton FL, 1980, CRC Press.
24. Tacker WA et al: Transchest defibrillation under conditions of hypothermia, *Crit Care Med* 9:390, 1981.
25. Wiggers CJ, Wegria R: Ventricular fibrillation due to single, localized induction and condenser shocks, applied during the vulnerable phase of ventricular systole, *Am J Physiol* 128:500, 1940.
26. Winkle RA et al: Measurement of cardioversion/defibrillation thresholds in man by truncated exponential waveform and apical patch-superior vena caval spring electrode configuration, *Circulation* 69:766, 1984.
27. Zipes DP et al: Termination of ventricular fibrillation in dogs by depolarizing a critical amount of myocardium, *Am J Cardiol* 36:37, 1975.

Chapter 2
Mechanisms of Defibrillation

Raymond E. Ideker
Patrick D. Wolf
Anthony S. L. Tang

BASIC ELECTRICAL EQUATIONS FOR DEFIBRILLATION

An electrical shock is thought to defibrillate by causing current to flow through the heart. The current (I) delivered by a defibrillation shock is directly proportional to the potential difference (V) and inversely proportional to the resistance (R) between the shocking electrodes according to Ohm's law.

$$V = I \cdot R \tag{2.1}$$

The voltage, current, and resistance (impedance) usually vary throughout the shock, as shown in Fig. 2-1, *A*, *B*, *C* for a shock delivered by a truncated capacitor discharge. The resistance increases as the shock voltage decreases.[52,56] The total charge delivered by the shock is the current integrated over the time of the shock (Fig. 2-1, *D*). Thus it is proportional to the area beneath the current curve shown in Fig. 2-1, *B*. The instantaneous power (P) is equal to the product of the voltage and the current (Fig. 2-1, *E*),

$$P = V \cdot I \tag{2.2}$$

which by Ohm's law can also be written as

$$P = \frac{V^2}{R} = I^2 \cdot R \tag{2.3}$$

Supported in part by the National Institutes of Health research grants HL-42760, HL-28429, HL-44066, HL-33637, and HL-40092, and National Science Foundation Engineering Research Center Grant CDR-8622201

15

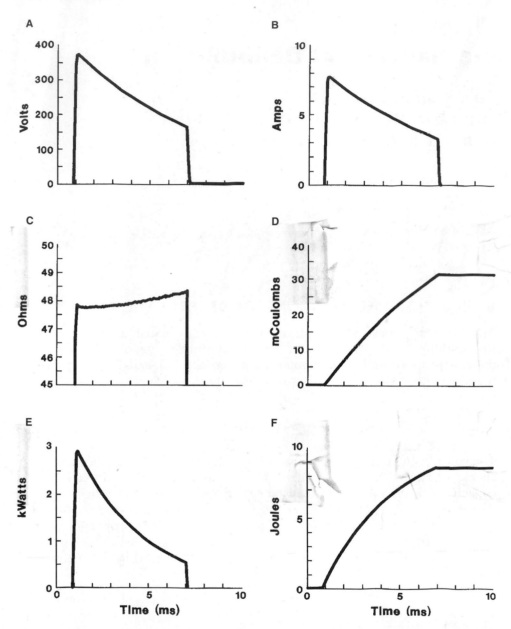

Fig. 2-1. Voltage (**A**), current (**B**), resistance (**C**), charge (**D**), power (**E**) and energy (**F**) for a defibrillation shock delivered by a truncated capacitor discharge. Time is shown horizontally and shock strength is shown vertically.

The energy is equal to the power times the duration of the waveform, which
for a waveform that varies with time can be calculated by integrating the
product of the voltage and current curves over the time of the shock (Fig.
2-1, *F*).

The voltage, energy, and charge stored in the defibrillator capacitor are
usually greater than that delivered during the shock because (1) part of the
shock voltage is expended within the defibrillator to overcome its internal
resistance and (2) the shock is usually truncated before all of the charge is
delivered as shown in Fig. 2-1. All of these quantities can be measured at or
inside the defibrillator and hence do not require measurements to be made
inside the body. However, these measurements outside the body do not indicate how current flow is distributed throughout the heart and thorax. Different amounts of current will traverse different parts of the heart and thorax
depending upon the geometry of the body and electrodes and the resistivity of
the various tissues. The relationship among voltage, current, and resistance in
different tissues is expressed by the form of Ohm's law that is applicable to
three-dimensional volume conductors.

$$\nabla V = \rho \cdot J \qquad (2.4)$$

where ∇V = potential gradient in volts/cm, ρ = resistivity in ohms/cm, and J
= current density in amps/cm^2. The resistivity to current flow is different in
different tissues; for example, it is about three times higher in cardiac muscle
than in blood.[45] Such differences in resistivity can have a large effect on the
distribution of current, as shown in Fig. 2-2 (Plate 1, **A**). Another property of
resistivity that can alter current flow in some tissues, such as cardiac and
skeletal muscle, is that the tissue resistivity is anisotropic, that is, it is different in different directions. In skeletal muscle, for example, the resistivity is
about ten times higher for current flow transverse to the long axis of the
fibers than current flow longitudinal to the long axis of the fibers, while in
cardiac muscle it is about three times higher across than along the long axis
of the fibers.[45]

The distribution of potential (that is, voltage) gradients and current densities generated throughout the heart by a particular strength shock given
through a particular electrode set can be estimated in two ways: by computer
modeling and by experimental measurement. While several different types of
computer modeling have been employed, including finite elements, finite differences, and integral equations,* all of them require estimates of the locations and sizes of the anatomic structures within the heart and thorax and of
the resistivities of these structures. Experimental measurements of potential
gradients to date have been invasive, requiring placement of electrodes at

---

*References 10, 17, 32, 43, 44, 47.

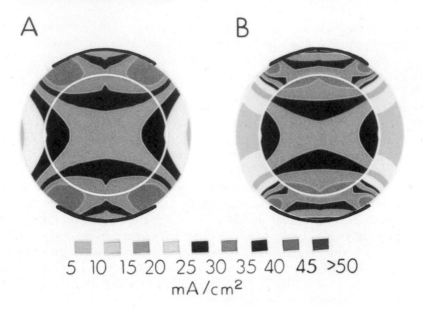

Fig. 2-2, **A** and **B**. Simulation demonstrating the effect of different resistivities on the distribution of current density during a shock. The left ventricular walls are idealized as a spherical shell surrounding a spherical left ventricular cavity. **A**, The resistivities of the muscle and the blood cavity are equal, 250 ohm/cm. **B**, The resistivity of the muscle is 333 ohm/cm and that of the blood cavity is 154 ohm/cm. In both cases a 100 V shock is given across the electrodes at the top and bottom of the idealized left ventricle. Colors represent different current densities according to the color code. The highly conductive blood in B shunts current away from the less conductive ventricular muscle, decreasing the current density in the portions (in yellow) of the idealized left ventricular muscle distant from the shocking electrodes. This figure is also shown in Plate 1, **A**.

locations on or in the heart with a fixed, predetermined spacing or at locations that are determined after the study.[6,53,56,59] Potentials generated by the shock are recorded from these electrodes, and the potential gradients are calculated from the potential differences between electrodes and the distances between electrodes. It is also possible to calculate current densities from the experimentally determined potential gradients using Eq. 2.4 if the resistivity of the tissue at each electrode site can be estimated and if it is assumed that resistivity in the tissue between the electrodes can be obtained by interpolation from that at the electrode sites.

The myocardium can be considered to consist of an extracellular and intracellular space, both of which have a much lower resistivity than the cell membrane that separates the two spaces.[21] Because individual cardiac cells and bundles of cells are longer than they are wide, and because there are fewer connections between cells and between bundles of cells at the sides of the individual cells and bundles than at their ends,[50] resistivity is anisotropic in both the extracellular and intracellular spaces. The anisotropies are different extracellularly and intracellularly, with the ratio of longitudinal to transverse resistivity much higher intracellularly than extracellularly.[11] The potential gradient distributions during defibrillation shocks that have been experimentally measured have been in the extracellular space since the recording electrodes are in this space.[6,53,56,59] Yet it is thought that the shocks defibrillate by changing the potential difference across the cell membrane, that is, the transmembrane potential.[25]

EFFECT OF THE SHOCK ELECTRIC FIELD ON THE TRANSMEMBRANE POTENTIAL

The relationship between the extracellular potential gradient distribution and the transmembrane potential is the subject of much ongoing research. For an isolated myocardial cell, modeling[29] and experiments[31,57] suggest that the end of the cell nearest the anode is hyperpolarized, the end of the cell nearest the cathode is depolarized, and the amount of hyperpolarization and depolarization is directly and linearly related to the extracellular potential gradient (Fig. 2-3). The relationship between the extracellular potential gradient and the transmembrane potential is not yet established for a syncytium of coupled myofibers as occurs in the heart. Some models predict that within approximately a centimeter of an anodal electrode all portions of all cells will be hyperpolarized and all portions of all cells will be depolarized at the cathode.[33,34,41,42] Another model predicts that because the anisotropy in resistivity along and across fibers is different in the extracellular and intracellular spaces, cells will be depolarized only a short distance away from the cathode along a line parallel to the long axis of the myofibers and passing through the electrode. All portions of the cells more than a millimeter away from the cathode along this line will be hyperpolarized (Fig. 2-4). Around the anode the location of hyperpolarized and depolarized regions will be reversed from that of the cathode. In the vast majority of the myocardium that is more than approximately 1 cm away from the defibrillation electrodes, this model predicts no simple relationship between the extracellular potential gradient and the changes in transmembrane potential.[46] Other models predict that the portion of the cells that are toward the anode are hyperpolarized and the portion toward the cathode are depolarized, similar to the case for an isolated myocardial cell, and that the amount of hyperpolarization and depolarization is directly and linearly proportional to the extracellular potential gradient (Fig. 2-5).[33,34,41,42]

For cases in which the stimulating electrodes are more than about 1 cm away, experimental results suggest that the threshold for stimulation of fully recovered myocardium occurs at a relatively constant extracellular potential gradient for a particular waveform independent of location of the myocardium with respect to the stimulating electrodes.[18] These experimental

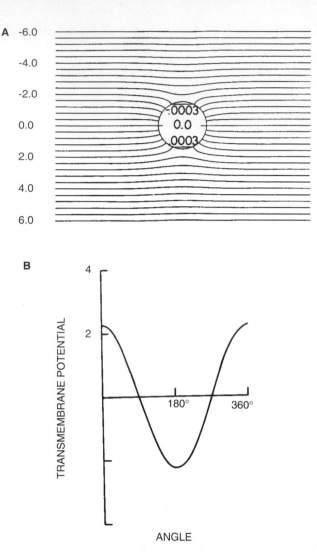

Fig. 2-3. Single spheroidal cell in a uniform extracellular potential gradient field. **A,** The cell is exposed to a uniform electrical field created by the cathode at the top and the anode at the bottom. Extracellular potentials are given in millivolts at the left, with isopotential lines spaced every 0.4 mV. The intracellular isopotential lines are spaced every 0.00003 mV. The potential difference across the inside of the cell is about 0.0007 mV. This is much less than the change in extracellular potential just outside the cell, which is more than 4 mV. **B,** The transmembrane potential in millivolts, which is equal to the difference between the intracellular and extracellular potentials in **A,** is shown as a function of the location on the surface of the cell, as expressed by the polar angle, with 0° at the top of the cell and 180° at the bottom. The top half of the cell toward the cathode is depolarized, and the bottom half toward the anode is hyperpolarized. (Adapted with permission from Klee M, Plonsey R: Stimulation of spheroidal cells—the role of cell shape, *IEEE Trans Biomed Eng* BME-23:347, 1976.)

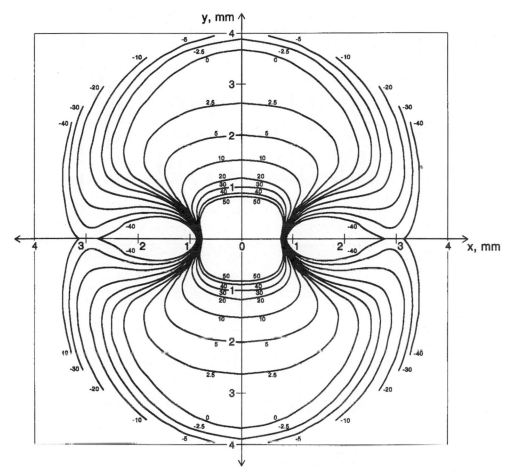

Fig. 2-4. Calculated transmembrane potential distribution for a bidomain model. The cathode is at the center of the figure at the origin of the coordinate system, and the anode is past the periphery of the figure in all directions. Isopotential contours are shown with values given in mV. The long axis of the myocardial fibers is parallel to the x axis. While the region beneath the cathode is depolarized, a region of hyperpolarization is present beginning slightly less than 1 mm away along fibers and almost 4 mm away across fibers. (Adapted with permission from Sepulveda NG, Barach JP, Wikswo JP: A three dimensional finite element bidomain model for cardiac tissue, *Proceedings of the Annual Conference of IEEE Engineering Med Biol Soc* 13:512, 1991.)

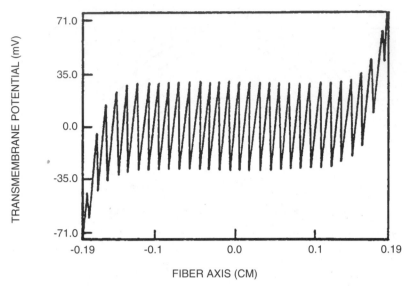

Fig. 2-5. Calculated transmembrane potential in a model that takes into account a high-resistance junction between cells. The transmembrane potential along a one-dimensional cylindrical strand of cardiac muscle, generated by an extracellular cathode at the right and an extracellular anode at the left, has two components: an aperiodic component, which causes hyperpolarization near the anode and depolarization near the cathode, and a periodic component, which oscillates with a period equal to the length of the individual cells of the strand, which is caused by the high resistance between cells. The aperiodic component has a significant value only close to the electrodes, whereas the periodic component dominates the transmembrane potential everywhere else. For increased visibility the periodic component has been exaggerated by making the junctional resistance between cells 17 times larger than its physiologic value. (Adapted with permission from Krassowska W, Pilkington TC, Ideker RE: Asymptotic analysis for periodic cardiac muscle, *Proceedings of the Annual Conference of IEEE Engineering Med Biol Soc* 8:255, 1986.)

results are consistent with a linear relationship between the extracellular potential gradient produced by a shock and the change in the transmembrane potential induced by the shock as predicted by some of the models.[33,34,41,42] However, the value of extracellular potential gradient needed to stimulate an action potential in diastole in the intact heart is much less than that needed for an isolated myofiber. The intact canine heart requires about 0.6 V/cm for stimulation with a 3 msec constant-current waveform when the electric field is oriented longitudinal to the long axis of the myofibers and about 1.8 V/cm when the field is oriented transverse to the long axis.[18] In contrast, isolated frog ventricular myocytes require approximately 1.5 V/cm for stimulation with a 3 msec rectangular waveform when the electric field is parallel to the long axis of the cells and approximately 9 V/cm when it is perpendicular to the long axis.[1,54] The ratio of the stimulation requirements along and across the cells approximately corresponds to the ratio of the length to the width of the cells (100 to 120 μm /10 to 20 μm). One possible reason for the difference in stimulation requirements for isolated cells and intact myocardium is that the myocardial cells are tightly coupled electrically so that a bundle of myofibers responds to an extracellular electric field as a single unit.[34] The end of this unit closer to the anode is hyperpolarized and the end closer to the cathode is depolarized. This electrical unit is estimated to be approximately 2000 μm long and 200 μm wide.[34] A width of 200 μm corresponds roughly to the distances between connective tissue septa observed in the ventricles.[49]

FIELD STIMULATION REQUIREMENTS FOR RELATIVELY REFRACTORY MYOCARDIUM

Myocardium that is relatively refractory requires a larger potential gradient field for stimulation of a new action potential than does fully recovered myocardium.[30] This is true for electric fields oriented along as well as across the long axis of the myocardial cells (Fig. 2-6). Below a strength of about 5 V/cm (the exact value depends upon the waveform and the orientation of the cells with respect to the electric field), a stimulus causes an all or none response.[30] If the myocardium is sufficiently recovered, the stimulus induces a new action potential; otherwise it has almost no effect (Fig. 2-6). Above 5 V/cm an intermediate or graded response can be produced if the cells are too refractory to undergo a complete new action potential (Fig. 2-6).[28] Such a graded response prolongs refractoriness and prolongs action potential duration, but less than that caused by a new action potential. Tissue stimulated to undergo a graded response usually does not give rise to a propagating activation front after the stimulus, probably because (1) the neighboring tissue is refractory and (2) a graded response has less stimulating ability than does a full action potential. The size and duration of the graded response vary directly with the size of the stimulus and the time since the tissue was last activated (Fig. 2-7). For sufficiently strong stimuli, action potential prolongation can be induced almost immediately after phase zero of the previous activation.

It has been proposed that this prolongation of refractoriness by the shock is important for defibrillation.* Prolongation of refractoriness by the shock is a part of the "upper limit of vulnerability" hypothesis for the mechanism of defibrillation dealing with how activation fronts arise after failed shocks. This hypothesis is discussed later in the chapter. It has also been suggested that prolongation of action potential duration by the shock is an important determinant of whether any activation fronts present just after the shock will block

*References 9, 14, 15, 22, 23, 48, 51.

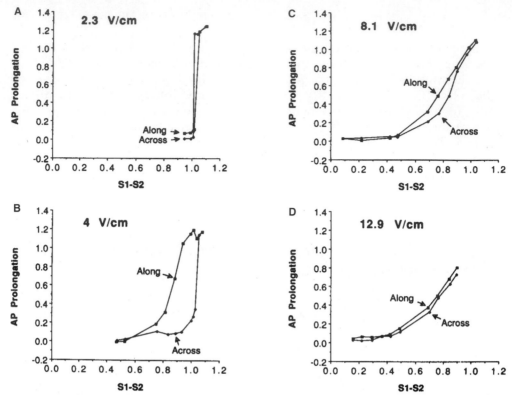

Fig. 2-6. Graphs showing action potential (AP) prolongation versus the stimulus
interval S1–S2 for electric field stimuli (S2) of 2.3, 4, 8.1, and 12.9 V/cm.
Each data point represents a different trial. The results were obtained from
one microelectrode cellular impalement in an isolated rabbit papillary muscle in a tissue bath. The muscle was paced (S1) at a regular rate of 0.5 Hz
and the premature S2 was a 2 ms duration square wave. The S1–S2 interval
and the AP prolongation are given as fractions of the control AP duration at
90% repolarization. The control AP duration, which had a mean value of
147 msec, was constant to within 4 msec. **A**, The 2.3 V/cm S2 given as late as
the time of 90% repolarization of the AP produced only a small AP prolongation. When S2 of this strength was given only 2–3 msec later, a new AP
was produced. **B**, When the 4 V/cm S2 was given as early as the midpoint of
the AP, S2 had no effect. When given late in relation to the AP repolarization, S2 produced a new AP. The 4 V/cm produced AP prolongation when
given at intermediate S1–S2 intervals. The AP prolongation was greater for
S2 oriented along compared with across the myocardial fibers. **C**, When the
S2 electric field strength was 8.1 V/cm, like the results for the 4 V/cm S2,
there was an intermediate range of S1–S2 intervals in which a greater AP
prolongation occurred for S2 oriented along the fibers compared with across
the fibers. **D**, When the S2 strength was 12.9 V/cm, AP prolongation occurred
for S2 given as early as the midpoint of the AP. For this S2 strength, the AP
prolongation was not markedly different for S2 along versus across the
fibers. (Adapted with permission from Knisley SB, Smith WM, Ideker RE:
Effect of field stimulation on cellular repolarization in rabbit myocardium—
implications for reentry introduction, *Circ Res* 70:707, 1992.)

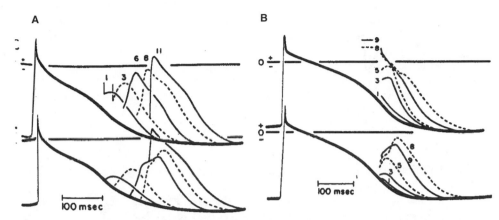

Fig. 2-7. Graded responses in a Purkinje fiber elicited by stimulation at different intervals (**A**) or different stimulus strengths (**B**). The top tracing in each panel is next to the stimulation site while the bottom tracing is farther away. **A**, As a fixed strength stimulus is given later and later during the action potential (complexes 1–8) a larger graded response is produced until finally a new action potential is produced (complex 11). **B**, Similar behavior occurs as the strength of the stimulus is increased at a fixed coupling interval. The two base lines are separated by 100 mV. (Adapted with permission from Kao CY, Hoffman BF: Graded and decremental response in heart muscle fibers, *Am J Physiol* 194:187, 1958.)

unidirectionally in regions of high refractoriness, followed by reentry, which leads to the resumption of fibrillation.[14] Even though different cells are in different portions of their action potential during fibrillation, a particular potential gradient within a certain range of shock potential gradients will prolong refractoriness of the cells in such a way that all the cells recover from refractoriness at almost the same time (Fig. 2-8). If all ventricular myocardium were exposed to the same potential gradient within this certain range, the dispersion of refractoriness present just before the shock would be almost totally obliterated by the shock. Since all cells would recover at about the same time, any activation fronts present would be much less likely to be blocked, and there would be less likelihood of reentry and the resumption of fibrillation.[14]

DETRIMENTAL EFFECTS OF STRONG ELECTRIC SHOCK FIELDS

At higher stimulus strengths signs of damage are seen, such as the transmembrane potential "hanging up" near the plateau voltage for long periods (Fig. 2-9).[38] Conduction block (Fig. 2-10)[61] and inhibition of normal automaticity (Fig. 2-11)[26,27,35] occur at extracellular potential gradients of approximately 60 V/cm or more. Shocks of 200 V/cm lasting 5 msec cause dielectric breakdown of the membranes of isolated chick embryo myocytes.[24] An extracellular potential gradient of 200 V/cm produces a voltage drop across the cell membrane of almost 1 volt, which, because the cell membrane is so thin, produces

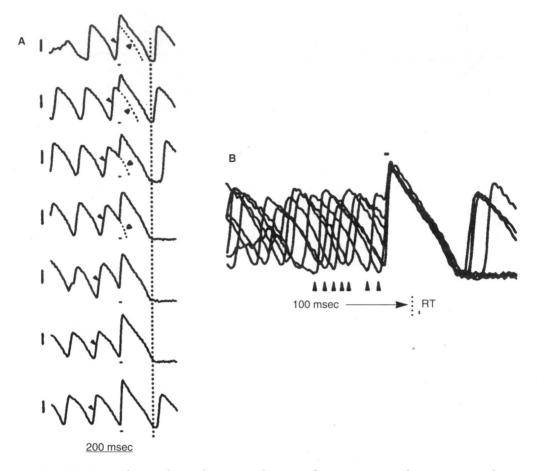

Fig. 2-8. Optical recordings showing induction of a constant repolarization time by a shock during fibrillation. **A**, Seven different tracings are shown. Shock times and durations are indicated by horizontal black bar underlying each trace. Filled arrowheads indicate upstroke immediately preceding shock. The dashed curves marked by arrowheads in traces a–d show likely time course of repolarization had the shock not been applied. Dashed curves were copied from the preceding action potential. Vertical dashed line indicates earliest repolarization time. Optical calibration bars on each trace show size of 1% fluorescence change. Shocks were 1.25 J. **B**, Optical recordings from **A** are superimposed. The horizontal line at the top shows the time and duration of the shock. Beginnings of preshock upstrokes are indicated by filled arrowheads. A constant repolarization time (RT) of 100 msec occurred in all traces. Recordings also show a high degree of overlap from the peak of the shock response to repolarization and give the impression that the shock evokes a single response at all levels of the action potential. (Adapted with permission from Dillon SM: Synchronized repolarization after defibrillation shocks—a possible component of the defibrillation process demonstrated by optical recordings in rabbit heart, *Circulation* 85:1865, 1992.)

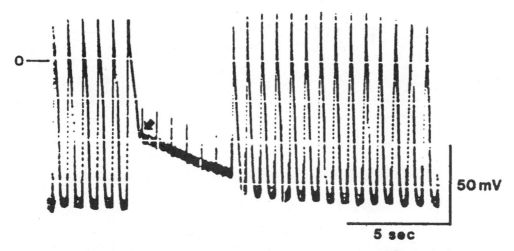

Fig. 2-9. Transmembrane potentials recorded from isolated Purkinje fiber demonstrating that a strong shock causes the potential to be elevated for several seconds. Total energy of the shock was 2.0 J. The energy was delivered as a truncated exponential 4 msec in duration. Note that the recovery of membrane potential was delayed. Pacing was attempted following the shock. The first pacing spike after the shock is indicated by the arrow. The Purkinje fiber was not excitable for about 5 sec after the shock. The horizontal bars note time and the vertical bars note millivolts. Zero potential is indicated. (Adapted with permission from Moore EN, Spear JF: Electrophysiologic studies on the initiation, prevention, and termination of ventricular fibrillation. In Zipes DP, Jalife J, editors: *Cardiac electrophysiology and arrhythmias,* Orlando, 1980, Grune & Stratton, pp 315–322.)

an extremely high potential gradient across the membrane. This extremely high potential gradient causes the cell membrane to break down and form holes through which ions redistribute indiscriminately.[24] The indiscriminate ion flow depolarizes the membrane, causing the potential to "hang up," conduction to be blocked, and automaticity to be inhibited. The number and size of the holes in the membrane and the length of time before they close increase as the potential gradient of the shock is increased.[24] When the potential gradient of the shock is more than 100 to 200 V/cm, cell death occurs.

Results from both computer modeling[10,17,43,44] and from experimental measurements[6,10,53,56,59] indicate that the potential gradient distribution is uneven throughout the heart for the electrode configurations used for defibrillation but is much more uneven for electrodes on and in the heart than for electrodes on the thorax (Fig. 2-12 [Plate 1, **B**]). For defibrillation configurations with one or both electrodes on or in the heart the ratio of the highest to the lowest potential gradients produced in the ventricles by a shock is approximately 20 to 1.[6,10,53,56,59] This ratio is approximately 4 to 1 for transthoracic defibrillation (Fig. 2-12, *C*).[10] For shocks that are just large enough to defibrillate, the lowest potential gradient observed in the ventricles ranges from 3 to 9 V/cm.[35,56,59,62]

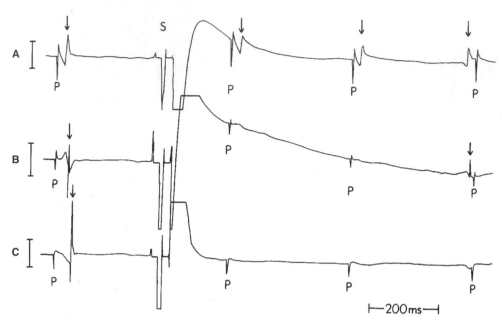

Fig. 2-10. Electrograms from three electrodes (**A, B**, and **C**) for an 850 V monophasic truncated exponential shock lasting 10 msec in which the trailing edge voltage was approximately 56% of the leading edge. The potential gradient during the fourth millisecond of the shock was 54 V/cm at electrode **A**, 63 V/cm at electrode **B**, and 114 V/cm at electrode **C**. No activation occurred in response to the first two postshock stimuli for electrode **B** and for all three stimuli at electrode **C**. The third postshock cycle was spontaneous, occurring before the pacing stimulus. *P*, pacing artifacts; *S*, shock; *arrows*, activations; *vertical bars*, 10 mV. (Adapted with permission from Yabe S et al: Conduction disturbances caused by high current density electric fields, *Circ Res* 66:1190, 1990.)

The minimum potential gradient needed for defibrillation is different for different waveforms. In dogs it is about 6 V/cm during the fifth msec of a monophasic truncated exponential waveform lasting 10 msec and with a time constant of approximately 7 msec.[62] For a similarly shaped biphasic waveform with each phase lasting 5 msec it is about 4 V/cm.[62] To achieve this minimum gradient, defibrillation configurations with electrodes on or in the heart produce gradients of 80 to 120 V/cm or more in the tissue adjacent to the electrodes. Thus conduction block and decreased wall motion may occur in this region for a short time after the shock.

THE "ELECTRICAL PARALYSIS" HYPOTHESIS OF DEFIBRILLATION

Some years before the results from cardiac mapping were available, it was hypothesized that the mechanism of defibrillation was electrical paralysis and

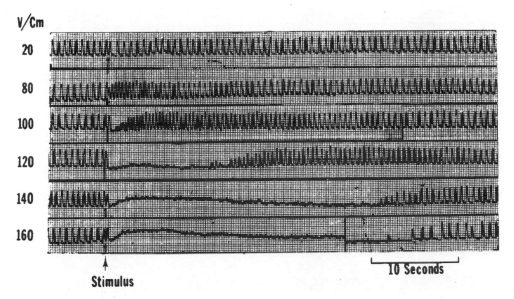

Fig. 2-11. Photocell mechanograms of a cultured myocardial cell before, during, and after 2 msec. time-constant capacitor discharges of increasing peak voltage gradient. Stimuli were administered at time indicated by arrow. Stimuli of 80 V/cm cause an increased rate of activation while stimuli of 100 V/cm inhibit activation for a short time. As the potential gradient increases, the period during which pacemaker activity is inhibited also increases. Ten seconds of arrest have been omitted from lowest strip chart recording (160 V/cm), as indicated by the vertical line. (Adapted with permission from Jones JL et al: Responses of cultured myocardial cells to countershock-type electric field stimulation, *Am J Physiol* 235:H214, 1978.)

conduction block throughout the ventricles lasting for several seconds after the shock.[40] Two findings have since indicated that this hypothesis is incorrect. First, successful shocks do not have to create such a strong potential gradient field (greater than 60 V/cm) throughout the ventricles to defibrillate (Fig. 2-13).[56,59] Second, one or two rapid activations frequently occur in the first 200 msec following a successful defibrillation shock.[8,39,63]

THE "CRITICAL MASS" HYPOTHESIS OF DEFIBRILLATION

This second finding led to the critical mass hypothesis of defibrillation.[39,63] It was assumed that the activation observed almost immediately following a successful defibrillation shock signified that it was not necessary for all fibrillation activation fronts to be halted by the shock for defibrillation to occur. It was hypothesized that for successful defibrillation fibrillation activation fronts had to be halted only within a certain critical mass of myocardium (perhaps 75% of the ventricular mass). Based on the concept of a critical mass of myocardium needed to sustain fibrillation,[20] it was assumed that any

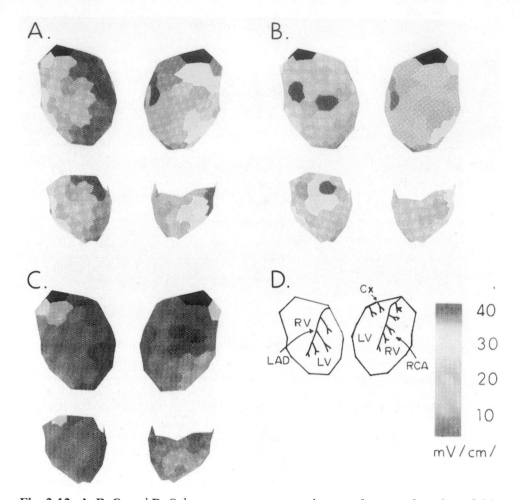

Fig. 2-12, A, B, C, and **D**. Color computer-generated maps of potential gradient fields generated by different defibrillation electrode configurations in a dog. **A**, The field for configuration (cathode→anode) V→P. **B,** The field for configuration V+O→P, where *V* represents a right ventricular apex catheter electrode, *A* a right atrial catheter electrode, *O* a right ventricular outflow tract catheter electrode, and *P* a cutaneous patch electrode on the left side of the thorax. **C,** The potential gradient field for a transthoracic shock given between electrodes on the right superior and left inferior portions of the anterior thorax in a dog. The endocardial surface of the heart is shown in the top two illustrations of each panel. The epicardial surface of the heart is shown in the bottom two illustrations of each panel. The two illustrations on the left show the anterior surface and the two illustrations on the right the posterior surface. The atria are not shown. The colors demonstrate the potential gradient distribution throughout the ventricular myocardium expressed in millivolts per centimeter per volt of shock. **D,** The color scale used to represent the potential gradient values. Black indicates a missing value. The difference between the highest and lowest potential gradient in the heart is much less in **C** for a transthoracic shock than for those electrode configurations shown in **A** and **B** in which at least one electrode is within the ventricles. This figure is also shown in Plate 1, **B**. *LAD*, left anterior descending coronary artery; *RCA*, right coronary artery; *CX*, circumflex coronary artery; *RV*, right ventricle; *LV*, left ventricle. (Adapted with permission from Tang ASL et al: Three-dimensional potential gradiant fields generated by intracardiac catheter and cutaneous patch electrodes, *Circulation* 85:1857, 1992.)

GRADIENT FIELD

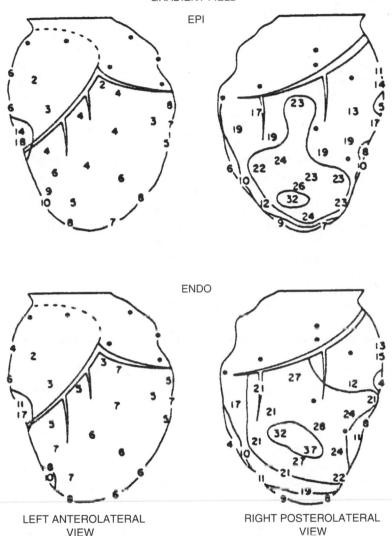

Fig. 2-13. The potential gradient field created in a dog heart by a 500 V defibrillation shock from a catheter electrode in the right ventricular apex and a cutaneous patch electrode at the left lower thorax. The numbers are the potential gradients at each recording site in volts per centimeter. Asterisks represent the top row of electrodes on the atria and the right ventricular outflow tract where potential gradients are not calculated because no recording sites are above them. Solid circles represent locations where potential gradients are not calculated, either because potentials at those locations are inadequate for interpretation or the exact location of that electrode is not known. Isogradient lines are separated by 10 V/cm. (Adapted with permission from Tang ASL et al: Measurement of defibrillation shock potential distributions and activation sequences of the heart in three dimensions, *Proc IEEE* 76:1176, 1988.)

activation fronts in the myocardium not included in this critical mass were incapable of maintaining fibrillation and died out after one or two cycles.[39,63]

Several recent observations from cardiac mapping are consistent with the critical mass hypothesis of defibrillation. Following very small shocks that are much weaker than needed to defibrillate and that are delivered from small defibrillation electrodes on the epicardium of dogs, activation fronts appear almost immediately after the shock in almost all portions of the ventricles.[48] This finding is consistent with the interpretation that the shock field is too weak to halt fibrillation activation fronts throughout the heart. As the shock strength is progressively increased, the region around the defibrillation electrodes in which the potential gradient exceeds approximately 6 V/cm (for a typical monophasic waveform) becomes larger, and activation fronts no longer arise from this region. This is consistent with the interpretation that a gradient of more than 6 V/cm is needed to halt the fibrillation activation fronts. For a shock just slightly weaker than that needed to defibrillate, only a portion of the ventricles is exposed to a potential gradient less than about 6 V/cm (Fig. 2-13),[56] and activation fronts following the shock arise principally from this region (Fig. 2-14). This is consistent with the interpretation that the shock was too weak to halt the fibrillation activation fronts in this region, which was just slightly larger than the minimum mass of myocardium needed to sustain fibrillation.

A second observation consistent with the critical mass hypothesis for defibrillation is the experimental finding that the earliest activation time recorded following an unsuccessful shock is approximately the time that this portion of myocardium would be predicted to activate during fibrillation if the shock had not been given.[59] This finding is consistent with the interpretation that the shock is so weak in this low gradient region that it has no effect on the activation sequence in that region (Fig. 2-15, *B*).

Recent cardiac mapping findings do not support the hypothesis that shocks slightly smaller than needed to defibrillate fail because they are too weak to alter the sequence of activation in those cardiac regions exposed to the lowest potential gradients.[9,62] While the first few activation sequences following such a failed defibrillation shock are sufficiently organized that they can be mapped with 128 electrodes spaced 1 to 2 cm apart throughout the ventricular free walls (Fig. 2-14), fibrillation just before the shock is much more complex and requires that the recording electrodes be more closely spaced to map the fibrillation activation sequences. Two studies have employed either plunge-needle electrodes spaced 5 mm apart to record the three-dimensional spread of activation[9] or epicardial electrodes spaced 3.8 mm apart to record the epicardial spread of activation[62] during ventricular fibrillation just before a defibrillation shock as well as the course of any activation fronts just after the shock. Fifteen seconds after the electrical induction of ventricular fibrillation in dogs fibrillation activation fronts followed pathways that were typically several centimeters in length, that could be tracked for up to 100 msec, and that frequently exhibited some similarity from cycle to cycle (Fig. 2-16).

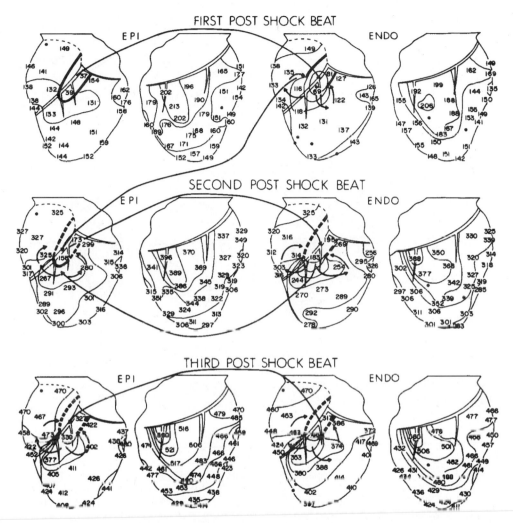

Fig. 2-14. The postshock activation sequence following an unsuccessful 500 V shock in the same animal as in Fig. 2-13. The first three postshock cycles leading to the resumption of ventricular fibrillation are presented. The numbers are the times in milliseconds of the local activations, timed from the beginning of the defibrillation shock. Isochronal lines are separated by 20 ms. Solid circles represent sites of electrodes where adequate recordings were not obtained. The solid bars signify conduction block; the dashed bars signify a frame shift from one isochronal map to the next. Such frame lines are necessary whenever a continuous process such as reentrant activation is illustrated by a series of static maps. (Adapted with permission from Tang ASL et al: Measurement of defibrillation shock potential distributions and activation sequences of the heart in three dimensions, *Proc IEEE* 76:1176, 1988.)

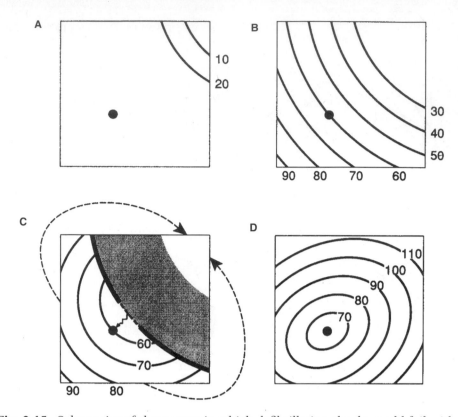

Fig. 2-15. Schematics of three ways in which defibrillation shocks could fail without altering the time interval between successive activations at an electrode site. The large black dot indicates site of earliest recorded postshock activation. Timings of activation and shock in subsequent panels are given with regard to the earliest activation registered in **A**. **A**, Passage of a VF activation front just before the shock with isochrones spaced every 10 msec. Activation traverses upper-right-hand corner of mapped region until shock is given at 20 msec. **B**, The shock is so weak that it does not alter the passage of the activation front so that activation continues smoothly across the mapped region. The electrode represented by the large dot activates at 60 msec. **C** and **D**, Two different mechanisms by which a shock could alter the VF activation front shown in **B** without altering the postshock activation time at marked electrode. **C**, The shock directly activates the shaded area. After the shock, a new activation front with a different activation sequence propagates away from the central portion of the lower-left-hand border of the directly activated region. Because tissue in this region is highly refractory, conduction velocity is very slow, as indicated by the jagged arrow, so the electrode at the large dot again records an activation at 60 msec. Two wide lines at the border of the directly activated area represent conduction block, caused by a graded response in these zones. As indicated by the two dashed lines, activation may then propagate around the lines of block to initiate reentry in a "figure-eight" pattern leading to the resumption of VF. **D**, The VF activation front is halted by the shock, but after a 40 msec pause, a new activation front with a focal activation pattern arises near the electrode shown by the large dot, which again activates at 60 msec and reinitiates VF. (Adapted with permission from Chen P-S, Wolf PD, Ideker RE: Mechanism of cardiac defibrillation—a different point of view, *Circulation* 84:913, 1991.)

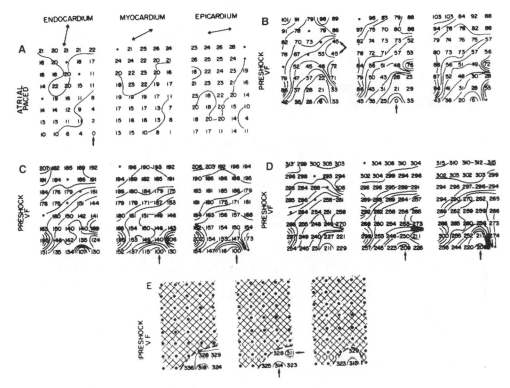

Fig. 2-16. Unidirectional conduction after an unsuccessful defibrillation shock. The three maps from left to right in each panel represent the endocardial, myocardial, and epicardial layers of recording electrodes, located in the right ventricular outflow tract of a dog. The electrodes in each map are 5 cm apart. Arrows indicate the site of early activation. Small closed circles indicate electrode sites where adequate recordings were not obtained. The isochronal lines are 10 msec apart. Occasionally, double activations were observed in certain channels, probably representing two activation fronts activating or electrotonically influencing either the same region or adjacent regions near the recording electrode. The timing of the second activation is shown under the first. The general direction of myocardial fiber orientation at each layer is parallel to the double-headed arrows above the isochronal maps of **A. A**, Patterns of activation during atrial paced rhythm. **B-E**, Consecutive activations during ventricular fibrillation (VF) immediately before the shock. Time zero is the time of the earliest activation in **B**. The shock occurred at 350 msec. The shock was delivered before the fourth mapped activation front had completely traversed the tissue **E**. The area not yet activated by this front at the time of the shock is crosshatched and the electrode location in this area are marked by asterisks. (Adapted with permission from Chen P-S et al: Comparison of activation during ventricular fibrillation and following unsuccessful defibrillation shocks in open-chest dogs, *Circ Res* 66:1544, 1990.)

Continued

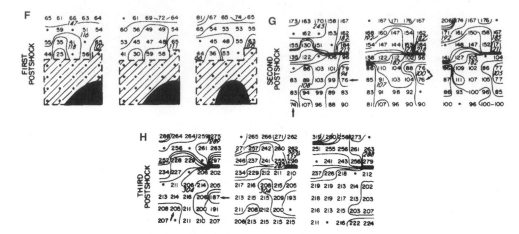

Fig. 2-16, cont'd.

F-H, The first three activations following the shock with the time of the shock as time zero. The region shown in black in **F** was probably refractory at the time of the shock because it activated just before the shock, whereas the hatched region with electrodes represented by dots may have been directly excited by the shock because it was the most recovered at the time of the shock. This response is similar to that diagrammed in Fig. 2-15, *C*.

Because of this moderate amount of organization during fibrillation, it was possible to predict to a certain extent what the sequence of activation should be for a few tens of milliseconds into the future if this sequence were not altered by a shock. In almost all cases an unsuccessful shock slightly weaker than needed to defibrillate was found to alter the sequence of activation in the ventricular regions exposed to the lowest potential gradients (Figs. 2-16, 2-17). This finding is controversial because the minimum electrode spacing necessary to map activation sequences during fibrillation is not yet definitely known.[2,60]

THE "UPPER LIMIT OF VULNERABILITY" HYPOTHESIS OF DEFIBRILLATION

If the finding illustrated in Fig. 2-16 is true, it can be explained by the upper limit of vulnerability hypothesis of defibrillation,[7] as illustrated in Fig. 2-15, *C*. The upper limit of vulnerability hypothesis for defibrillation states that for a shock to defibrillate, it must not only halt activation fronts by directly exciting or prolonging the refractoriness of the myocardium just in front of these activation fronts but must also not give rise to new activation fronts at the border of the directly excited region that reinitiate fibrillation. Since the shock field in this region ranges from about 3 to 9 V/cm, which is higher than the approximately 1 V/cm needed to excite fully recovered myocardium, most tissue that is relatively refractory should be directly excited by the shock field

ENDOCARDIUM   MYOCARDIUM   EPICARDIUM

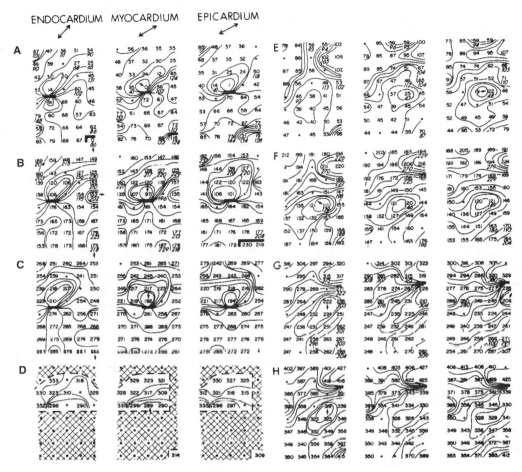

Fig. 2-17. Early postshock cycles exhibiting a repeating focal pattern of activation. Symbols are the same as for Fig. 2-16. **A-D,** Activation before the shock repeats in a "figure-eight" pattern of reentry. The shock occurred at 343 msec. **E-H,** Repeating focal patterns of activation after the shock. This response is similar to that diagrammed in Fig. 2-15, *D*. (Adapted with permission from Chen P-S et al: Comparison of activation during ventricular fibrillation and following unsuccessful defibrillation shocks in open-chest dogs, *Circ Res* 66:1544, 1990.)

(shaded region in Fig. 2-15, *C*). Myocardium that is too refractory to be directly excited by the shock, but which is exposed to a potential gradient less than about 5 V/cm, will be largely unaffected by the shock. After the shock, an activation front will form at the border between this tissue and the tissue that was directly excited by the shock and slowly propagate into the tissue that was not directly excited by the shock as this tissue becomes less refractory with time after the shock (Fig. 2-15, *C*). Myocardium that is just a little too refractory to be excited by the shock and that is exposed to a potential gradient greater than about 5 V/cm will have its refractoriness prolonged by the shock. Therefore, activation after the shock cannot propagate into this tissue from the border of the region directly excited by the shock (Fig. 2-15, *C*). After this region recovers, activation fronts arising in tissue exposed to a potential gradient of less than 5 V/cm can propagate into the region, form reentrant pathways, and reinduce fibrillation. According to the upper limit of vulnerability hypothesis for defibrillation, even though the shock field was sufficiently strong (1) to directly excite myocardium at all points in front of the advancing activation fronts during fibrillation and (2) to alter the activation sequence throughout the region, the shock still failed to defibrillate because it gave rise to new activation fronts that reinitiated fibrillation.[8] According to this interpretation, earliest sites of activation following shocks that are not quite strong enough to defibrillate first appear in the regions exposed to the lowest shock potential gradient. This occurs because the potential gradient in this region is less than the critical value of approximately 5 V/cm so that activation fronts appear at the border of the regions directly excited by the shock and not because the shock was too weak to affect the preshock activation fronts in this region. The reason that this site of earliest postshock excitation activates at approximately the same time as if the shock had not been given is that, whether or not the shock is given, this site activates almost as soon as it passes out of its refractory period and its refractory period is only slightly changed by the shock.

The manner in which the shock reinduces fibrillation in Fig. 2-15, *C*, is similar to the mechanism by which a large premature stimulus is thought to induce fibrillation when given during the vulnerable period of regular rhythm (Fig. 2-18).[5,19] This mechanism was predicted by Winfree,[58] based on an analysis of certain nonlinear systems. These results suggest that if the stimulus field is everywhere above the critical value of approximately 5 V/cm, refractory periods will be prolonged everywhere adjacent to all directly excited regions, and no activation fronts will form following the stimulus. Thus if a shock is sufficiently strong (but not so strong that it damages tissue, giving rise to activation fronts in the tissue exposed to very high gradients), it will not initiate fibrillation no matter when it is given during the vulnerable period of regular rhythm. This exact result has been found experimentally.[4,16,36] The shock strength above which fibrillation is not induced is called the upper limit of vulnerability.

The upper limit of vulnerability hypothesis predicts that since the critical potential gradient that leads to the induction of fibrillation during the vulnerable period of regular rhythm is about the same as that which leads to fibrillation (about 5 V/cm for a typical monophasic waveform in both cases), then the shock strength at the upper limit of vulnerability in regular rhythm should be approximately the same as the minimum shock strength needed to defibrillate. Several different studies have found this to be true in animals (Fig. 2-19).[3,4,16,36,55]

An experimental finding not explained by the upper limit of vulnerability

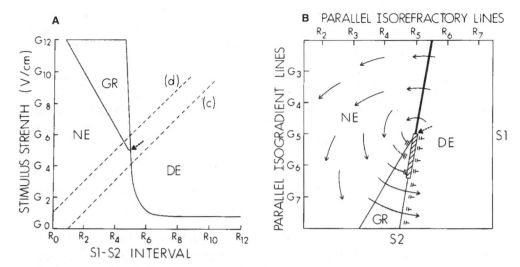

Fig. 2-18. Graded response theory for reentry. **A,** Strength-interval curve. A modified strength-interval curve is shown, with stimulus strength in volts per centimeter on the y-axis and S1-S2 interval, or refractoriness, on the x-axis. On the y-axis, G_{12} represents the largest potential gradient and G_0 the smallest. On the x-axis, R_{12} represents the most recovered tissue and R_0 the most refractory. R_0 does not represent phase 0 of the action potential, but merely tissue fully refractory to a premature stimulus. Interaction of the isorecovery and isogradient lines produces either direct excitation (*DE*), graded response (*GR*), or neither effect (*NE*). The potential gradient at G_5 is ~ 5 V/cm while the potential gradient at rheobase is 0.8 V/cm for a typical monophasic waveform.[24] The site where the three regions, *DE, NE,* and *GR,* intersect is called the critical point. The dashed arrow represents the position of the critical point in this panel and in **B. B,** Diagrammatic representation of reentry induced in the presence of perpendicular isorecovery and isogradient lines. The row of pacing wires (S1) on the right creates parallel isorecovery lines (R_7 through R_2), with R_7 the least refractory and R_2 the most refractory. The S2 from the bottom creates parallel isogradient lines (G_7 through G_3), with G_7 the largest gradient and G_3 the weakest. The solid and hatched lines are the frame and block lines, respectively. The II— represents areas of temporary unidirectional conduction block. For this idealized diagram, the S1-S2 interval equals the recovery period (preshock interval equals the critical refractory period) at R_5, and the S2 voltage creates a potential gradient of 5 V/cm at G_5. The S2 shock directly excites the area near the S1 site (DE) and produces a region of graded response (GR). Activation fronts only propagate away from part of the directly excited area, activation fronts do not propagate away from the directly excited area abutting regions of graded response, thus forming an area of temporary unidirectional conduction block. An activation front conducting toward the S2 site from the early sites of activation produces another region of conduction block (*hatched area*) when it enters tissue insufficiently repolarized from graded response or direct excitation. When the myocardium has recovered, activation can conduct through this area and from a reentrant circuit, as shown by the arrows spanning the GR zone and entering the DE zone. (Adapted with permission from Frazier DW et al: Stimulus-induced critical point—mechanism for electrical initiation of reentry in normal canine myocardium, *J Clin Invest* 83:1039, 1989.)

hypothesis for defibrillation is that in approximately half of unsuccessful defibrillation episodes with shocks slightly weaker than needed to defibrillate, activation spreads in all directions away from the site of earliest activation in a focal pattern (Figs. 2-15, *D*, 2-17) rather than spreading in primarily one direction as would be expected if activation is spreading away from the border of a region directly excited by the shock.[9] It is not clear the focal patterns observed experimentally represent activity triggered by the shock or whether they represent small reentrant pathways that are missed because the electrode spacing is too great.

If the upper limit of vulnerability hypothesis is correct, then the one or two rapid activations sometimes observed following a successful defibrillation shock[8,39,63] may be the equivalent of the one or two rapid responses that are frequently seen when a large premature stimulus is given in an attempt to induce fibrillation.[37] It is possible for the same strength and timing of premature stimulus in the same animal to sometimes induce fibrillation and other times induce repetitive responses, probably because of slight changes in autonomic and metabolic states between stimulation trials. The same reasons may explain why a defibrillation shock of a given strength may sometimes succeed and other times fail in the same patient or animal.[13] Instead of the existence of a discrete defibrillation threshold value for shocks in which all shocks greater or equal to this value always succeed and shocks less than this value always fail, there appears to be a range of shock strengths that may sometimes defibrillate for which the probability of successful defibrillation increases as the shock strength increases (Fig. 2-20).[12] Another reason that a defibrillation shock of a particular strength may succeed during some fibrillation episodes but not others in the same patient is that the distribution of

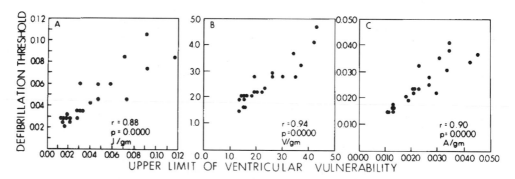

Fig. 2-19. Relationship between defibrillation threshold and the upper limit of vulnerability for defibrillation electrodes with the right atrium as anode and the ventricular apex as cathode in 22 dogs. Results are expressed in units of energy (**A**), voltage (**B**), and current (**C**). All units are divided by the heart weight. (Adapted with permission from Chen P-S et al: Comparison of the defibrillation threshold and the upper limit of ventricular vulnerability, *Circulation* 73:1022, 1986.)

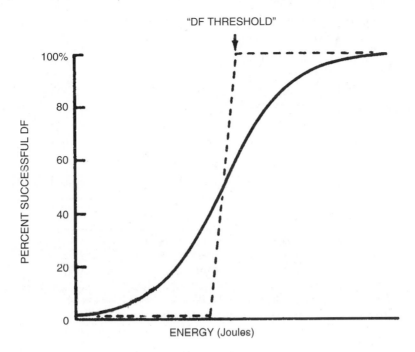

Fig. 2-20. Comparison of the defibrillation threshold and defibrillation curve concepts. A defibrillation threshold (*dashed line*) implies a clear-cut distinction between effective and ineffective energies, while a curve (*solid line*) implies a dose-response relationship with increasing energies associated with greater percentages of success. *DF*, defibrillation. (Adapted with permission from Davy JM et al: The relationship between successful defibrillation and delivered energy in open-chest dogs: reappraisal of the "defibrillation threshold" concept, *Am Heart J* 113:77, 1987.)

activation fronts and refractoriness at the time of the shock is different for every episode of fibrillation.

CONCLUSION

Whichever proposed mechanism for defibrillation is true, almost all of them imply that a certain change in transmembrane potential should be created by the shock in all or in a critical mass of the ventricles. If the change in transmembrane potential is linearly related to the extracellular potential gradient, then a minimum potential gradient is needed throughout all or a critical mass of the ventricles. However, most electrode configurations create an uneven gradient distribution throughout the heart (Fig. 2-12). An uneven shock field is not only wasteful, since much of the shock strength is used to increase the potential gradient to values that are higher than needed in most cardiac regions just to increase the lowest gradients to the minimum level required for defibrillation (Fig. 2-21), but it can cause damage in the high gradient

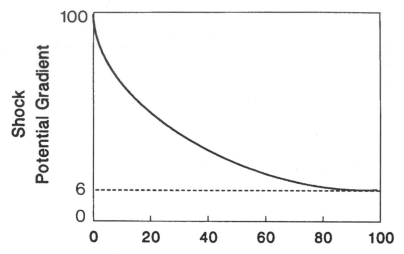

Fig. 2-21. Idealized diagram of distribution of ventricular potential gradients in V/cm generated by shocks from small epicardial defibrillation electrodes demonstrating that most of the shock field is wasted. Every tick mark on the abscissa represents 20% of the ventricular volume. If the same minimum potential gradient is required throughout the ventricular myocardium for defibrillation (indicated by the dashed line), then that portion of the shock field above the dashed line is wasted. (Adapted with permission from Ideker RE et al: Current concepts for selecting the location, size and shape of defibrillation electrodes, *PACE* 14:227, 1991.)

regions. According to these concepts, the best defibrillation field is the one that is the most even that can be created with the smallest shock voltage and energy. As shown in Fig. 2-12, it is not always easy to produce such a field. One of the regions of low potential gradient shown in Fig. 2-12, *A*, is at the anterior base of the right and left ventricles. While the addition of another electrode into the right ventricular outflow tract, used as a common cathode with the electrode in the right ventricular apex, increases the potential gradient in this region, it creates a new region of low gradient between the two common cathodes, since both are at the same voltage (Fig. 2-12, *B*).

Though much has been learned about the mechanism of defibrillation in the last few years, much is still unknown. Indeed, the fundamental questions listed below have not yet been definitively answered. What is the effect of the extracellular electric field produced by a defibrillation shock on the transmembrane potential? How do these changes in transmembrane potential halt fibrillation? Why are some biphasic waveforms superior for defibrillation? Why do identical defibrillation shocks given at different times in the same individual sometimes succeed and other times fail? While we have learned bits and pieces about the answers to these questions and several hypotheses have been advanced to answer them, we do not yet completely understand the mechanism of defibrillation. Much progress is being made in this area of research, however, and there is reason to hope these questions will be answered in the next few years.

REFERENCES

1. Bardou AL et al: Directional variability of stimulation threshold measurements in isolated guinea pig cardiomyocytes: relationship with orthogonal sequential defibrillating pulses, *PACE* 13:1590, 1990.

2. Bayly PV et al: Minimum electrode spacing for mapping ventricular fibrillation using spatial sampling theory, *Proc Computers in Cardiology*, Alamitos, CA, IEEE Computer Society Press, 1992, pp 5-8.

3. Chen P-S: Effects of pacing rate and timing of defibrillation shock on the relation between the defibrillation threshold and the upper limit of vulnerability in open chest dogs, *J Am Coll Cardiol* 18:1555, 1991.

4. Chen P-S et al: Comparison of the defibrillation threshold and the upper limit of ventricular vulnerability, *Circulation* 73:1022, 1986.

5. Chen P-S et al: Mechanism of ventricular vulnerability to single premature stimuli in open-chest dogs, *Circ Res* 62:1191, 1988.

6. Chen P-S et al: The potential gradient field created by epicardial defibrillation electrodes in dogs, *Circulation* 74:626, 1986.

7. Chen P-S: Mechanism of cardiac defibrillation: a different point of view, *Circulation* 84:913, 1991.

8. Chen P-S et al: Activation during ventricular defibrillation in open-chest dogs: evidence of complete cessation and regeneration of ventricular fibrillation after unsuccessful shocks, *J Clin Invest* 77:810, 1986.

9. Chen P-S et al: Comparison of activation during ventricular fibrillation and following unsuccessful defibrillation shocks in open chest dogs, *Circ Res* 66:1544, 1990.

10. Claydon FJ III et al: A volume conductor model of the thorax for the study of defibrillation fields, *IEEE Trans Biomed Eng* BME-35:981, 1988.

11. Clerc L: Directional differences of impulse spread in trabecular muscle from mammalian heart, *J Physiol* 255:335, 1976.

12. Davy JM: The relationship between successful defibrillation and delivered energy in open-chest dogs: reappraisal of the "defibrillation threshold" concept, *Am Heart J* 113:77, 1987.

13. Deale OC: Nature of defibrillation: determinism versus probabilism, *Am J Physiol* 259:H1544, 1990.

14. Dillon SM: Synchronized repolarization after defibrillation shocks: a possible component of the defibrillation process demonstrated by optical recordings in rabbit heart, *Circulation* 85:1865, 1992.

15. Dillon SM: Optical recordings in the rabbit heart show that defibrillation strength shocks prolong the duration of depolarization and the refractory period, *Circ Res* 69:842, 1991.

16. Fabiato A: Le seuil de réponse synchrone des fibres myocardiques. Application à la comparaison expérimentale de l'efficacité des différentes formes de chocs électriques de défibrillation, *Arch des Mal du Coeur* 60:527, 1967.

17. Fahy JB: Optimal electrode configurations for external cardiac pacing and defibrillation: an inhomogeneous study, *IEEE Trans Biomed Eng* BME-34:743, 1987.

18. Frazier DW et al: Extracellular field required for excitation in three-dimensional anisotropic canine myocardium, *Circ Res* 63:147, 1988.

19. Frazier DW et al: Stimulus-induced critical point: Mechanism for electrical initiation of reentry in normal canine myocardium, *J Clin Invest* 83:1039, 1989.

20. Garrey WE: The nature of fibrillatory contractions of the heart—its relation to tissue mass and form, *Am J Physiol* 33:397, 1914.

21. Henriquez CS: Simulating the electrical behavior of cardiac tissue using the bidomain model, *CRC Crit Rev Biomed Eng* 21:1, 1993.

22. Ideker RE et al: Basic mechanisms of ventricular defibrillation. In Glass L, Hunter P, McColloch A, editors: *Theory of the heart*, New York, 1991, Springer-Verlag, p 533.

23. Ideker RE et al: Ventricular defibrillation: basic concepts. In El-Sherif N, Samet P,

editors: *Cardiac pacing and electrophysiology*, Orlando, 1991, Saunders, p 713.

24. Jones JL: Microlesion formation in myocardial cells by high-intensity electric field stimulation, *Am J Physiol* 253:H480, 1987.

25. Jones JL: Improved cardiac cell excitation with symmetrical biphasic defibrillator waveforms, *Am J Physiol* 253:H1418, 1987.

26. Jones JL, Jones RE: Determination of safety factor for defibrillator waveforms in cultured heart cells, *Am J Physiol* 242:H662, 1982.

27. Jones JL: Response of cultured myocardial cells to countershock-type electric field stimulation, *Am J Physiol* 235:H214, 1978.

28. Kao CY, Hoffman BF: Graded and decremental response in heart muscle fibers, *Am J Physiol* 194:187, 1958.

29. Klee M, Plonsey R: Stimulation of spheroidal cells—the role of cell shape, *IEEE Trans Biomed Eng* BME-23:347, 1976.

30. Knisley SB: Effect of field stimulation on cellular repolarization in rabbit myocardium: implications for reentry induction, *Circ Res* 70:707, 1992.

31. Knisley S et al: Transmembrane potential changes measured optically during field stimulation of ventricular cells, *J Am Coll Cardiol* 19:122A, 1992 (abstract).

32. Kothiyal KP: Three-dimensional computer model of electric fields in internal defibrillation, *Proc IEEE* 76:720, 1988.

33. Krassowska W: Periodic conductivity as a mechanism for cardiac stimulation and defibrillation, *IEEE Trans Biomed Eng* BME-34:555, 1987.

34. Krassowska W: Potential distribution in three-dimensional periodic myocardium. Part II. Application to extracellular stimulation, *IEEE Trans Biomed Eng* BME-37:267, 1990.

35. Lepeschkin E: Local potential gradients as a unifying measure for thresholds of stimulation, standstill, tachyarrhythmia and fibrillation appearing after strong capacitor discharges, *Adv Cardiol* 21:268, 1978.

36. Lesigne C et al: An energy-time analysis of ventricular fibrillation and defibrillation thresholds with internal electrodes, *Med Biol Eng* 14:617, 1976.

37. Moe GK: Analysis of the initiation of fibrillation by electrographic studies, *Am J Physiol* 134:473, 1941.

38. Moore EN, Spear JF: Electrophysiologic studies on the initiation, prevention, and termination of ventricular fibrillation. In Zipes DP, Jalife J, editors: *Cardiac electrophysiology and arrhythmias*, Orlando, 1985, Grune & Stratton, p 315.

39. Mower MM: Patterns of ventricular activity during catheter defibrillation, *Circulation* 49:858, 1974.

40. Peleska B: Cardiac arrhythmias following condenser discharges and their dependence upon strength of current and phase of cardiac cycle, *Circ Res* 13:21, 1963.

41. Plonsey R: One-dimensional model of cardiac defibrillation, *Med Biol Eng Comp* 29:465, 1991.

42. Plonsey R, Barr RC: Inclusion of junction elements in a linear cardiac model through secondary sources: application to defibrillation, *Med Biol Eng Comp* 24:137, 1986.

43. Ramirez IF: Effects of cardiac configuration, paddle placement and paddle size on defibrillation current distribution: a finite-element model, *Med Biol Eng Comp* 27:587, 1989.

44. Rush S: Current distribution from defibrillation electrodes in a homogeneous torso model, *J Electrocardiol* 2:331, 1969.

45. Rush S: Resistivity of body tissues at low frequencies, *Circ Res* 12:40, 1963.

46. Sepulveda NG, Wikswo JP Jr: Electric and magnetic fields from two-dimensional anisotropic bisyncytia, *Biophys J* 51:557, 1987.

47. Sepulveda NG: Finite element analysis of cardiac defibrillation current distributions, *IEEE Trans Biomed Eng* BME-37:354, 1990.

48. Shibata N et al: Epicardial activation following unsuccessful defibrillation shocks in dogs, *Am J Physiol* 255:H902, 1988.

49. Sommer JR, Scherer B: Geometry of cell and bundle appositions in cardiac muscle: light microscopy, *Am J Physiol* 248:H792, 1985.

50. Spach MS et al: The discontinuous nature of propagation in normal canine cardiac muscle. Evidence for recurrent discontinuities of intracellular resistance that affect

the membrane currents, *Circ Res* 48:39, 1981.

51. Swartz JF: Conditioning prepulse of biphasic defibrillator waveforms enhances refractoriness to fibrillation wavefronts, *Circ Res* 68:438, 1991.

52. Tacker WA Jr et al: Recommendations of the conference. IV. New directions in defibrillation, *Med Instrum* 12:49, 1978.

53. Tang ASL et al: Three-dimensional potential gradient fields generated by intracardiac catheter and cutaneous patch electrodes, *Circulation* 85:1857, 1992.

54. Tung L: Influence of electrical axis of stimulation on excitation of cardiac muscle cells, *Circ Res* 69:722, 1991.

55. Wharton JM et al: Electrophysiologic effects in vivo of monophasic and biphasic stimuli in normal and infarcted dogs, *PACE* 13:1158, 1990.

56. Wharton JM et al: Cardiac potential and potential gradient fields generated by single, combined, and sequential shocks during ventricular defibrillation, *Circulation* 85:1510, 1992.

57. Windisch H et al: Optical monitoring of excitation patterns in single cardiomyocytes, *Proc 12th Annual Conf of the IEEE Engineering in Medicine and Biology Society* 12:1641, 1990.

58. Winfree AT: *When time breaks down: The three-dimensional dynamics of electrochemical waves and cardiac arrhythmias*, Princeton, NJ, 1987, Princeton University Press.

59. Witkowski FX: Mechanism of cardiac defibrillation in open-chest dogs with unipolar DC-coupled simultaneous activation and shock potential recordings, *Circulation* 82:244, 1990.

60. Witkowski FX, Penkoske PA: Activation patterns during ventricular fibrillation. In Jalife J, editor: *Mathematical approaches to cardiac arrhythmias*, New York, 1990, The New York Academy of Sciences, p 219.

61. Yabe S et al: Conduction disturbances caused by high current density electric fields, *Circ Res* 66:1190, 1990.

62. Zhou X et al: Epicardial mapping of ventricular defibrillation with monophasic and biphasic shocks in dogs, *Circ Res* 72:145, 1993.

63. Zipes DP et al: Termination of ventricular fibrillation in dogs by depolarizing a critical amount of myocardium, *Am J Cardiol* 36:37, 1975.

Chapter 3
Waveforms for Implantable Cardioverter Defibrillators (ICDs) and Transchest Defibrillation

Janice L. Jones

CELLULAR BASIS FOR DEFIBRILLATION

The first waveform used for ventricular defibrillation was the 60 Hz AC current that is used as standard household current. The delivered shock was a sine wave that alternated between positive and negative polarity every 17 msec, as shown in Fig. 3-1, and lasted for up to 1 second. However, because defibrillation was associated with significant cardiac damage, the delivered waveform evolved to a single undamped capacitor discharge, sometimes called DC, or direct current, defibrillation because the shock consists of a single pulse in one direction rather than the oscillating pulses characteristic of AC defibrillation. The undamped capacitor discharge is described mathematically by a curve called an "undamped exponential," so the waveform is frequently called by this name. The significant damage that was still produced by the undamped capacitor discharge waveform led to the addition of an inductor, which rounded the initial, sharp, high-voltage peak thought to be responsible for the dysfunction. It is this "damped exponential" waveform that is now used clinically for transthoracic defibrillation. Depending on the capacitance, inductance, and resistance of a particular model of defibrillator and the impedance of the subject, the waveform is either "critically damped" (Edmark waveform) so that it does not oscillate, or "underdamped" (Lown waveform) so that it does oscillate (has one or more negative components). Lown believed the polarity reversal might further reduce dysfunction.

With the advent of internal defibrillators, new waveforms were required because the large inductors used for transthoracic defibrillation were not suitable for small implanted devices. In order to avoid the dysfunction-inducing, high-voltage, sharp peaks associated with the undamped capacitor dis-

46

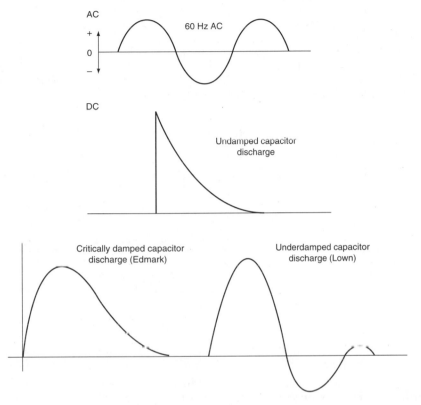

Fig. 3-1. Transthoracic defibrillator waveforms.

charge, these devices use an undamped discharge with a much longer time constant and then truncate it at about 5 msec so that it closely resembles a square (or low-tilt, trapezoidal) wave, which is currently the best-known monophasic waveform for defibrillation.[8,23,24,39] A sample of this "monophasic truncated exponential" is shown in Fig. 3-2. This waveform has performed satisfactorily with epicardial patch electrode systems, although a few patients have unacceptably high thresholds.

New transvenous lead systems, which do not require a thoracotomy, hold great promise for expanding the number of patients who can take advantage of internal defibrillators. However, the very uneven electric fields produced by these lead systems resulted in very high thresholds, precluding implantation in a significant number of patients, and increased the probability for dysfunction in high electric field areas near the electrodes. Therefore, there has been increasing interest in developing new waveforms with lower thresholds. Development of new waveforms requires a better understanding of mechanisms underlying defibrillation. Therefore, mechanisms underlying defibrillation and defibrillator-induced dysfunction have been the topic of intense research.

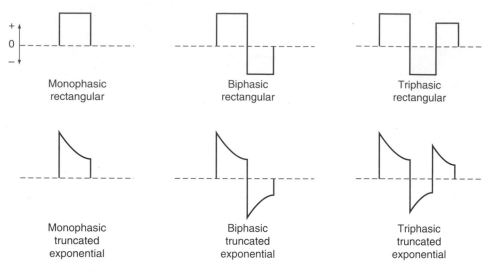

Fig. 3-2. Experimental defibrillator waveforms.

Several hypotheses are currently under investigation. The critical mass hypothesis states that an adequate mass of cells in a given mass of fibrillating myocardium must be depolarized to make them nonexcitable.[70,93] The upper limit of vulnerability hypothesis states that low-intensity shocks defibrillate, but that the shock must be strong enough to avoid inducing vulnerable period fibrillation.[13] The extension of refractoriness hypothesis states that the defibrillating shock interacts primarily with cells during their refractory period and prolongs refractoriness in most of the myocardium so that fibrillation wavefronts cannot propagate and fibrillation ceases.[55,58,59,79,81] These three hypotheses are not mutually exclusive.

The extension of refractoriness hypothesis is based on results using monophasic action potential (MAP) recordings in humans during internal defibrillator implants, as shown in Fig. 3-3. This figure shows that cells are seldom stimulated during diastole.[80] Rather, a new fibrillation wavefront re-stimulates cells as soon as they are out of their refractory period. As shown in Fig. 3-3, the defibrillation shock interacts with ventricular cells during their refractory period. The subsequent refractory period extension makes cells refractory at the time of arrival of the next fibrillation wavefront. Therefore, refractory period extension in a large mass of the ventricle stops fibrillation. This finding lends support to recent studies exploring the ability of defibrillating shocks to produce refractory period extension.[81,83,91]

Under the extension of refractoriness hypothesis, high-intensity monophasic waveforms delivered during the refractory period produce responses that prolong the total action potential duration. Action potential prolongation by high-intensity stimuli is clearly demonstrated by computer simulations of the ventricular action potential.[44] In Fig. 3-4, *A*, cells are stimulated during their refractory period with monophasic stimuli of increasing intensity. The first

HUMAN DEFIBRILLATION

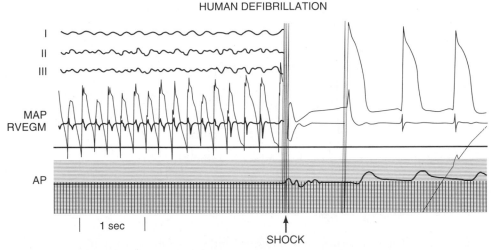

Fig. 3-3. Recordings taken during clinical testing of an implantable defibrillator (Swartz JF, Jones JL, Fletcher RD: Characterization of ventricular fibrillation based on monophasic action potential morphology in the human heart, *Circulation* 87:1907, 1993). Upper three tracings are leads I, II, and III of the electrocardiogram. *MAP* is a monophasic action potential recording from the right ventricular apex. *RVEGM* is a bipolar electrogram recorded from the sensing lead of the defibrillator. *AP* is the aortic pressure. On the left side of the figure, the heart is in fibrillation. At the arrow, a successful defibrillation shock is given that restores a normal rhythm (right side of figure).

action potential (*F1*) represents a fibrillation action potential. The defibrillation shock (*D*) produced a response that prolonged the action potential. The time when a second fibrillation wavefront could normally restimulate the cell is shown by the dotted line at *F2*. For a stimulus at 1 times diastolic threshold, only a small response is produced, which cannot prevent the second fibrillation wavefront from reexciting the cell. However, after stronger stimulus of three and five times diastolic threshold, a large response was produced, which extended the refractory period of the cell and prevented the fibrillation wavefront from continuing. Fig. 3-4, *B*, shows that the shock-induced response duration increases with shock intensity up to approximately three times diastolic threshold. The probability of successful defibrillation also increases sigmoidally with shock intensity, suggesting that for successful defibrillation shock intensities of approximately three times diastolic threshold must be achieved in regions of the heart exposed to the weakest electric field intensities.

The requirement for relatively high shock intensities of greater than three times diastolic threshold to produce refractory period prolongation occurs in experimental models ranging from isolated cells to canine,[83] rabbit,[16] and human[79,82] hearts. In the isolated cell model, low intensity shocks of 1.5 times diastolic threshold failed to prolong the action potential when delivered dur-

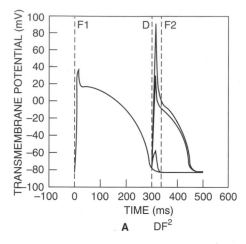

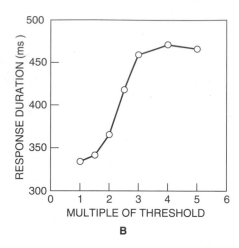

Fig. 3-4. A, Three superimposed action potential tracings generated by a computer model of the ventricular action potential. The tracings show an initial control action potential (*F1*), which simulates a fibrillation action potential. During the relative refractory period of the *F1* action potential, a simulated defibrillation shock (*D*) is given. The figure shows graded responses produced by *D* at 1, 3, and 5 times diastolic threshold when a 10 msec monophasic rectangular waveform is used at an *F1-D* coupling interval of 300 msec. *F1* is a 10 msec monophasic rectangular waveform at 1.5 times diastolic threshold. No response is produced at 1 times threshold. However, high-intensity pulses produce a graded response. The dashed line at *F2* shows the time at which a new fibrillation wavefront would be expected to reexcite the cell in the absence of a shock. **B,** Total *F1-D* response duration as a function of *D* stimulus intensity. (Modified from Jones JL, Jones JE: Effects of monophasic defibrillator waveform intensity on graded response duration in a computer simulation of the ventricular action potential, *Proc IEEE Eng Med Biol Soc* 13:598, 1991.)

ing the refractory period.[81] In the canine model,[83] 1 V/cm monophasic shocks, which are approximately 1 times diastolic threshold, also failed to produce refractory period extension. In contrast, significant refractory period extension was produced in the canine model with higher intensity (5-10 V/cm) shocks delivered 25 msec prior to the end of the refractory period. In clinical studies during invasive electrophysiological testing, refractory period extension occurred with stimuli that were four times greater than diastolic threshold but not with stimuli two times greater than threshold.[79,82]

These results suggest that monophasic stimuli can prolong the refractory period sufficiently to prevent reentry loops and produce defibrillation if they are sufficiently strong, that is, greater than about three times diastolic threshold in regions of the heart receiving the lowest current densities. Since diastolic threshold is 1 to 2 V/cm with 5 to 10 msec monophasic waveforms,[48,65] voltage gradients of 4 to 8 V/cm would be required for successful defibrillation. In agreement with this hypotheses, minimum voltage gradients that occur in the dog heart during successful defibrillation with monophasic waveforms are approximately 5 to 7 V/cm.[87,92]

DYSFUNCTION IN HIGH STIMULUS INTENSITY REGIONS OF THE HEART

Because of the uneven current distribution produced by defibrillation electrodes, some regions of the heart, especially those near the electrodes, receive a much higher shock intensity than regions far from the electrodes. For internal defibrillation this electric field is more even with large epicardial patch electrodes than with transvenous electrodes. The deleterious effects of nonuniform fields are accentuated because stimulating partially refractory cells in the fibrillating heart requires three to four times more voltage and current than stimulating the cells of a normally beating heart.

With the epicardial patch-to-patch configuration used for internal defibrillation, the pacing (excitation) threshold is usually less than 5V whereas defibrillation is accomplished with approximately 800V (for the monophasic truncated exponential waveform). Due to the large ratio between pacing and defibrillation thresholds, cells in regions of the heart near the electrodes, which are exposed to the highest current densities, are subjected to a shock intensity up to 150 times their excitation threshold (150 V/cm) during defibrillation using the same electrode system. For small epicardial electrodes in one canine study, maximum voltage gradients of approximately 182 V/cm were measured near the defibrillation electrodes at defibrillating intensities.[87] Therefore, successful defibrillation is dependent not only on electric fields in the low current density regions of the heart, but also on effects in high current density regions of the heart. High current density causes dysfunction. With transvenous defibrillation, the electric fields are most nonuniform, and dysfunction near the electrodes is an even more important consideration.

IN VIVO EFFECTS OF HIGH STIMULUS INTENSITIES

Several experimental studies confirm that defibrillation shocks induce postshock dysfunction.[64,65] Postshock, intensity-dependent, conduction block lasting several seconds is produced in high current density areas near the defibrillation electrodes beginning at approximately 65 V/cm.[89] High-intensity shocks also have produced postshock ventricular standstill,[23,24] decreased contractility,[27] and irreversible fibrillation that was different from "vulnerable period" fibrillation produced at lower shock intensities and that could not be corrected by additional defibrillation shocks.[71] Very-high-intensity shocks caused morphologic injury and shock-induced death within 15 minutes.[3] With internal defibrillators, even after short fibrillation durations lasting only 15 seconds, pacing thresholds are increased for several seconds following the shock.[25,26]

In one study, where epicardial potential gradients were measured directly in dogs defibrillated with a 14 msec truncated exponential waveform, 11 of 67 successful defibrillations were followed by episodes of nonsustained, monomorphic ventricular tachycardia that arose from near the defibrillation electrodes where voltage gradients were high. The mean voltage gradient at the site of earliest epicardial activation was 47 V/cm.[87] This study also showed a maximum epicardial voltage gradient of 182 V/cm in regions near the electrodes when the minimum gradient was 7.3 V/cm, a ratio of 25 to 1.

The role of shock-induced dysfunction in reducing probability of successful defibrillation has also been shown using transthoracic defibrillation of the 100 Kg calf following 30 seconds of fibrillation. Fig. 3-5, *A*, redrawn from Schuder et al.,[75] shows the percentage of fibrillation episodes in which the first shock defibrillates successfully as a function of shock intensity for the clinically used Edmark waveform. At low shock intensities the probability of successful defibrillation increases with stronger intensity. However, as intensity continues to increase, the percent success decreases. Therefore, the percent success that can be achieved on the first shock, even at optimal intensity, never reaches 100%. The decrease in percent success with increasing intensity is probably caused by immediate, shock-induced refibrillation due to transient postshock dysfunction to myocardial cells.[37,51] Following successful transthoracic defibrillation in the calf model, another type of dysfunction may occur, which is transient, postshock A-V block, or ventricular standstill.[23,24] Arrhythmia severity and duration are dependent on shock intensity.

The overall relationship between (1) shock intensity and waveform, outcomes of defibrillation (2) success or (3) failure, and (4) occurrence of postshock arrhythmias is shown in Fig. 3-5, *B*. The probability of successful defibrillation is plotted as a function of postshock dysfunction following successful defibrillation for monophasic rectangular waveforms having waveforms durations ranging from 0.5 to 40 msec. Each point represents a particular combination of shock waveform (duration of rectangular wave in msec) and intensity (amps) compiled using data from Schuder's laboratory.[23,24] The ordinate shows the percent success for a particular combination and the abscissa represents the time to normal sinus rhythm for successful defibrillations induced by that specific combination. Independent of waveform, region *A* shows a range where defibrillation success increases with increasing intensity due to the ability to directly stimulate a greater amount of ventricular tissue. These low-intensity shocks produce few arrhythmias. Shocks of higher intensities form the general region (*B*) where the percent success decreases with increasing "time to normal sinus rhythm" following the successful defibrillations. Region B suggests that shocks that induce significant postshock arrhythmias also produce a low percent success, presumably due to immediate shock-induced refibrillation.

These results show that a high probability of successful defibrillation can be produced with little dysfunction by some waveforms and that defibrillation with dysfunction is produced by other waveforms. Electric waveform is not

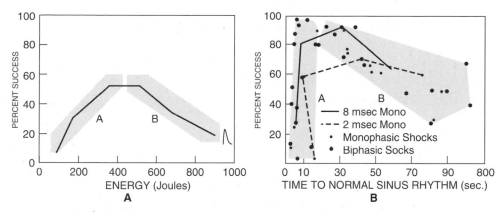

Fig. 3-5. A, Probability of success as a function of stimulus intensity for transthoracic defibrillation in the calf using the damped sine wave (Edmark) waveform. Starting at low intensities, probability of success increases with stimulus intensity, reaches a maximum, then decreases at higher shock intensities. Figure is modified from reference 75. **B,** Probability of defibrillation as a function of postshock time to return of normal sinus rhythm after high-intensity shocks that produce a postshock ventricular standstill (symptom of shock-induced dysfunction). (Data collated from Gold HJ et al: Transthoracic ventricular defibrillation in the 100 kg calf with unidirectional rectangular pulses, *Circulation* 56:745, 1977; Schuder JC et al: Transthoracic ventricular defibrillation in the calf with symmetrical one-cycle bidirectional rectangular wave stimuli, *IEEE Trans Biomed Eng* 30:415, 1983.)

only a determinant of defibrillation but is also an important determinant of successful resuscitation. This chapter later discusses the concept that a waveform's *safety factor* (ratio of shock intensity producing postshock dysfunction to that producing excitation or defibrillation) predicts the maximum percent success that that waveform can achieve *in situ* at its optimal shock intensity.[37,39,40,41,52]

IN VITRO EFFECTS OF HIGH STIMULUS INTENSITIES

The mechanism underlying postshock dysfunction has been examined using myocardial cells *in vitro*. When spontaneously contracting myocardial cell monolayers are subjected to electric field stimulation, a typical pattern of response occurs with increasing shock intensity. Low-intensity shocks of approximately 1 V/cm produce excitation or pacing. Higher-intensity shocks produce a transient postshock tachyarrhythmia. At still higher intensities beginning at about 50 V/cm, a postshock arrest occurs and the duration of postshock arrest is dose-dependent. At shock intensities above 150 to 200 V/cm contracture and cellular fibrillation occur. Postshock arrhythmias are

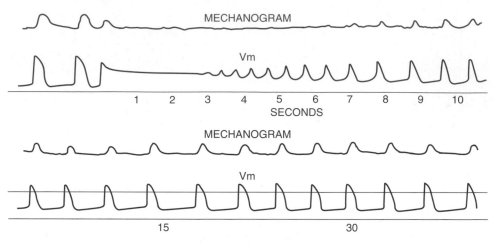

Fig. 3-6. Transmembrane potential (V_M) and mechanograms from a spontaneously contracting myocardial cell monolayer before, during, and following a high-intensity electric field stimulus similar to that which occurs in regions near the internal defibrillator electrodes.[89] (Modified from Jones JL et al: Response of cultured myocardial cells to countershock-type electric field stimulation, *Am J Physiol* 235:H214, 1978.)

due to a severe depolarization of the myocardial cell membrane lasting up to several minutes,[37-40,42,51] as shown by the tracings in Fig. 3-6. The upper tracing shows the cellular mechanogram and indicates an approximately 8 second postshock contractile arrest. The second tracing shows the corresponding transmembrane potential and demonstrates the prolonged, shock-induced membrane depolarization responsible for the arrest of contractile activity. The lower two tracings show complete recovery approximately 20 seconds following the shock. Ionic exchanges causing this prolonged depolarization probably occur through transient sarcolemmal microlesions, approximately 50 Å in diameter, that are produced by the shock.[49] Nondiscriminate ionic exchange through these microlesions causes a transient cytoplasmic sodium[28,29] and calcium[50] overload as well as postshock myocardial potassium loss.[62] The resulting ionic imbalance causes severe ultrastructural injury at 30 seconds following shocks of 200 V/cm, but only minor, potentially reversible alterations following shocks of 80 V/cm.[54]

These cellular studies suggest that membrane depolarization, which leads to inexcitability, activation of ectopic foci, slowed conduction velocity, and conduction block in those areas of the ventricle receiving the highest current densities, is probably the common mechanism underlying both postshock arrhythmias following successful defibrillation and postshock refibrillation leading to unsuccessful defibrillation following high-intensity shocks in the transthoracic calf model. Similar cellular depolarization could produce the transient conduction block observed in regions near the electrodes in the canine model, and the transient increased pacing threshold following internal defibrillation.

SINGLE SHOCK MONOPHASIC WAVEFORM DEFIBRILLATION

Because defibrillation shocks can induce myocardial dysfunction, an important concept has emerged to describe defibrillator waveforms, that of a *safety factor*.[37,39,40,41,52] The safety factor is defined as the ratio of the shock intensity required to produce postshock dysfunction (dysfunction threshold) to that required to produce defibrillation *in vivo* or to produce a cellular response in *in vitro* myocardial cells under fibrillation conditions.[48]

Fig. 3-7 combines the relationship of *in vivo* transthoracic defibrillation of the calf with cellular excitation, arrhythmia production, and the safety factor *in vitro*. The solid lines are defibrillation probability of success contours (strength-duration curves for a specific probability of success).[24] For a waveform duration of 6 msec (shown by the vertical line), the probability of success increases from 25% to 90%, then begins to decrease with increasing shock intensity, as explained in Fig. 3-5, *A*. This waveform has a high safety factor, as shown by the high probability of success that can be achieved at optimum intensity and the large ratio between intensities producing a specific probability of defibrillation at low intensities (defibrillation threshold) and the same probability of defibrillation at high intensities where postshock refibrillation decreases the probability of success (dysfunction threshold). In contrast, a 1 msec duration waveform can achieve a maximum of only 25% success at any intensity. Because of this waveform's low safety factor, dysfunction begins to occur below the defibrillation threshold.

The lower dotted line in Fig. 3-7 is the excitation threshold strength-duration curve for partially refractory isolated cells.[18] Note that it closely parallels the lower defibrillation contour for 50% successful defibrillation (defibrillation threshold) for waveform durations that do not show significant postshock dysfunction. The upper dotted line is the voltage gradient producing the 4 sec postshock arrest for each waveform duration in the isolated cell model (dysfunction strength-duration curve). Note that it closely parallels the upper dysfunction contour, which represents decreasing probability of success at each waveform duration. The dysfunction strength-duration curves and the defibrillation or excitation strength-duration curves differ in shape rather than by a scaling factor, because mechanisms underlying postshock dysfunction (microlesion formation)[49,51] differ from those producing defibrillation (stimulation of partially refractory cells).[39,44,48]

Fig. 3-8 shows correlations between results from the cultured cell model and the transthoracic calf model[23,24] in more detail and further confirms that the results obtained in the cultured cell model are consistent with those obtained *in situ*. To make these correlations it is necessary to set criteria to quantitate defibrillation success. Fig. 3-5, *A*, showed that the probability of successful defibrillation increases with shock intensity for low-amplitude

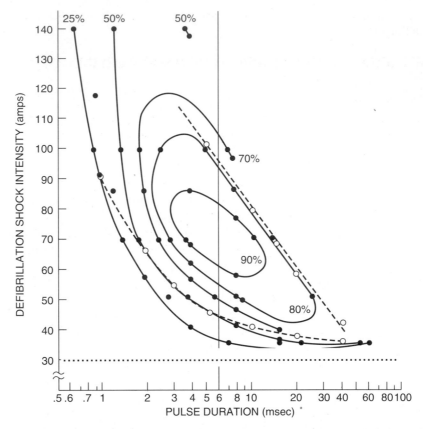

Fig. 3-7. Transthoracic strength-duration contours for a specific probability of successful defibrillation using monophasic rectangular waves having durations ranging from 0.7 to 60 msec in the calf model.[24] The lightly dotted horizontal line shows the apparent rheobase. The lower dashed curve shows the excitation strength-duration curve for rectangular wave field stimulation for partially refractory cells[48] normalized to the defibrillation threshold at 40 msec. The upper dotted line is the strength-duration curve for postshock dysfunction (4-second postshock arrest of spontaneous contraction) in the cultured cell model[37] normalized to the 80% success defibrillation curve at 20 msec. (Reproduced from Jones JL, Jones RE: Post-shock arrythmias—a possible cause of unsuccessful defibrillation, *Crit Care Med* 8:167, 1980.

shocks, reaches a maximum, then decreases, probably because the strong shock produces transient dysfunction leading to immediate refibrillation.[37] For waveforms that exceed a specific success criterion, for example, 80%, an *in vivo safety factor* similar to that defined *in vitro* can be defined using 80% success as the arbitrary criterion. The 80% success point on the ascending portion of the curve represents the "defibrillation threshold" and the 80% success on the descending portion of the curve represents the "dysfunction threshold." The safety factor for an 80% rate of transthoracic defibrillation, shown on the vertical axis of Fig. 3-8, *A*, then becomes the ratio of the "dysfunction threshold" to the "defibrillation threshold." The horizontal axis of Fig. 3-8, *A*, is the safety factor obtained in the cultured cell model.[39] Fig. 3-8, *A*, demonstrates that for monophasic rectangular waveforms the *in vivo* safety factor is directly proportional to the *in vitro* safety factor. Fig. 3-8, *B*, shows the close correlation between the *in vitro* safety factor and the maximum percent success obtainable in the transthoracic defibrillation of the calf using monophasic rectangular waveforms of several durations. In Fig. 3-8, *B*, the 1 msec rectangular wave, which has a relative *in vitro* safety factor of 70,[39] produces only a maximum of 40%[23,24] success in the calf; the 4 to 5 msec rectangular waveform, which has an *in vitro* safety factor of 100, produces a maximum of 93% success. Fig. 3-8, *C*, shows the relationship between 50% success on the ascending (low shock intensity) portion of the bell shaped probability of defibrillation curve (defibrillation threshold for those monophasic rectangular waveforms that can exceed 50% success) and the *in vitro* stimulation threshold for partially refractory myocardial cells under fibrillation conditions.[39,48] This figure shows that waveforms that have low defibrillation thresholds are also able to stimulate relatively refractory cells with a low shock intensity.

The predictive value of the *in vitro* safety factor has been validated for several waveforms other than monophasic rectangular waves. The Edmark waveform now used for transthoracic defibrillation, which has a low *in vitro* safety factor of approximately 80[39] can achieve only a 53% success in the calf model.[75] Untruncated exponentials, which are known to induce dysfunction *in situ*, have lower safety factors than rectangular waveforms at all waveform durations.[39] The symmetrical biphasic waveform to be discussed in the next section, which has a safety factor of 120 *in vitro*,[40] achieves a 99% success in the calf.[73]

A second measure of waveform safety similar to the safety factor, the *therapeutic index*,[3] has been defined as the ratio of shock intensity (current) causing morphologic damage or immediate postshock death when shocks are given in sinus rhythm to the defibrillation threshold for that waveform. For the damped sinusoidal waveform, the *therapeutic index*[3] is 5 for morphologic injury and 22 for death. However, dysfunction expressed by arrhythmia production has not been studied with the therapeutic index approach.

Fig. 3-9 diagrammatically summarizes the relationship between defibrillation success and the waveform safety factor. For waveforms with low safety factors, as shown in Fig. 3-9, *A*, dysfunction occurs at voltages lower than those producing 100% defibrillation and only a low maximum probability of success can be achieved. In contrast, waveforms with large safety factors, such as those diagrammed in Fig. 3-9, *B*, reliably produce 100% success under optimum conditions, due to the lack of shock-induced dysfunction at defibrillating intensities and maintain virtually 100% success over a range of

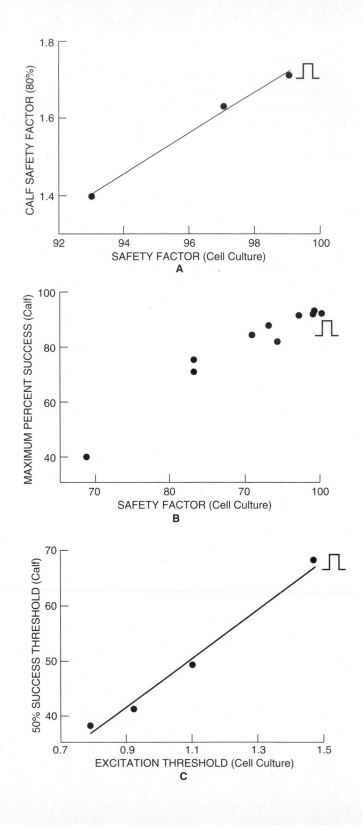

Fig. 3-8. Correlations between data from cell culture model and from the transthoracic calf model. **A**, Safety factor for monophasic rectangular defibrillator waveforms in the calf model computed from reference 24 correlates closely with safety factor determined in the cultured cell model as determined from references 37 and 39. **B**, The maximum probability of success that can be obtained at the optimum shock intensity for a specific duration monophasic rectangular waveform[24] also correlates closely with its *in vitro* safety factor,[39] suggesting that postshock dysfunction may limit the maximum probability of success obtainable with a specific waveform. **C**, The shock intensity that produces a 50% probability of success on the ascending limb of the bell-shaped defibrillation curve[24] corresponds closely with the excitation threshold for partially refractory cells in the cultured cell defibrillation model,[39] suggesting that stimulation of partially refractory cells may be a significant factor underlying defibrillation.

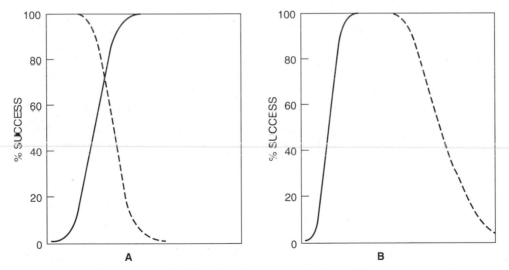

Fig. 3-9. Theoretical probability of defibrillation curves as a function of shock intensity for waveforms having low (**A**) and high (**B**) safety factors. The solid line represents the theoretical defibrillation curve if dysfunction were not produced. The dashed line represents the decreasing probability of success at high intensities due to postshock dysfunction. The overall probability of success is determined by the superposition of these two curves.

shock intensities. This produces a greater margin of safety for operator error or for a heart "traumatized" by prolonged fibrillation. Waveforms with high safety factors also produce fewer postshock hemodynamic changes. For example, left ventricular dP/dt following defibrillation was shown to be lower with a 2 msec, 80% tilt waveform having a low safety factor than with a 10 msec, 50% tilt waveform having a high safety factor, and the time to recovery of normal sinus rhythm was increased from 40 seconds to 70 seconds.[27]

BIPHASIC DEFIBRILLATOR WAVEFORMS

DEFIBRILLATION THRESHOLD REDUCTION

Monophasic waveforms are defined as having a single polarity, as shown in Figs. 3-1 and 3-2. To create a biphasic waveform the waveform polarity is switched part way through the pulse so that the first part of the waveform is delivered with one polarity and the second part of the waveform is delivered with the opposite polarity. Some biphasic waveforms decrease defibrillation threshold energy to about one half that required by monophasic waveforms with the same total pulse duration. For example, defibrillation thresholds obtained in one canine study using a right ventricular catheter/subcutaneous patch electrode system showed a threshold of 19.5 J with the monophasic waveforms and 9.7 J using a biphasic waveform.[11] Similar results have been obtained in several other animal[12,20,21,56,60] and clinical[5,88] studies.

Detailed studies to determine the best shape for biphasic waveforms have been carried out in animal models.[17,73,74,85] Because truncated exponentials are the easiest waveforms to produce for internal defibrillators, most research has concentrated on these waveforms. Fig. 3-10, which is redrawn from Dixon et al.,[17] shows defibrillation thresholds for truncated exponential waveforms having a total duration of 10 msec. Threshold for the monophasic waveform was approximately 160 V. In this study, when the first pulse duration was equal to or larger than the second pulse, threshold decreased significantly to approximately 90 V. When the first pulse duration was smaller than the second pulse, the biphasic waveform actually increased threshold to approximately 270 V. Therefore, thresholds for the biphasic versions of this waveform can be either higher or lower than that for the monophasic waveform, depending on the time at which the pulse is reversed. In general, even with rectangular waveforms, biphasic waveforms where the first pulse is equal to or greater in duration or intensity compared with the second pulse seem to work best. This brings out an important aspect of biphasic waveforms that must be considered by every physician if future implantable defibrillators allow selection of pulse shape. *Biphasic waveforms do not necessarily lower threshold. They must be carefully specified based on an understanding of defibrillation mechanisms.*

Although truncated exponentials are used clinically and are therefore desirable for experiments designed to produce the lowest thresholds, it is very difficult to determine mechanisms underlying threshold reduction, because

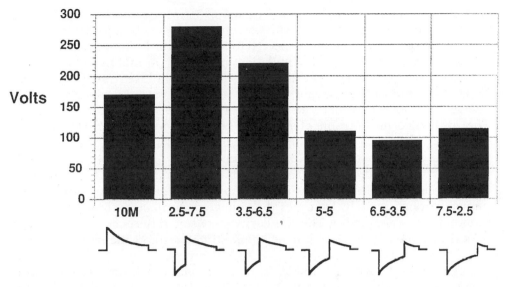

Fig. 3-10. Defibrillation threshold for monophasic and biphasic truncated exponential defibrillator waveforms with a total duration of 10 msec. Defibrillation threshold for biphasic waveforms is a function of the duration of the positive and negative pulses. It can be either higher (2.5/7.5 waveform) or lower (6.5/3.5 waveform) than that for the monophasic waveform.) (Reproduced from Dixon EG et al: Improved defibrillation thresholds with large contoured epicardial electrodes and biphasic waveforms, *Circ Res* 69:842, 1991.)

several parameters change at the same time. For example, as can be seen in Fig. 3-10, when the duration of the first pulse is changed, the transition voltage between the first and second pulse and the duration of the second pulse are also changed. Therefore rectangular waveforms are used in some laboratories to separate these variables[73,74] and to explore defibrillation mechanisms,[56,81] as described below. With development of new technologies, it may also become possible to create rectangular waveforms for use in both transthoracic and internal clinical defibrillators.

MECHANISM OF THRESHOLD REDUCTION WITH BIPHASIC DEFIBRILLATOR WAVEFORMS

Biphasic waveforms that are approximately 10 msec in duration can be selected to decrease defibrillation threshold to approximately one half of that required with monophasic waveforms having the same duration.[11,12,17,56] Fig. 3-4 showed that monophasic waveforms, when delivered during the refractory period, may produce defibrillation by extending the cellular refractory period so that new fibrillation wavefronts cannot reexcite the cells. However, monophasic waveforms were only able to prolong the refractory period when delivered at relatively high intensity (about 3 times diastolic threshold. If other waveforms could produce similar refractory periods at lower intensities near threshold, they would be expected to lower defibrillation threshold.

Studies using electric field stimulation in humans[79,82] and in isolated cells[58] showed that low-intensity (1.5 times diastolic threshold) symmetrical biphasic stimuli produced significantly greater refractory period prolongation than control monophasic waveforms having similar total duration and intensity. The difference in duration of response between monophasic and biphasic waveforms disappeared with higher intensity shocks of four times diastolic threshold because both waveforms could now prolong the refractory period.[44,82] This finding is consistent with the finding that both monophasic and biphasic waveforms have high defibrillation efficacy at higher shock intensity approximately 1.4 times the voltage defibrillation threshold for the monophasic waveform.[56] The similarity between differences in refractory period prolongation at low but not high stimulus intensities and threshold differences between monophasic and biphasic waveforms is consistent with the hypothesis described below that the additional refractory period prolongation produced by low-intensity biphasic waveforms is responsible for their lower defibrillation thresholds.

During defibrillation ventricular cells are exposed to an electric field stimulus that simultaneously depolarizes one pole of the cell while hyperpolarizing the other,[61,63,72] as shown in Fig. 3-11, A. This complex interaction makes it difficult to separate the electrophysiologic effects of hyperpolarization and depolarization in different portions of the sarcolemma. One cannot determine which prolongs response duration during refractory period stimulation. Therefore current injection stimulation, which hyperpolarizes or depolarizes all portions of the cell membrane uniformly, as shown in Fig. 3-11, B, is useful in determining mechanisms underlying graded response prolongation by biphasic waveforms.[81]

Refractory period extension (response duration) similar to that observed with field stimulation also occurs with current injection. Fig. 3-12 shows the total response duration (TRD) produced by a second stimulus (S2, similar to the defibrillating stimulus D in Fig. 3-4), given during the refractory period of the first stimulus (S1, similar to the F1 stimulus in Fig. 3-4), as a function of coupling interval (S1-S2) for monophasic (Fig. 3-12, A) and biphasic (Fig. 3-12, B) stimulation. Ten S2 responses for different S1-S2 coupling intervals are superimposed on each figure. For the monophasic waveform, total response duration increased with S1-S2 coupling interval only after the refractory period (the last three responses shown). Only a very short action potential prolongation was produced when the stimulus was given during the refractory period. The biphasic waveform (Fig. 3-12, B) produced prolonged responses at earlier S1-S2 coupling intervals during the monophasic waveform refractory period (the last six responses) and produced longer response durations at specific coupling intervals during the cellular refractory period.

Fig. 3-13 shows the difference in response duration produced by biphasic

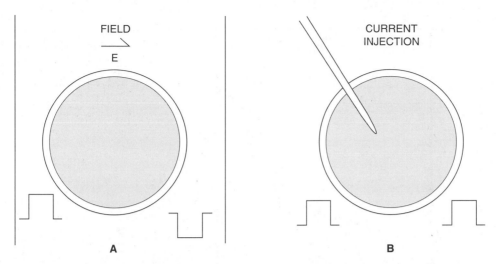

Fig. 3-11. Diagram contrasting electric field stimulation with current injection stimulation of a myocardial cell. With field stimulation (**A**), one portion of the cell membrane is hyperpolarized while the opposite portion is depolarized. With current injection stimulation (**B**), all portions of the membrane are either hyperpolarized or depolarized.

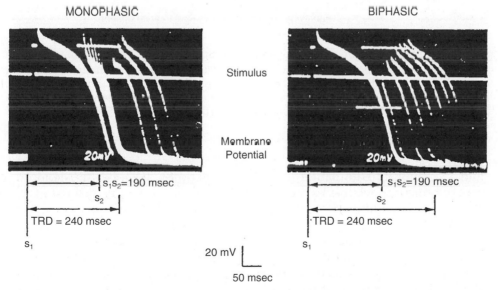

Fig. 3-12. Superimposed action potential recordings showing membrane responses to 1.5 times diastolic threshold current injection stimuli delivered at different S1-S2 coupling intervals during and following the relative refractory period. The biphasic waveform produces graded responses further into the refractory period than does the monophasic waveform. (Reproduced from Swartz JF et al: Conditioning prepulse of biphasic defibrillator waveforms enhances refractoriness to fibrillation wavefronts, *Circ Res* 68:438, 1991.)

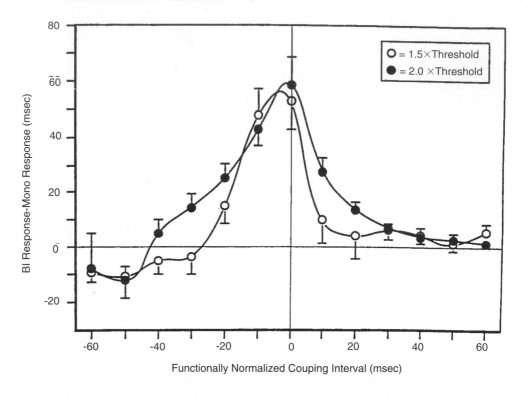

Fig. 3-13. Mean difference in total response duration at specific S1-S2 coupling intervals between monophasic and biphasic S2 stimuli as a function of the S1-S2 coupling interval normalized to the end of the S1 refractory period. (Reproduced from Swartz JF et al: Conditioning prepulse of biphasic defibrillator waveforms enhances refractoriness to fibrillation wavefronts, *Circ Res* 68:438, 1991.)

and monophasic stimulation at 1.5 and 2.0 times diastolic threshold as a function of time relative to the end of the refractory period (defined as 0).[81] The maximum difference in response duration of 62 msec occurred just before the end of the refractory period (at time equals 0). The difference in response duration disappeared at diastolic coupling intervals when both waveforms were effective in producing action potentials. The improved refractory period graded responses produced by biphasic waveforms occurred because the first hyperpolarizing portion of the biphasic waveform altered the membrane such that the subsequent depolarizing pulse produced a significantly larger response than could the depolarizing pulse alone. For current injection stimulation this response was specific to membrane hyperpolarization by the prepulse since prolonged responses did not occur when the polarity of the biphasic waveform was reversed.[81] (With electric field stimulation the direction of current through the electrodes is not important because the field produces opposite effects on opposite sides of the cells and responses are produced by the biphasic waveform at intensities below the response threshold for the monophasic waveform.) Therefore biphasic waveforms improve refractory period responses because the first hyperpolarizing phase repolarizes portions of the cell membrane. This allows time- and voltage-dependent excitation channel recovery and terminates the refractory period. The second phase then produces a longer response, which prolongs total cellular refractoriness, blocks fibrillation wavefronts, and terminates fibrillation.

Computer models of the ventricular action potential may improve our understanding of the ionic mechanisms underlying threshold reduction with biphasic waveforms by allowing a detailed examination of the underlying ionic currents.[43-47] A very simple model that contains sodium and calcium inward currents to describe the action potential upstroke and two potassium currents to describe repolarization can adequately describe action potential shape and define the cellular refractory period.[7,18] The primary characteristic defining the cellular refractory period is sodium channel inactivation, which occurs immediately following the upstroke of the action potential. Recovery from inactivation during and following repolarization is a time- and voltage-dependent process. With monophasic waveform S2 stimulation the model shows that no sodium current can be produced during the refractory period (Fig. 3-14, A, C). With low intensity biphasic waveforms (Fig. 3-14, A, B) the enhanced responses that occur correlate with increased sodium channel activity. This finding suggests that increased recovery of sodium channels from the inactivated to the resting state during the hyperpolarizing prepulse allows a larger sodium current to be produced during the subsequent depolarization. The larger sodium current produces greater slow calcium channel activation and is therefore indirectly responsible for prolonging response duration. Consistent with this hypothesis, enhanced refractory period responses, which are produced by biphasic waveforms at 1.5 times diastolic threshold (Fig. 3-15, A), do not occur when sodium channels are blocked as shown in Fig. 3-15, B.[45]

EFFECTS OF FIBRILLATION DURATION ON DEFIBRILLATION THRESHOLD

Several studies show that the probability of successful conversion of ventricular fibrillation to normal sinus rhythm decreases significantly with the long fibrillation durations associated with out-of-hospital resuscitations.[2,14,86,90] Although most hearts are relatively easy to defibrillate within the first 30 seconds of fibrillation, both clinically and in experimental models, defibrillation threshold increases even during this period, at least in animal models.[19,56,78] For example, recent studies in the biventricular working rabbit heart model[56] showed that the voltage threshold for monophasic waveforms (V_{50}) increased with fibrillation duration from 5 to 30 seconds (Fig. 3-16).

In the transthoracic calf model,[78] waveforms having high safety factors,

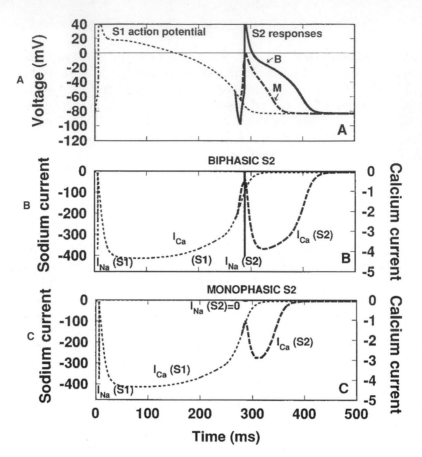

Fig. 3-14. Simulated action potentials (**A**) with associated inward sodium and calcium membrane currents (**B** and **C**) obtained from a computer model of
the ventricular action potential. In **A**, *B*-biphasic, *M*-monophasic. In **B** and
C, I_{Na} (S1)-Sodium current response to S1 stimulus; I Ca (S1)-calcium current response to S1 stimulus; I_{Na}(S2)-sodium current response to S2 stimulus; I_{Ca} (S2)-calcium current response to S2 stimulus. **A**, S2 refractory
period stimulation at an S1-S2 coupling interval of 280 msec (to the depolarizing pulse) with a hyperpolarizing/depolarizing 10 msec biphasic (*B*)
and a 10 msec monophasic (*M*) intracellular current injection waveform.
The refractory period response to the biphasic waveform is longer than the
response to the monophasic waveform. **B**, S2 sodium current following
biphasic waveform stimulation is almost as large as the control S1 sodium
current and is accompanied by a large S2 calcium current. **C**, Following
monophasic stimulation at the same coupling interval there is almost no
sodium current and the calcium current is very small. (Data adapted from
Jones R, Jones J: Refactory period stimulation with biphasic defibrillator
waveforms prolongs S1S2 response duration in the B-R computer model of
the ventricular action potential, *PACE* 13:93, 1990; Jones JL, Jones RE:
Enhanced graded response duration and sodium current with biphasic
defibrillator waveforms in a ventricular action potential computer model,
Circulation 84:II 610, 1991 [abstract].)

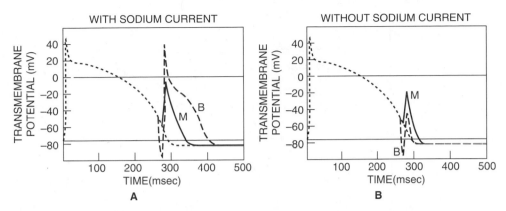

Fig. 3-15. Simulated action potentials resulting from stimulation of a computer model of the ventricular action potential. The control S1 action potential is shown by a dotted line. S2 refractory period stimulation using biphasic (*dashed line*) and monophasic (*solid line*) waveforms in the presence of sodium current (**A**) and in the absence of sodium current (**B**) (simulating blocked sodium channels). **A,** The biphasic waveform produces longer responses when normal sodium currents are allowed. However, when the sodium currents are blocked (**B**), the biphasic waveform fails to produce longer responses. These results strengthen the hypothesis that sodium channel recovery following early repolarization underlies increased biphasic waveform efficacy. (Data from Jones JL, Jones RE: Sodium channel blockade inhibits refactory period extension produced by biphasic defibrillator waveforms in a computer model of the ventricular action potential, *J Am Coll Cardiol* 17:335, 1991 [abstract].)

which produced a 100% success following 30 seconds of fibrillation, achieved only a 70% success following 1 minute of fibrillation. Therefore the criteria for a good defibrillator waveform become more stringent as the duration of fibrillation increases.

Clinically, no increase in defibrillation threshold was observed between 10 and 20 seconds fibrillation.[4] However, clinical studies place severe limitations on the methods that can ethically be used to determine defibrillation thresholds, and potentially small increases in threshold between these close time intervals may not have been revealed with these less precise methods.

Biphasic waveforms (10 msec duration, 50% undershoot) reduce defibrillation threshold compared to monophasic waveforms in both clinical and experimental models for fibrillation durations between 5 and 30 seconds, as discussed in the preceding sections. However, the relative efficacy of the biphasic waveform increases with increasing fibrillation duration because, while monophasic waveform threshold increases, biphasic waveform threshold remains relatively stable in rabbits as shown by the lower, more horizontal line for the biphasic waveform in Fig. 3-16.[56] Therefore B/M (the ratio of biphasic waveform threshold to monophasic waveform threshold) appears

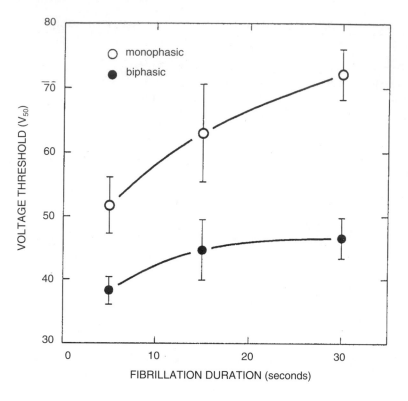

Fig. 3-16. Effects of fibrillation duration on defibrillation threshold in the isolated biventricular working rabbit heart using rectangular, 5 msec duration, monophasic and asymmetric biphasic (50% undershoot) defibrillator waveforms. (Modified from Jones JL et al: Increasing fibrillation duration enhances relative asymmetrical biphasic versus monophasic defibrillator waveform efficacy, *Circ Res* 67: 376, 1990.)

inversely proportional to monophasic waveform threshold as shown in Fig. 3-17, *A*. This figure combines data from 5, 15, and 30 seconds of fibrillation in the isolated, biventricular, working rabbit heart, and shows B/M as a function of monophasic waveform threshold. B/M decreases as monophasic threshold (M) increases. Stabilization of threshold by biphasic waveforms may be due to their combined ability to stimulate cells during their refractory period (valid at all fibrillation durations) and their ability to stimulate potassium depolarized cells (important for longer fibrillation durations), as discussed below.

Monophasic action potential recordings in humans (see Fig. 3-3) show that defibrillation shocks are delivered evenly throughout the cellular refractory periods of different cells no matter how long the fibrillation duration.[81] Therefore, the enhanced refractory period responses produced by biphasic waveforms are consistent with their ability to decrease defibrillation threshold at all fibrillation durations ranging from 5 to 30 seconds.[56]

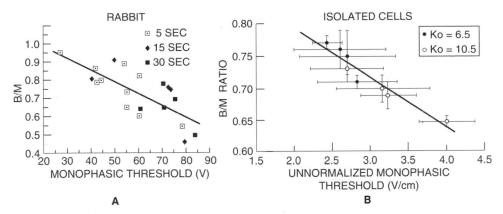

Fig. 3-17. A, Defibrillation threshold ratio for biphasic and monophasic waveforms as a function of monophasic waveform defibrillation threshold for fibrillation durations of 5, 15, and 30 seconds in the isolated, biventricular working rabbit heart. (Reproduced from reference 56). **B,** Biphasic to monophasic waveform excitation threshold ratio for myocardial cell aggregates as a function of monophasic waveform threshold under conditions of high extracellular potassium and short cycle length encroaching on the refractory period which simulate fibrillation. (Reproduced from Jones JL, Jones RE, Balasky G: Improved cardiac cell excitation with symmetrical biphasic defibrillator waveforms, *Am J Physiol* 253:H1418, 1987.)

However, as fibrillation duration increases within the 5 to 30 second range, myocardial cells become ischemic due to the lack of blood flow, and the frequency of the fibrillation lead II ECG decreases, suggesting lower activation rates.[2] Extracellular potassium accumulates in the interstitial spaces, causing the membrane to become depolarized to approximately −60 mV.[1] It is under these conditions that biphasic waveform threshold remains low while monophasic threshold increases. The mechanism for threshold stabilization has been examined in isolated myocardial cells. In this model, monophasic waveform excitation threshold increases when cells are made partially refractory through combinations of potassium depolarization and short cycle length encroaching on the refractory period.[48] The stabilization of excitation threshold by biphasic waveforms under these conditions is similar to the stabilization of defibrillation threshold by biphasic waveforms described above. Therefore the B/M ratio observed for excitation in isolated cells is very similar to that observed for defibrillation threshold in the rabbit heart, as shown in Fig. 3-17, *B*. These results are in agreement with the hypothesis that electric stimulation produces defibrillation by enhancing responses produced in partially refractory cells. The ventricular cell computer model[46] shows that when the initial membrane potential is depolarized to −60 mV, the ability of biphasic waveforms to decrease threshold is associated with improved availability of sodium channels following hyperpolarization by the first pulse.

IMPROVED DEFIBRILLATION EFFICACY WITH SHORT-DURATION BIPHASIC WAVEFORMS

In the canine model short-duration symmetrical biphasic waveforms, 3 msec in total duration, also improve defibrillation efficacy compared to similar short-duration monophasic waveforms.[15] However, in the canine[15,91] and isolated cell[36,55,59] models short-duration biphasic waveforms do not enhance the refractory period prolongation compared to similar-duration monophasic waveforms as do the long-duration biphasic waveforms. The ventricular cell computer model gives insight into the mechanism underlying this lack of improved efficacy. In this model 2 msec biphasic waveforms were also less able to prolong response duration than the corresponding monophasic waveform, as shown in Fig. 3-18,[55] which shows a very short period of membrane hyperpolarization during the short first phase of the biphasic waveform. Because sodium channel recovery is both a time- and voltage-dependent process, it is likely that this time is too short to allow sufficient sodium channel recovery to enhance the duration of the response to the subsequent depolarizing pulse.

At short durations it is likely that biphasic waveforms increase the probability of success by a different mechanism. An examination of the defibrillation strength-duration curves for monophasic waveforms[23] shows that the voltage (or current) required for defibrillation increases sharply for short-duration waveforms. Because such high-intensity stimuli are required, it is likely that cellular dysfunction is produced in regions of high current density.* Short-duration waveforms also have a lower safety factor (ratio of dysfunction threshold to excitation threshold for partially refractory cells) than do long-duration waveforms.[39,40] Therefore, as discussed earlier in this chapter, dysfunction is more likely to occur in high current density regions near the electrodes, even at defibrillation threshold intensities. Cellular dysfunction in high current density regions may lead to secondary refibrillation, causing a decreased probability of success.

As shown in Fig. 3-19, *A*, a small second pulse following the defibrillation shock shortens the duration of postshock arrest produced by the "defibrillation pulse" in the isolated cell model, even though it slightly increases delivered energy.[42] In this example the second pulse is 5 msec in duration and 10% in amplitude of the first pulse. Dysfunction reduction is very prominent for short-duration second pulses that are 1 msec in duration and 10% to 70% in amplitude of the first pulse, as shown in Fig. 3-19, *B*. The relative amplitude and duration of these second pulses are similar to the 40% to 60%, 2 msec undershoot or second phase of short-duration defibrillator waveforms that improve defibrillation efficacy but do not improve refractory period stimulation. Since the transient, shock-induced membrane depolarization that underlies this postshock arrest *in vitro* may also underlie postshock ventricular standstill and conduction block observed *in situ*, decreased postshock dysfunction produced with short-duration biphasic waveforms[42] would reduce

*References 23, 37-40, 42, 49, 50, 66, 73, 89.

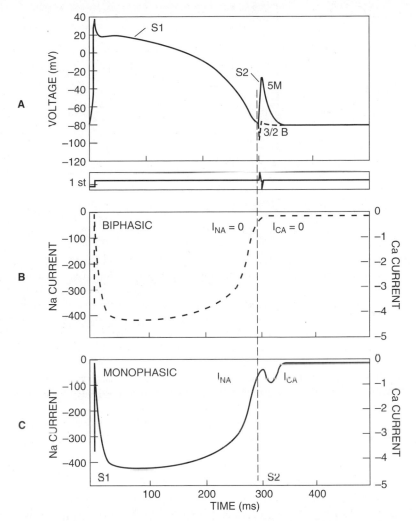

Fig. 3-18. Simulated refractory period responses (**A**) and associated sodium and calcium membrane currents (**B** and **C**) obtained from a computer model of the
ventricular action potential using an S1-S2 coupling interval of 300 msec.
In contrast to Fig. 3-14, which showed responses to long-duration waveforms of 10 msec, this figure shows responses to short-duration (5 msec
total duration) waveforms delivered at 1.5 times diastolic threshold for the
monophasic waveform. The control S1 action potential is shown to the left
of the figure. The refractory period stimulus, shown by S2, is delivered near
the end of the S1 action potential. The monophasic S2 waveform is a 5
msec rectangular pulse, and the biphasic S2 waveform is a 3 msec hyperpolarizing pulse followed by a 2 msec depolarizing pulse. **A,** The monophasic
S2 stimulus (*solid line*) produces a small graded response that correlates
with the small S2 sodium and calcium currents in **C**. The biphasic S2 stimulus (*dashed line*) produces only a hyperpolarizing shock artifact but no
actual response. The lack of membrane response to the short-duration
biphasic stimulus correlates with the lack of S2 sodium or calcium current
observed in **B**. (Data adapted from Jones JL et al: Short duration biphasic
defibrillator waveforms inhibit refractory period responses, *Circulation* 82:
2552, 1990 [abstract].)

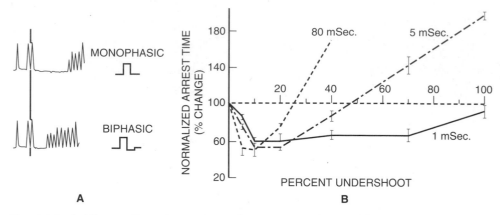

Fig. 3-19. A, Photocell mechanograms showing contractions of a spontaneously contracting cultured myocardial cell monolayer. Following a high-intensity electric field stimulus delivered at the time indicated by the arrow, there is a transient shock-induced arrest of contractile activity. The arrest following a biphasic shock (5 msec rectangular wave followed by a 5 msec reverse pulse with 10% undershoot) is shorter than that following the monophasic shock (5 msec rectangular waveform) of the same intensity. **B,** Shock-induced arrest time for biphasic waveforms as a function of percent undershoot of the second phase for second phases of different durations. Arrest times are normalized to those obtained with a control 5 msec waveform at the same intensity. (Jones JL, Jones RE: Decreased defibrillator induced dysfunction with biphasic rectangular waveforms, *Am J Physiol* 247:H792, 1984.)

the probability for secondary arrhythmias and improve defibrillation efficacy at specific shock intensities.

Even with longer-duration biphasic waveforms with a total duration of 10 msec the second pulse of biphasic waveforms may be important in preventing postshock dysfunction in high current density regions, especially with transvenous catheter systems or with transthoracic defibrillation. When both pulses of the biphasic waveform are 5 msec in duration, the asymmetrical waveform with 50% undershoot increases dysfunction threshold by about 15% while the symmetrical waveform does not alter dysfunction compared to the monophasic control waveform.[53]

TRIPHASIC WAVEFORMS

As shown in the previous sections, specifically shaped biphasic waveforms with relatively long first and second pulses greater than about 3 msec decrease the defibrillation threshold. This effect appears to be related to their improved ability to produce prolonged refractory period responses in myocardial cells under fibrillation conditions.[81] Differently shaped biphasic waveforms, which have a second negative portion 5 to 20 msec in duration and 5% to 20% in amplitude of the first portion, do not substantially improve cellular responses but reduce shock-induced dysfunction produced at specific shock intensities.[42] Similar biphasic waveforms decrease the duration of post-shock ventricular standstill in the calf model[74] and reduce the duration of conduction block in high current density regions near the defibrillating electrode in the canine model.[89] These two independent mechanisms for improving defibrillation efficacy could be combined into a single triphasic waveform.[41] The first pulse would lower threshold (by converting fast excitation channels to the resting state); the second pulse would produce the prolonged cellular response responsible for defibrillation; and the third pulse would help ameliorate dysfunction produced by the first two pulses. Triphasic waveforms with relative amplitudes of 100%/100%/10% (5 msec duration for each pulse) ameliorate dysfunction and increase safety factor *in vitro*.[41] Compared to monophasic rectangular waves, which have safety factors that peak at 100 with durations of 5 to 10 msec, biphasic waveforms increase the safety factor to 120 and triphasic waveforms to 130.

Similar truncated exponential triphasic waveforms decreased defibrillation threshold in the canine model[57] and reduced postshock arrhythmias in the calf model.[76] Other experiments to confirm the improved defibrillating ability of triphasic waveforms and optimize their shape have yet to be performed.

MULTIPLE PULSES AND PATHWAYS

The major recent research emphasis has been on biphasic waveforms because they reduce defibrillation significantly without requiring specialized lead systems. However, several other experimental waveforms and electrode configurations are also being tested to improve defibrillation efficacy. These include sequential pulses, overlapping pulses, and double pulse defibrillation.

SEQUENTIAL PULSE DEFIBRILLATION

During defibrillation the electric field produced between the two defibrillation electrodes is very uneven. Because the ability to defibrillate depends on producing a field of specific intensity (approximately 6 to 7 V/cm for a 14 msec truncated exponential)[87] in regions of weakest field intensity that are distant from the electrodes, any arrangement of electrodes that makes the electric field more uniform should reduce defibrillation threshold. One way in which the field can be made more uniform is by using three or four electrodes instead of two electrodes. However, if the shock is delivered through all electrodes simultaneously, "cold spots" are produced between the electrodes of the same polarity. Therefore, two shocks are usually delivered "sequentially" between different electrode pairs with a very short time interval separating the shocks.[9,87] Fig. 3-20 shows four electrodes on the surface of the heart during a clinical study to determine whether delivery of two sequential pulses through opposite pairs of the electrodes lowers defibrillation threshold compared to delivery of a single comparable shock through only one electrode pair using the waveforms shown in Fig. 3-20, *B*. For single shock defibrilla-

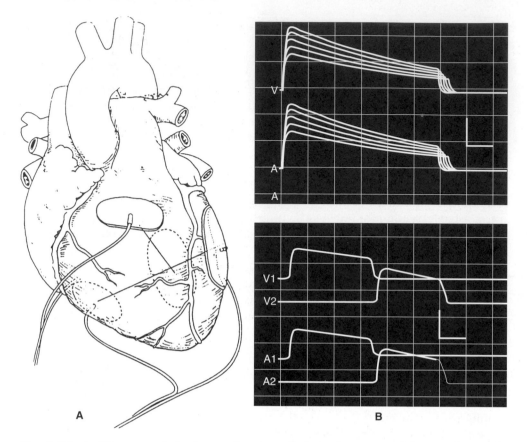

Fig. 3-20. A, Diagram of the heart showing clinical placement of four orthogonal
defibrillation electrodes used for sequential pulse defibrillation. **B,** Waveforms used for this clinical study of orthogonal sequential pulse defibrillation. (Modified from Jones DL, Klein GJ, Kallok MJ: Improved internal
defibrillation with twin pulse sequential energy delivery to different lead
orientations, *Am J Cardiol* 55: 821, 1985.)

tion the 5 msec truncated exponential pulse was delivered between a mesh
electrode on the posterior left ventricle (the anode) and the anterior right ventricle (the cathode). The first pulse of the sequential pulse shock was also
delivered through this pathway but was followed by a second pulse delivered
between the mesh electrode on the anterior left ventricle (anode) and the posterior right ventricle (cathode). In different trials large and small defibrillator
electrodes were tested. Summary results from this protocol are shown in Fig.
3-21, which shows the mean total energy required for both electrode
configurations for the large and small electrodes. With the small electrodes
(circles), defibrillation threshold for single shocks was very high, in agreement with the small surface area covered and the presumably large area of
"cold spots." The use of sequential pulses decreased defibrillation energy

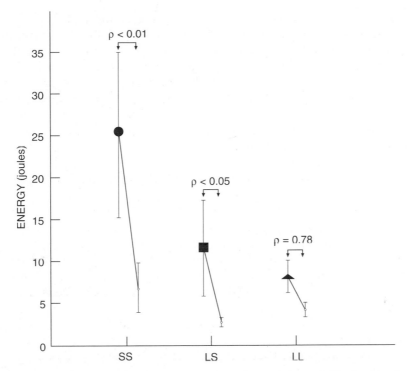

Fig. 3-21. Results from the clinical protocol used to compare defibrillation thresholds for single-pulse defibrillation with that using sequential pulses through orthogonal electrodes. (Modified from Jones DL, Klein GJ, Kallok MJ: Improved internal defibrillation with twin pulse sequential energy delivery to different lead orientations, *Am J Cardiol* 55: 821, 1985.)

threshold by about a factor of 5, consistent with the more uniform current delivery expected from these electrodes. When large electrodes, which produced a more uniform electric field, were used, defibrillation threshold for single pulses was reduced significantly. In this case the use of sequential pulses produced a significant though less impressive threshold reduction. Similar results have been obtained in several other animal[10,32] and clinical studies[6,9,31] and the optimal separation between the pulses is approximately 0.2 msec.[35]

In a recent study the potential gradients produced by sequential and simultaneous shocks delivered through a three-electrode system with electrodes placed on the lateral right atrium (R), the lateral left ventricular base (L), and the left ventricular apex (V) were directly compared with those produced by a single shock through two of the electrodes. The results showed that with a single pulse, minimum and maximum voltage gradients (V/cm) were 5.8/106 (R:V) and 7.3/182 (L:V), whereas the simultaneous pulse through all electrodes (R + L):V produced gradients of 5.7/130 and the sequential pulse (R:V

– L:V) produced gradients of 6.6/99. Using the sequential pulse protocol, electric fields were more uniform. As seen from this data the maximum voltage gradient produced by shocks having similar minimum intensities was lower.[87] Therefore sequential pulses also reduce the probability of shock-induced dysfunction in regions near the electrodes.[37,49,89] A recent animal study comparing sequential pulse defibrillation using three electrodes with biphasic waveform defibrillation through two electrodes showed that, with some electrode configurations and waveforms, sequential monophasic pulses may be more effective than biphasic waveforms.[34] Carefully adjusted combinations of sequential pulsing through multiple electrodes and biphasic waveforms may produce further reductions in defibrillation threshold as discussed below.[30]

DOUBLE DEFIBRILLATOR PULSES

Several investigators have tried to reduce defibrillation threshold by taking into account the cellular refractory period.* Rather than delivering a single high-intensity shock that would "stimulate" even refractory cells, two lower-intensity shocks are delivered, but with a separation that approximates the cell's action potential duration. The timing of the shocks is set so that the first shock stimulates cells that are at the end of their refractory period. The second shock stimulates cells that were refractory to the first shock. This technique proved useful in reducing the peak voltage for each shock, but did not reduce the total energy required to defibrillate. Even though total energy is not reduced with the double shock protocol, it may still be useful because it reduces peak voltage/current of the shock and thus may reduce the probability of postshock dysfunction.

The concept of double and sequential pulse defibrillation has been tested with biphasic waveforms with the first pulse delivered from the right ventricular apex catheter to a left lateral thorax patch and the second shock from a left ventricular apex patch to a catheter electrode in the right ventricular outflow tract.[30] The results, shown in Fig. 3-22, show that defibrillation threshold is increased significantly when the shocks are given 50 msec apart, compared to shocks through either electrode system alone (long arrows at left of figure), but that threshold is reduced when the pulses are given 90 to 100 msec apart or when the shock interval is approximately 90% to 110% of the fibrillation cycle length. These results suggest that biphasic waveforms combined with either the sequential-pulse technique or with the double-pulse technique behave like monophasic waveforms under similar defibrillation protocols and may still further reduce the voltage required for defibrillation.

CONCLUSIONS

Nonthoracotomy implantation of either right ventricular catheter/ subcutaneous patch or catheter-only systems produce much less uniform electric

*References 22, 67-69, 77, 84.

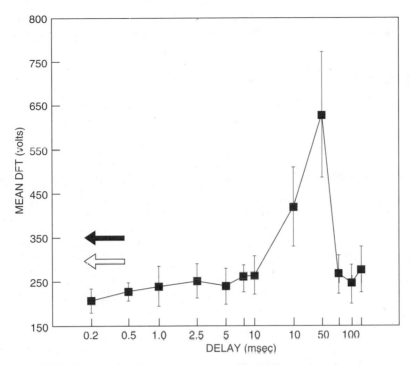

Fig. 3-22. Defibrillation voltage threshold for double biphasic pulses as a function of delay between the pulses. The arrows represent thresholds for the first or second shock alone from another study. (Modified from Johnson EE et al: Effect of pulse separation between two sequential biphasic shocks given over different lead configurations on ventricular defibrillation energy, *Circulation* 85:2267, 1992.)

fields. Consequently they require development of waveforms with much higher safety factors and lower defibrillation thresholds in order to reduce the probability of dysfunction in high current density regions near the defibrillation electrodes when intensities required for defibrillation are achieved in weak current density regions far from the electrodes. In addition, development of smaller generators with longer lifetimes requires development of waveforms with lower defibrillation thresholds. New experimental work in animal and clinical models, which is investigating mechanisms underlying defibrillation, is leading to the desired improved waveforms. However, because defibrillation mechanisms are still only poorly understood, many decisions concerning waveforms for implantable and transthoracic defibrillators must still be made on an empirical basis. This concept was elegantly put by Kugelberg in 1975[67] when he said:

> The exact nature of fibrillation is not yet known and therefore the ideal defibrillation cannot be performed. The double pulses have not presented a solution to the problem, but when such a solution finally is found—I am convinced that it

will be a low-energy combination of pulses. Anyhow, I would like to make this comparison—if a locked door has to be passed dynamite can be used, if one doesn't have the key.

REFERENCES

1. Akiyama T: Intracellular recording of in situ ventricular cells during ventricular fibrillation, *Am J Physiol* 240:H465, 1981.
2. Allen JD et al: Fibrillation frequency and ventricular defibrillation, *Proc IEEE Eng Med Biol Soc* 14:655, 1992.
3. Babbs CF et al: Therapeutic indices for transchest defibrillator shocks: effective, damaging, and lethal electrical doses, *Am Heart J* 99:734, 1980.
4. Bardy GH et al: A prospective, randomized evaluation of effect of ventricular fibrillation duration on defibrillation thresholds in humans, *J Am Coll Cardiol* 13:1362, 1989.
5. Bardy GH et al: A prospective randomized evaluation of biphasic versus monophasic waveform pulses on defibrillation efficacy in humans, *J Am Coll Cardiol* 14:728, 1989.
6. Bardy GH et al: Prospective comparison of sequential pulse and single pulse defibrillation with use of two different clinically available systems, *J Am Coll Cardiol* 14:165, 1989.
7. Beeler GW, Reuter H: Reconstruction of the action potential of ventricular myocardial fibres, *J Physiol* 268:177, 1977.
8. Bourland JD, Tacker WA Jr, Geddes ME: Strength-duration curves for trapezoidal waveforms of various tilts for transchest defibrillation in animals, *Med Instrum* 12:38, 1978.
9. Bourland JD et al: Sequential pulse defibrillation for implantable defibrillators, *Med Instrum* 20:138, 1986.
10. Chang MS: Double and triple sequential shocks reduce ventricular defibrillation threshold in dogs with and without myocardial infarction, *J Am Coll Cardiol* 8:1393, 1986.
11. Chapman PD et al: Comparative efficacy of monophasic and biphasic truncated exponential shocks in nonthoracotomy internal defibrillation in dogs, *J Am Coll Cardiol* 12:739, 1988.
12. Chapman PD et al: Comparison of monophasic with single and dual capacitor biphasic waveforms for nonthoracotomy canine internal defibrillation, *J Am Coll Cardiol* 14:242, 1989.
13. Chen PS et al: Activation during ventricular defibrillation in open-chest dogs: evidence of complete cessation and regeneration of ventricular fibrillation after unsuccessful shocks, *J Clin Invest* 77:810, 1986.
14. Dalzell GWN, Adgey AAJ: Determinants of successful transthoracic defibrillation and outcome in ventricular fibrillation, *Br Heart J* 65:311, 1991.
15. Daubert JP et al: Response of relatively refractory canine myocardium to monophasic and biphasic shocks, *Circulation* 84:2522, 1991.
16. Dillon SM: Optical recordings in the rabbit heart show that defibrillation strength shocks prolong the duration of depolarization and the refractory period, *Circ Res* 69:842, 1991.
17. Dixon EG et al: Improved defibrillation thresholds with large contoured epicardial electrodes and biphasic waveforms, *Circulation* 76:1176, 1987.
18. Drouhard J, Roberge FA: Revised formulation of the Hodgkin-Huxley representation of the sodium current in cardiac cells, *Comp Biomed Res* 20:333, 1987.
19. Echt DS, Barbey JT, Black JN: Influence of ventricular fibrillation duration on defibrillation energy in dogs using bidirectional pulse discharges, *PACE* 11:1315, 1988.
20. Fain ES, Sweeney MB, Franz, MR: Improved internal defibrillation efficacy with a biphasic waveform, *Am Heart J* 117:358, 1989.
21. Flaker GC et al: Superiority of biphasic shocks in the defibrillation of dogs by epicardial patches and catheter electrodes, *Am Heart J* 118:288, 1989.
22. Geddes LA, Tacker WA Jr, McFarlane JR: Ventricular defibrillation with single and twin pulses of half-sinusoidal current, *J Appl Physiol* 34:8, 1973.

23. Gold HJ et al: Transthoracic ventricular defibrillation in the 100 kg calf with unidirectional rectangular pulses, *Circulation* 56:745, 1977.

24. Gold JH, HC Schuder, H Stoeckle: Contour graph for related percent success in achieving ventricular defibrillation to duration, current, and energy content of shock, *Am Heart J* 98:207, 1979.

25. Guarnieri T et al: Increased pacing threshold after an automatic defibrillator shock in dogs: effects of Class I and Class II antiarrhythmic drugs, *PACE* 11:1324, 1988.

26. Huagui GL et al: Defibrillation shocks increase myocardial pacing threshold: an intracellular microelectrode study, *Am J Physiol* 260:H1973, 1991.

27. Holmes HR et al: Hemodynamic responses to two defibrillating trapezoidal waveforms, *Med Instrum* 14:47, 1980.

28. Holt RW, GM Saidel, JL Jones: Sodium diffusion from cardiac cell aggregate after defibrillation, *Proc AIChE Meeting*, 1988.

29. Holt RW, RE Jones, JL Jones: Increased cytosolic sodium following defibrillator-type electric field stimulation, *Circulation* 78 (Part II), abstract 46, 1988.

30. Johnson EE et al: Effect of pulse separation between two sequential biphasic shocks given over different lead configurations on ventricular defibrillation energy, *Circulation* 85:2267, 1992.

31. Jones DL et al: Internal cardiac defibrillation in man: pronounced improvement with sequential pulse delivery to two different lead orientations, *Circulation* 73:484, 1986.

32. Jones DL, Klein GJ, Kallok MJ: Improved internal defibrillation with twin pulse sequential energy delivery to different lead orientations in pigs, *Am J Cardiol* 55:821, 1985.

33. Jones DL et al: Sequential pulse defibrillation in humans: orthogonal sequential pulse defibrillation with epicardial electrodes, *J Am Coll Cardiol* 11:590, 1988.

34. Jones DL, Klein GJ, Wood GK: Biphasic versus sequential pulse defibrillation: a direct comparison in pigs, *Am Heart J* 124:97, 1992.

35. Jones DL et al: Internal ventricular defibrillation with sequential pulse countershock in pigs: comparison with single

pulses and effects of pulse separation, *PACE* 10:497, 1987.

36. Jones J: Effect of waveform duration on cellular responses to monophasic and biphasic defibrillation waveforms, *Proc AAMI 26th Annual Meeting*, 1991.

37. Jones JL, Jones RE: Post-shock arrhythmias—a possible cause of unsuccessful defibrillation, *Crit Care Med* 8:167, 1980.

38. Jones JL, Jones RE: Postcountershock fibrillation in digitalized myocardial cells in vitro, *Crit Care Med* 8:172, 1980.

39. Jones JL, Jones RE: Determination of safety factor for defibrillator waveforms in cultured heart cells, *Am J Physiol* 242:H662, 1982.

40. Jones JL, Jones RE: Improved defibrillator waveform safety factor with biphasic waveforms, *Am J Physiol* 245:H60, 1983.

41. Jones JL, Jones RE: Improved safety factor with triphasic defibrillator waveforms, *Circ Res* 64:1172, 1989.

42. Jones JL, Jones RE: Decreased defibrillator induced dysfunction with biphasic rectangular waveforms, *Am J Physiol* 247:H792, 1984.

43. Jones R, Jones J: Refractory period stimulation with biphasic defibrillator waveforms prolongs S1S2 response duration in the B-R computer model of the ventricular action potential, *PACE* 13:93, 1990.

44. Jones JL, Jones RE: Effects of monophasic defibrillator waveform intensity on graded response duration in a computer simulation of the ventricular action potential, *Proc IEEE Eng Med Biol Soc* 13:598, 1991.

45. Jones JL, Jones RE: Sodium channel blockade inhibits refractory period extension produced by biphasic defibrillator waveforms in a computer model of the ventricular action potential, *J Am Coll Cardiol* 17:335, 1991 (abstract).

46. Jones JL, Jones RE: Threshold reduction with biphasic defibrillator waveforms: role of excitation channel recovery in a computer model of the ventricular action potential, *J Electrocardiol* 23:30, 1991.

47. Jones JL, Jones RE: Enhanced graded response duration and sodium current with biphasic defibrillator waveforms in a ventricular action potential computer model, *Circulation* 84:II610, 1991 (abstract).

48. Jones JL, Jones RE, Balasky G: Improved cardiac cell excitation with symmetrical biphasic defibrillator waveforms, *Am J Physiol* 253:H1418, 1987.

49. Jones JL, Jones RE, Balasky G: Microlesion formation in myocardial cells by high-intensity electric field stimulation, *Am J Physiol* 253:H480, 1987.

50. Jones J: Defibrillator induced dysfunction and calcium overload, *Fed Proc* 46:409, 1987.

51. Jones JL et al: Response of cultured myocardial cells to countershock-type electric field stimulation, *Am J Physiol* 235:H214, 1978.

52. Jones JL, Milne K, Jones R: Improved safety factor with long duration symmetrical biphasic defibrillator waveforms, *PACE* 15:529, 1992.

53. Jones JL, Milne K, Jones RE: Postshock dysfunction induced by simulated one- and two-capacitor defibrillator waveforms, *Proc IEEE Eng Med Biol Soc* 14:638, 1992.

54. Jones JL et al: Ultrastructural injury to chick myocardial cells in vitro following "electric countershock," *Circ Res* 46:387, 1980.

55. Jones JL et al: Short duration biphasic defibrillator waveforms inhibit refractory period responses, *Circulation* 82:2552, 1990 (abstract).

56. Jones JL et al: Increasing fibrillation duration enhances relative asymmetrical biphasic versus monophasic defibrillator waveform efficacy, *Circ Res* 67:376, 1990.

57. Jones JL et al: Triphasic waveforms increase defibrillation efficacy over biphasic waveforms with catheter/subcutaneous patch electrodes, *J Am Coll Cardiol* 13:218, 1989.

58. Jones JL et al: Extracellular field stimulation with symmetrical biphasic defibrillator waveforms enhances refractory period responses, *Proc AAMI 25th Ann Meeting* 1990, p 46 (abstract).

59. Karasik P, Jones R, Jones J: Effect of waveform duration on refractory period extension produced by monophasic and biphasic defibrillator waveforms, *PACE* 14:715, 1991 (abstract).

60. Kavanagh KM: Comparison of the internal defibrillation thresholds for monophasic and double and single capacitor biphasic waveforms, *J Am Coll Cardiol* 14:1343, 1989.

61. Klee M, Plonsey R: Stimulation of spheroidal cells—the role of cell shape, *IEEE Trans Biomed Engineering* BME-23:347, 1976.

62. Koning G, Veefkind AH, Schneider H: Cardiac damage caused by direct application of defibrillator shocks to isolated Langendorff-perfused rabbit heart, *Am Heart J* 4:473, 1980.

63. Krassowska W, Pilkington TC, Ideker RE: Periodic conductivity as a mechanism for cardiac stimulation and defibrillation, *IEEE Trans Biomed Eng* BME-34:555, 1987.

64. Lepeschkin E et al: Analysis of cardiac damage following elective cardiac defibrillation, *Proc Cardiac Defibrillation Conference*, W Lafayette, Indiana, 1975, Purdue University, pp 85-90.

65. Lepeschkin E et al: Local potential gradients as a unifying measure for thresholds of stimulation, standstill, tachyarrhythmia and fibrillation appearing after strong capacitor discharges, *Adv Cardiol* 21:268, 1977.

66. Li HG et al: Defibrillation shocks increase myocardial pacing threshold: an intracellular microelectrode study, *Am J Physiol* 260:H1973, 1991.

67. Kugelberg J: Multiple pulse defibrillation, *Proc Cardiac Defibrillation Conference*, W Lafayette, Indiana, 1975, Purdue University, p 81.

68. McFarlane J et al: Ventricular defibrillation with single and multiple half sinusoidal pulses of current, *Cardiovasc Res* 5:286, 1971.

69. Moore TW, DiMeo FN, Dubin SE: The effect of shock separation time on multiple-shock defibrillation, *Med Instrum* 12:31, 1978.

70. Mower MM et al: Patterns of ventricular activity during catheter defibrillation, *Circulation* 49:858, 1974.

71. Peleska B: Cardiac arrhythmias following condensor discharges and their dependence upon strength of current and phase of cardiac cycle, *Circ Res* 13:21, 1963.

72. Rush S et al: Field modeling for defibrillation studies, *Proc Cardiac Defibrillation Conference*, W Lafayette, Indiana, 1975, Purdue University, pp 103-107.

73. Schuder JC et al: Transthoracic ventricular defibrillation in the 100 kg calf with sym-

metrical one-cycle bidirectional rectangular wave stimuli, *IEEE Trans Biomed Eng-* 30:415, 1983.

74. Schuder JC, McDaniel, WC, Stoeckle H: Defibrillation of 100kg calves with asymmetrical, bidirectional, rectangular pulses, *Cardiovasc Res* 18:419, l984.

75. Schuder JC, McDaniel, WC, Stoeckle H: Transthoracic ventricular defibrillation of 100 kilogram calves with critically damped sinusoidal shocks, *Proc AAMI 21st Annual Meeting*, 1986.

76. Schuder, JC, McDaniel, WC, Stoeckle H: Triphasic rectangular waveforms: a comparison with biphasic wave shocks in the defibrillation of 100 kilogram calves, *Proc AAMI 24th Annual Meeting*, 1989.

77. Schuder JC et al: Transthoracic ventricular defibrillation in the dog with unidirectional rectangular double pulses, *Cardiovasc Res* 4:497, 1970.

78. Schuder JC et al: Relationship between duration of ventricular fibrillation and effectiveness of therapuetic shock, *Proc ACEMB*, 1972.

79. Swartz JF, Jones JL, Fletcher RD: Symmetrical biphasic defibrillator waveforms enhance refractory period stimulation in the human heart, *J Am Coll Cardiol* 17:335, 1991 (abstract).

80. Swartz JF, Jones JL, Fletcher RD: Characterization of ventricular fibrillation based on monophasic action potential morphology in the human heart, *Circulation* 87:1907, 1993.

81. Swartz JF et al: Conditioning prepulse of biphasic defibrillator waveforms enhances refractoriness to fibrillation wavefronts, *Circ Res* 68:438, 1991.

82. Swartz JF et al: Field stimulation with symmetrical biphasic waveforms prolongs refractoriness to simulated refibrillation in human hearts, *PACE* 14:192, 1991 (abstract).

83. Sweeney RJ: Ventricular refractory period extension caused by defibrillation shocks, *Circulation* 82:965, 1990.

84. Sweeney RJ, Gill RM, Reid PR: Use of the fibrillation cycle length to effectively combine multiple defibrillation shocks, *Circulation* 84:II-610, 1991 (abstract).

85. Tang ASL et al: Ventricular defibrillation using biphasic waveforms: the importance of phasic duration, *J Am Coll Cardiol* 13:207, 1989.

86. Weaver WD et al: Factors influencing survival after out-of-hospital cardiac arrest, *J Am Coll Cardiol* 7:752, 1986.

87. Wharton JM et al: Cardiac potential and potential gradient fields generated by single, combined, and sequential shocks during ventricular fibrillation, *Circulation* 85:1510, 1992.

88. Winkle RA et al: Improved low energy defibrillation efficacy in man with the use of a biphasic truncated exponential waveform, *Am Heart J* 117:122, 1989.

89. Yabe S et al: Conduction disturbances caused by high current density electric fields, *Circ Res* 66:1190, 1990.

90. Yakaitis RW et al: Influence of time and therapy on ventricular defibrillation in dogs, *Crit Care Med* 8:157, 1980.

91. Zhou X et al: Prolongation of repolarization time by electric field stimulation with monophasic and biphasic shocks in open-chest dogs, *Circ Res* 68:1761, 1991.

92. Zhou X et al: Potential gradient needed for defibrillation with monophasic and biphasic shocks, *PACE* 12:66, 1989 (abstract).

93. Zipes DP et al: Termination of ventricular fibrillation in dogs by depolarizing a critical amount of myocardium, *Am J Cardiol* 36:37, 1975.

Chapter 4
Electrodes for Transchest and ICD Defibrillation and Multifunctional Electrodes

L. A. Geddes

Electrical defibrillation is achieved by the passage of a current pulse through electrodes; three types of electrodes are used: (1) transthoracic, (2) heart-surface, and (3) intracardiac. There are two types of transthoracic electrodes: handheld and preapplied (which are self-adhering). There are two types of direct-heart electrodes: handheld and implantable. Implantable electrodes are used with the implantable cardioverter-defibrillator (ICD) and consist of combinations of electrodes that are either patches applied to the heart surface, intracavity catheter-mounted rings or coils, or subcutaneous patches.

The ideal electrode system requires that a uniform defibrillating current must reach almost all of the myocardial tissue to render it refractory, thereby extinguishing the reentrant excitation that sustains fibrillation.

TRANSTHORACIC ELECTRODES

HANDHELD ELECTRODES

Fig. 4-1 shows a typical handheld electrode used for transchest defibrillation. A button (x) on the handle allows the operator to deliver the shock. Such electrodes are applied to the chest after the metal part is covered with a low-resistivity electrode gel, or after a low-resistivity pad is applied to the metal. The gel-coated electrode was used early in defibrillation and is still in widespread use because of its low cost, simplicity, and low impedance. Use of low-resistivity gel, specifically designed for defibrillation, is important. Ultrasonic coupling gel or K-Y jelly should never be used, because these preparations are poor conductors of electric current. Sirna et al.[45] reported that ultrasonic coupling gel produced a 20% higher impedance than low-resistivity gel.

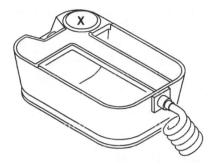

Fig. 4-1. Hand-held transthoracic electrode.

There is an American National Standard for the size of defibrillating electrodes published in 1989 by the Association for the Advancement of Medical Instrumentation (AAMI); it recommends:

3.2.1.21 Paddle Electrode Contact Area: The minimum contact area per electrode shall be:
1) 50cm² for adult transthoracic use
2) 32cm² for adult internal use
3) 15cm² for pediatric transthoracic use
4) 9cm² for pediatric internal use

The standard does not specify a shape; most electrodes are either circular or rectangular with rounded corners. Many electrodes are larger than the 50 cm² minimum, often being 80 to 100 cm².

In addition to proper size, it is necessary to use electrodes located in the proper sites to achieve an adequate current-density distribution within the ventricles. The optimum locations for thoracic electrodes were determined empirically from animal and human studies. In the early days of defibrillation two electrode configurations were used: chest-to-back and precordial. The former array was used for atrial cardioversion but was found to be effective for ventricular defibrillation with a large back-plate electrode. The anterior (precordial) chest location is most frequently used today for emergency defibrillation because it allows quick and easy application.

Advantage has been taken of the anatomic distribution of low- and high-conducting tissues in the thorax to select the optimum locations for precordial electrodes. Location is clearly important, as shown by Geddes et al.,[26] who determined the effect of electrode site on defibrillation threshold in dogs using 5 msec damped sine-wave current applied to a small (3.2 cm diameter) exploring electrode paired with a large electrode. First, a large (12 cm diameter) electrode was sutured to the right chest and the defibrillation threshold was mapped on the left hemithorax with the 3.2 cm diameter electrode. Second, a large (23 × 30cm) electrode was placed on the back and the anterior thorax was mapped with the 3.2 cm electrode. Third, the 12 cm diameter electrode was sutured to the left chest and the right chest was mapped with the 3.2 cm electrode. From the threshold defibrillating current values measured at uniformly spaced sites, isodose (amps/kg) contours were plotted. Fig. 4-2, *A*, shows the results for the left-chest (3.2 cm) right-chest (12cm) study. Fig. 4-2, *B*, shows the results for the anterior (3.2cm) chest-to-back (23 × 30 cm) study. Figure 4-2, *C*, shows the results for the right-chest (3.2 cm) to left-chest (12 cm) study. The shaded areas identify the locations for the different thresholds, the darker areas representing the lowest defibrillating current thresholds.

With the large electrode on the right chest and the small electrode on the left (Fig. 4-2, *A*), it is clear that the lowest current for defibrillation was found with the small electrode over the apex-beat area. With the small electrode on the anterior chest and the large (23 × 30 cm) electrode on the back (Fig. 4-2, *B*), the lowest current for defibrillation was just central to the apex-beat area. With the 12 cm electrode on the left chest and the 3.2 cm electrode used to map the right chest (Fig. 4-2, *C*), the threshold for defibrillation was higher and the region for the minimum was in the head-tail direction and appeared to follow the inferior vena cava, indicating that much of the current may be conducted to the heart by the venous blood. Clearly, defibrillation success will depend on electrode location. From the size of the thoracic-current windows, it is likely that electrodes that are too large will be less effective in delivering current to the ventricles. Similarly electrodes that are too small will result in inadequate current to some of the ventricular mass.

Many electrical models have been reported for the thorax with the goal of studying the effect of electrode size and location on myocardial current density. Although such studies do give a good insight into the variables, they run into complexity because of the anatomic arrangement of tissues and fluids, all with differing conducting properties. Moreover, most tissues have different conductivity values in the transverse and longitudinal directions.

PREAPPLIED, ADHESIVE ELECTRODES

Certain patients are identifiable as being at high risk of fibrillation, and for them there are several types of preapplied electrodes. All contain a conducting medium backed by a metal foil, which in turn is backed by a pliable insulating material. In some cases the conducting medium consists of a gel pad impregnated with electrolyte; in others the gel is a conducting adhesive. Around the conducting medium is an adhesive perimeter, which is usually an extension of the insulating backing. All such electrodes have a plastic peel-off cover that protects the electrode from drying during storage. Additional protection is afforded by a hermetically sealed package. Both features provide a long shelf-life for these liquid-containing electrodes.

Fig. 4-3 illustrates four types of electrodes; Figs. 4-3, *A*, and 4-3, *B*, show

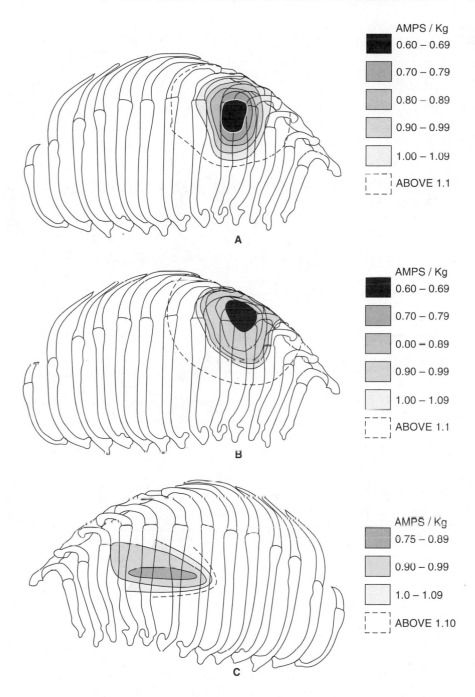

Fig. 4-2. Isocurrent contours for defibrillation obtained by mapping the chest with a small (3.2 cm) electrode paired with a large indifferent electrode. **A,** Left chest. **B,** Anterior chest. **C,** Right chest. (Redrawn from Geddes LA et al: The thoracic windows for electrical ventricular defibrillation current, *Am Heart J* 94:67, 1977.

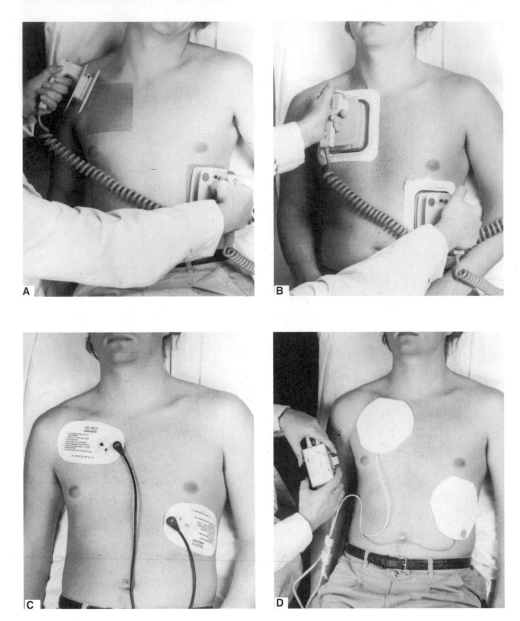

Fig. 4-3. Preapplied electrodes. **A**, 3-M defib pads. **B**, AMI pads and preapplied electrodes. **C**, Self-adhering Physio-Control pads. **D**, Darox pads with Darox coupler for the defibrillator. (From *Health Devices* 19:33, 1990. By permission ECRI, Plymouth Meeting, PA 19462.)

handheld electrodes in the anterior chest location (*A* and *B* are 3M and AMI electrodes, respectively). Fig. 4-3, *C*, illustrates Physio-Control, self-adhering electrodes with lead wires for connection to the defibrillator. Fig. 4-3, *D*, illustrates Darox electrodes and also shows the adapter required for connection to the defibrillator.

The preapplied, self-adhering, disposable electrode has some advantages over handheld electrodes. They can be made conformable and can be applied prophylactically in the correct locations. Because the conducting gel is contained inside the electrode by the adhesive perimeter, the exposed parts of the chest are dry, making it easy to apply CPR without the hands slipping from liquid gel that is applied when paddle electrodes are used. Another important feature is that the operator is prevented from using the incorrect coupling gel. Preapplied electrodes can be used for repeated shocks over a prolonged period. Usually, with preapplied electrodes, separate ECG recording electrodes are used. With the self-adhering type, operator safety is enhanced because it is not necessary to be near the subject when the defibrillating shock is delivered.

There are some disadvantages to preapplied electrodes. The first is that a defibrillator coupling device is needed and in some designs a means must be provided for discharging the defibrillator. Contact may not be as good with preapplied, self-adhering electrodes because manual pressure is not applied by the operator. This is partly the reason that the impedance of preapplied electrodes is slightly higher than that for handheld paddles. Also, self-adhering electrodes do not adhere as well to diaphoretic subjects or to subjects with very hairy skin. The adhesive may stick to the hair more than to the skin. Preapplied electrodes should never be removed and reapplied, because the adhesive will be less effective. Instead, new electrodes should be used. Also, if the electrode is stiff, "tenting," that is, buckling of the electrode, can occur so that a portion does not contact the skin. With buckling, the effective electrode area is decreased, the impedance is high, and less current may flow; consequently higher defibrillator output is required and arcing is more likely to occur under such an electrode. Finally, for semisolid gels, if the storage package is punctured, the electrolyte can dry out and result in poor contact when applied to the subject.

There is no special performance standard for semisolid gel pads or preapplied electrodes. However, the AAMI/ANSI Defibrillator and ECG standards of performance apply to these electrodes.

Electrophysiologic studies carry the risk of ventricular fibrillation. In some instances, right- or left-ventricular catheterization is used to perform angiographic studies, and there is some risk of precipitating ventricular fibrillation during these procedures. To permit prompt defibrillation in such circumstances, several manufacturers provide x-ray transparent, preapplied, precordial defibrillating electrodes. With a defibrillator connected to the electrodes during fluoroscopy, any tachyarrhythmia can be treated promptly.

IMPEDANCE OF PREAPPLIED ELECTRODES

When preapplied electrodes first appeared, there was considerable interest in their impedance compared to that exhibited by handheld paddle electrodes coated with low-resistivity electrode gel. Ewy et al.[17] conducted a 24-dog study in which the impedance of paddles coated with low-resistivity gel was compared to that offered by two types of preapplied electrodes (SAF-D-FIB and DEFIB-PADS). Damped sinusoidal current at 100 and 400 J was applied. At both energy levels the preapplied electrodes exhibited a higher impedance than that with the paddle electrodes coated with low-resistivity gel. In the case of the SAF-D-FIB electrodes the impedances were 28% and 20% higher at the 100 and 400 J levels. The impedances for the DEFIB-PADS were 14% and 17% higher at the 100 and 400 J levels. In a similar 8-dog study Ewy and Taren[16] found that CDC electrode gel cups offered a higher impedance than handheld paddles. Tacker and Paris[49] undertook an 8-dog study to compare the impedance and percent successful defibrillation between paddle electrodes coated with a low-resistivity gel and the same electrodes used with a semisolid DEFIB-PAD placed between each electrode and the skin. Damped sinusoidal current was used with both types, and 10kg of force pressed the electrodes against the chest. With the gel-coated paddles the average impedance was 37 ohms and with the DEFIB PADS between the electrodes and skin the average impedance was 44 ohms. However, the defibrillation percent success with the paddles was 77.5% and that with the DEFIB PADS was 87.5%. The authors stated that DEFIB-PADS were as good as gel but not better since the difference in success was not statistically significant. They also stated that the slightly higher percent success may be due to slightly improved current distribution under the DEFIB-PAD.

Indirect evidence for a different current-density distribution under preapplied electrodes comes from a human study by Jakobson et al.[35] who compared the CK skeletal-muscle specific enzyme release following cardioversion in humans using paddle electrodes and DEFIB-PADS under standard paddle electrodes. It was found that DEFIB-PADS were associated with only one half the CK release compared to standard electrodes and electrode gel. Decreased CK levels suggest less muscle tissue damage, and perhaps that is due to more even current distribution under the electrodes.

The issue of whether the higher impedance of preapplied electrodes affected percent successful defibrillation aroused considerable interest and produced clinical studies focused on this subject. Kerber et al.[38] reported an 80-patient study using preapplied electrodes that contained stannous chloride electrode gel. Three different damped sine wave defibrillators were used for cardioversion and defibrillation. The authors reported a mean impedance of 75 +/− 21 ohms offered to the defibrillating current and also reported that the preapplied electrodes were equally effective with precordial or chest-to-back positions. From earlier studies with hand-held paddle electrodes, Kerber had reported a chest impedance of 67 +/− 36 ohms. In an 11-dog study with the same defibrillators, impedance was compared with preapplied electrodes and handheld electrodes coated with low-resistivity gel. Shocks of 50, 75, 100, 125, and 150 J were delivered and the current was measured. The preapplied electrodes were placed on the anterior chest as well as on the chest and back. Although the impedances with the handheld electrodes were slightly lower, the percent successful defibrillation was essentially the same. It was also noted that the impedance for all electrodes decreased with increasing current and energy. This subject will be discussed later in this chapter.

Using dogs, Aylward et al.[4] investigated the effect of different coupling agents on the thoracic impedance as well as the percent successful defibrillation. They used handheld paddle electrodes coated with a low-resistivity gel and two types of gel pads under the electrodes. They found that although the thoracic impedance was slightly lower with the handheld paddles coated with low-resistivity gel, the percent successful defibrillation was essentially the same for all three types of electrodes.

The foregoing shows clearly that preapplied electrodes and gel pads function well for defibrillation and cardioversion, if they conform and adhere snugly to the chest, despite the fact that they exhibit a slightly higher impedance than handheld paddle electrodes. Obviously, if they do not conform and adhere well because of hairy or wet skin or electrode stiffness, they will not maintain adequate contact for effective current flow.

When considering the impedance of the electrode-subject circuit, it is well to remember that where the current flows is equally important. Therefore when comparing electrode types, it is important that they be placed in the same locations and equally important is the comparative percent successful defibrillation data.

ELECTRODES FOR THE IMPLANTED CARDIOVERTER DEFIBRILLATOR (ICD)

For the ICD many electrode configurations have been investigated. In the early days of ICD research it was hoped that it would be possible to use the same implantation technique used for cardiac pacemakers. Therefore animal studies using right-heart catheter bipolar electrodes were undertaken to determine the voltage, current, and energy required for defibrillation. Because the implant had to be as small as possible, the truncated exponential wave rather than the damped sine wave was used, because the latter requires inclusion of a heavy inductor. The major design goal was achievement of defibrillation with the lowest voltage to enable the use of space-efficient electrolytic capacitors in the implant. These early studies were reviewed in a book by Tacker and Geddes.[47]

The first investigations using right-heart catheter electrodes employed the configuration shown in Fig. 4-4, A. Heilman et al.[33] introduced the superior-vena cava (SVC) and right-ventricle apex (RVA) catheter electrode array. The two electrodes in the right ventricle (MV and RV) could be used to detect the

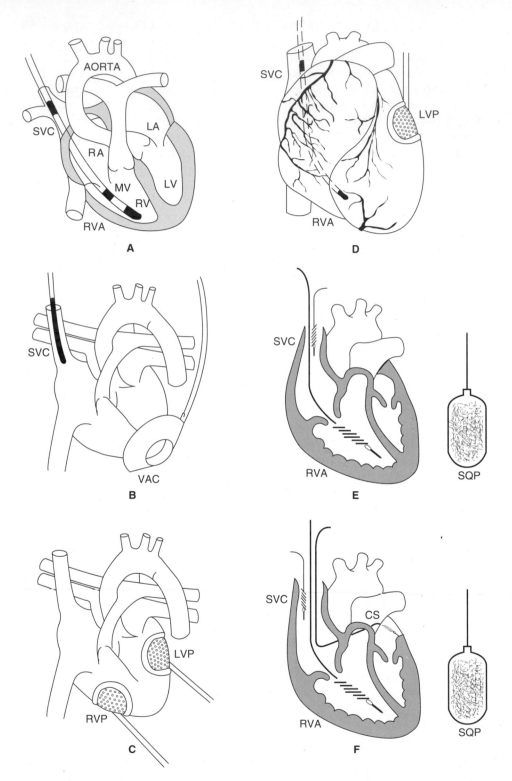

Fig. 4-4. Electrodes for the automatic implantable cardioverter defibrillator (ICD).

ventricular electrogram and the stroke-volume induced impedance change.[28] Several investigators developed right-heart catheters with electrodes of different sizes and spacings to determine the configuration that provided defibrillation with the least energy. Heilman then devised a conical electrode to fit over the apex of the ventricles (VAC), as shown in Fig. 4-4, *B*. However, all these electrode arrays required more current, voltage, and energy for defibrillation than is required with transventricular electrodes. In a 41-patient study, Troup et al.[51] showed that the energy required with transventricular patch electrodes was significantly less than with a SVC–left-ventricular apex electrode. In retrospect, this result should have been apparent because blood resistivity is about one third of that of myocardium and current injected by a bipolar catheter electrode tends to flow along the blood in the vena cava and heart chambers around the catheter. This was one reason that high current and energy were needed for defibrillation, especially with two electrodes in the right heart. The first commercially available ICD employed transventricular, epicardial patch electrodes (RVP, LVP), as shown in Fig. 4-4, *C*, the electrodes being of a titanium screen backed with silicone.

Guse et al.[30] investigated the optimum electrode array using a single pulse of defibrillating current in dogs. Electrodes were placed in the RV apex, RV outflow tract, LV, and four cutaneous patches (anterior, posterior, and left and right chest). The lowest defibrillation energy was encountered when the current pulse was delivered between the LV electrode and the four chest-patch electrodes joined together.

SEQUENTIAL PULSE DEFIBRILLATION

Bourland et al.[6] reported a different strategy for reducing the current, voltage, and hence the energy required for defibrillation. The technique involves the delivery of a first pulse of current to one pair of electrodes. Then at a very short interval later a second pulse of current is delivered to a second pair of electrodes. Note that there are two current pathways at different instants and so there is no electrical interference between the two current pulses.

The two-current path, sequential-pulse method described by Bourland et al.[6] was implemented in dogs using three electrodes (SVC, RVA, LVP), as shown in Fig. 4-4, *D*. A 5 msec pulse was delivered between the SVC and RVA electrodes, and 1 msec later a second 5 msec pulse was delivered between the RVA and LVP electrodes. Defibrillation threshold was compared to a single 10 msec pulse delivered between the RVA-SVC catheter electrodes. The two-path, sequential-pulse method defibrillated with 56% less energy than the single-pulse single-path method.

Jones et al.[36] used Bourland's method and electrode array in pigs to investigate the importance of separation of the two pulses. They found that of three separations (1, 10, and 100 msec) the 1 msec separation achieved defibrillation with the lowest energy. They also found that the two-current path, sequential-pulse method defibrillated with 57% less energy than when the SVC-RVA catheter electrode was used with a single current pulse.

To eliminate the need for a thoracotomy with the Bourland method, Budde et al.[7] replaced the LVP electrode by a subcutaneous patch (SQP) electrode over the cardiac apex or over the 2–3 or 3–4 intercostal space (Fig. 4-4, *E*). Several variables were investigated in this study, and the conclusion was that acceptably low-energy defibrillation could be obtained with the subcutaneous electrode using the two-path, sequential-pulse method, thereby eliminating the need for a thoracotomy.

A different electrode array was investigated by Walcott et al.[52] to compare the energy required for defibrillation with a single-current path and two-current paths using sequential pulses. Electrodes were placed in the right-ventricular outflow tract, the apex of the right ventricle, the apex of the left ventricle, and on the left chest. The threshold for defibrillation was significantly lower with the sequential pulses delivered first between the left ventricular apex and right ventricular outflow tract and the second between the right ventricular apex and left chest electrode.

Fig. 4-4, *F*, shows the principal electrode locations that can be used without a thoracotomy and with a preference for venous access. It has been found that it is not very difficult to place an electrode in the coronary sinus (CS). Therefore this and the RVA electrode can be used for pulse 1 and the RVA and SQP electrodes can be used for pulse 2 with the 2-pulse, 2-current-path method. However, with intraventricular electrodes, whether used for a single current path or two current paths, the areas of the electrodes must be large enough to carry the defibrillating current pulse without bubble production or arcing. This topic is covered at the end of this chapter.

All who are developing ICDs are seeking electrode sites and sizes that will allow defibrillation with the least energy and without a thoracotomy. At present neither the optimum size or site for transventricular patch electrodes are known. However, the location and size should not interfere with coronary artery flow or ventricular-wall motion. The electrodes should be small enough so that their edges are not too close to each other, yet large enough to have most of the ventricular mass between them. Dixon et al.[14] showed in a 20-dog study that substantially less energy was required for defibrillation with large contoured-patch electrodes on the ventricles, compared to flat-patch electrodes of about one third to one fourth of the area. The edges of large electrodes should not be so close that current is shunted away from the myocardial mass. Many of these factors have been discussed by Ideker et al.[34]

Some of the ICDs include a VVI pacemaker, but the electrode for pacing is not used for defibrillation. A large-area pacing electrode is inefficient electrically, as reported by Furman et al.[18] The optimum pacing electrode is one that is small in area and therefore unable to carry adequate current to defibrillate.

A lesson learned from cardiac pacing may apply to the ICD, namely that after electrode implantation the threshold current for pacing increases as fibrous tissue surrounds the electrode or as tissue-edema fluid accumulates around the electrodes. Encapsulation of the electrodes with fibrous tissue can increase the impedance and change the current-density distribution. Both effects are likely to increase the energy required for defibrillation, because fluid accumulation in the fibrous pockets could shunt current away from the higher resistivity tissue pathways of the myocardium. Also, if inflammation increases the volume of pericardial fluid, current may be shunted around the heart. Those who investigate this effect should monitor both the threshold defibrillating current and impedance to identify the mechanism of the increase in defibrillation energy threshold.

HANDHELD ELECTRODES USED WITH THORACOTOMY

During surgery, or occasionally during emergency defibrillation, concave, disc-shaped electrodes are applied to the heart surface to supply the electric shock. The principles for electrode performance for this procedure are similar to those for epicardial ICD electrodes. A typical handheld electrode is shown in Fig. 4-5.

CURRENT DENSITY

Electrode size and location determine current density in the heart. In selecting the sites it is important to recognize that the objective is to obtain a uniform current density distribution in all of the fibrillating myocardium. If there is a region where the current is poorly distributed, that region will not be defibrillated and can serve as a source of excitation to refibrillate the ventricles after the shock is terminated. Whereas transventricular electrodes may produce a fairly uniform current-density distribution, such a distribution is less likely with intraventricular or transchest electrodes. Complicating the sit-

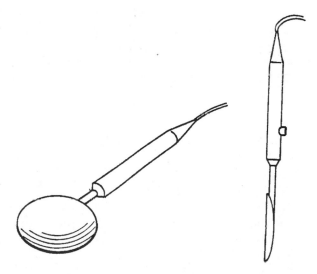

Fig. 4-5. Hand-held transventricular electrodes.

uation is the fact that between the heart and electrodes are tissues, for example, muscle, bone, lung, and fat, each of which has a different conductivity and anatomic distribution.

EVIDENCE OF UNEVEN CURRENT DENSITY

It is not uncommon to observe red rings on the chest following defibrillation with paddle electrodes. Such marks are the result of the high current density under the perimeters of the two electrodes. It has been shown theoretically and experimentally by Caruso et al.[8] that the current density under the perimeter of a skin-surface electrode is about three times higher than the current density under the center of the electrode, as shown in Fig. 4-6, *A*. Proof that this condition exists can be obtained from skin-temperature measurement using high-speed thermography. Because heating is proportional to the square of current density, heating under the perimeter of an electrode will be most prominent. Fig. 4-6, *B*, illustrates a thermogram made using a pediatric defibrillating electrode applied to the shaved chest of a dog, the electrode being removed immediately after delivery of the pulse of current. Observe the white ring, indicating the heated region of the skin under the electrode perimeter. In the section of this chapter that deals with the decrease in impedance due to successive shocks, there is a discussion of the tissue response to high current density.

FRACTION OF THORACIC CURRENT REACHING THE VENTRICLES

Because of the complex distribution of conducting tissues surrounding the heart, it is clear that a substantial percentage of the injected current is shunted around the ventricles. It is possible to estimate the percentage of thoracic current that reaches the ventricles by using threshold-current data obtained from direct-heart and transchest defibrillation of animals. Geddes et al.[23] showed that the defibrillation threshold for damped sine wave current applied to transventricular electrodes over a wide range of heart weight is $I = 0.021w^{1.098}$, where I is in amps (pk) and w is the heart weight in grams. For the same type of current applied to thoracic electrodes on animals of widely differing weights, the peak current $I = 1.87W^{0.88}$, where W is the body weight in kilograms. By knowing the relationship between heart weight and body weight, it is possible to estimate the percent of thoracic current that achieves defibrillation. Table 4-1 shows the heart weight as a function of body weight for different species. Using the foregoing information, Fig. 4-7 shows the relationship between the percent of thoracic current that flows through the ventricles versus body weight, for heart weights of 0.3%, 0.5%, and 0.7% of body weight. Although these studies were performed on animals, the concept is applicable to humans and the results are consistent with the data from transventricular and transchest defibrillation studies.

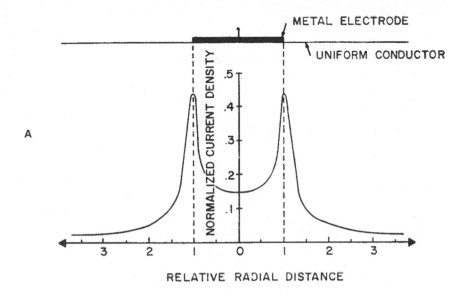

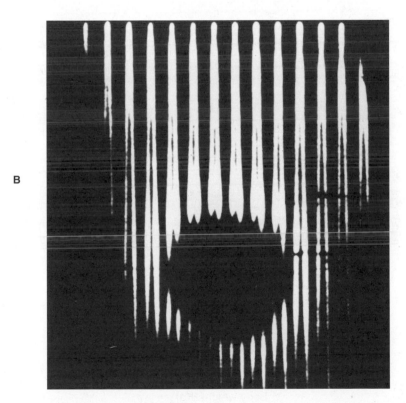

Fig. 4-6. Current-density distribution under a skin-surface electrode (**A**) and thermogram of the skin after the passage of a current pulse through the electrode (**B**). **B**, The heated perimeter (*white*) is clearly shown as is expected from the high perimeter current density. (From Geddes LA, Baker LE: *Principles of applied biomedical instrumentation*, New York, 1989, Wiley Interscience. By permission.)

Table 4-1
Heart Weight (w) as a Function of Body Weight (W)*

Species	Equation	% Body Weight
Simian	4.187W + 0.761	0.42
Canine	8.397W − 14.55	0.84
Porcine	3.412W + 49	0.314
Large felines	5.32W + 56	0.53
Equine	6.972W + 221.6	0.697
Bovine	3304W + 212.4	0.32

*Derived from Geddes LA, Tacker WA: Engineering and physiological considerations of direct capacitor-discharge ventricular defibrillation, *Med Biol Eng Comput* 9:185, 1971.

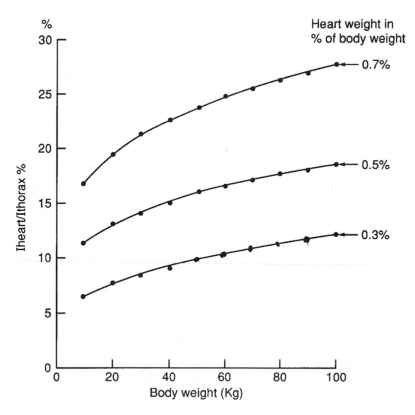

Fig. 4-7. Percent of thoracic current that flows through the ventricles versus body weight (kg) for hearts weighing 0.7, 0.5 and 0.3 percent of body weight.

ELECTRICAL PROPERTIES OF ELECTRODES

Appearing between the electrode terminals there are two electrical components: that representing the two electrode-electrolyte interfaces and that representing the living tissues. The latter is simpler electrically than the electrode-electrolyte interface. For defibrillating current levels the living tissue is almost purely resistive. However, the electrical nature of the electrode-electrolyte interface at each electrode is far from simple and is infrequently discussed. In the following paragraphs we will develop the nature of the circuit appearing between the terminals of the electrodes and show how the magnitudes depend on current density and electrode size.

ELECTRODE-ELECTROLYTE INTERFACE

When a metallic electrode comes into contact with an electrolyte, a charged interface is developed. It is across this interface that the current, which is a flow of electrons in the metal conductor, is converted to a flow of ions in the electrolyte. Helmholtz[32] showed that this interface consists of a double layer of charge, that is, charges of one sign at the metal electrode surface and charges of the opposite sign in the electrolyte. Fig. 4-8, *A*, illustrates this concept. Such a charged layer has interesting properties and resembles a charged capacitor as well as a voltage source. Because current can be passed through the interface, it must have the properties of resistance; Fig. 4-8, *B*, collects these components.

From much experimental evidence, Fig. 4-9, *A*, illustrates a simple equivalent circuit for an electrode-electrolyte interface. The voltage $E_{1/2}$ is called the half-cell potential that depends on the species of metal, the type of electrolyte,

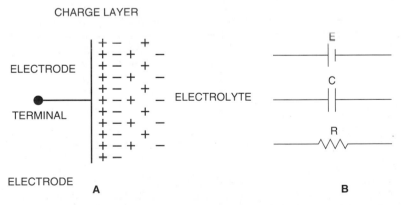

Fig. 4-8. An idealized charge distribution at an electrode-electrolyte interface and the three components that can be used to create an electrical model: a voltage source (*E*), a capacitance (*C*) and resistance (*R*).

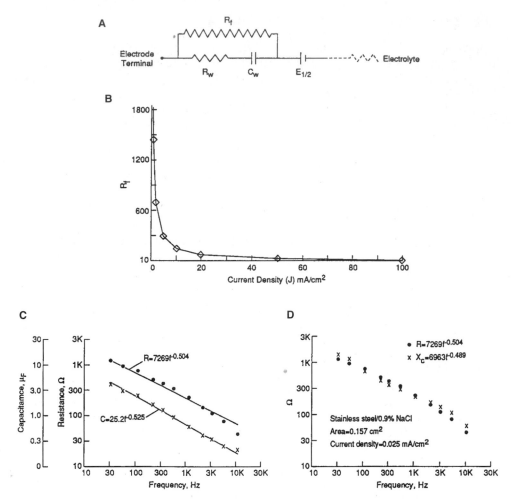

Fig. 4-9. Equivalent circuit for a single electrode-electrolyte interface, consisting of the faradic resistance (R_f), the Warburg resistance (R_w), and capacitance (C_w), the half-cell potential ($E_{1/2}$), and the manner in which these components vary. (**A** redrawn from Mayer et al: A new method for measuring the Faradic resistance of a single electrode-electrolyte interface, *Australasian Phys Eng Sci in Med* 15:38, 1992; **B** and **C** redrawn from Geddes LA et al: The impedance of stainless steel electrodes, *Med Biol Eng Comput* 9:511, 1971.)

and its temperature. Half-cell potentials are tabulated with respect to the potential of the standard hydrogen electrode (SHE). We will discuss the significance of the half-cell potential later.

The faradic resistance (R_f) accounts for the direct-current properties of the electrode-electrolyte interface. The magnitude of R_f decreases with increasing surface area. However, the striking feature of R_f is that it is extremely dependent on the current density used to measure it; R_f decreases dramatically with increasing current density (Fig. 4-9, B). This is partly why an ohmmeter cannot be used to estimate the resistance offered to defibrillating current. The nature of the decrease in R_f with increasing current density was reported by Mayer et al.[43] and Fig. 4-9 B shows the type of relationship for stainless steel (scaled to 1 cm^2) in contact with saline at room temperature.

The capacitance (C_w) and resistance (R_w) are called the Warburg components of the interface (Warburg[53,54]). Although represented by the symbols for resistance (R_w) and capacitance (C_w), they are polarization elements, the magnitudes of which depend on the area of the electrode, the species of metal, the type of electrolyte and its temperature, the frequency of the current used for measurement and the current density.

For low-current density, an increase in frequency decreases the Warburg resistance (R_w) and capacitance (C_w), as shown in Fig. 4-9, C. The reactance of C_w, namely $1/2\pi f C_w$, decreases with increasing frequency, as shown in Fig. 4-9, D. In fact, for many metals, R_w is almost equal to X_w, as shown in Fig. 4-9, D. Ragheb and Geddes[44] tabulated the values for R_w and C_w for commonly used electrode metals in contact with saline at room temperature. Both R_w and X_w = $\frac{1}{2}\pi f C_w$ vary as $1/f^\alpha$, where α is approximately 0.5. Therefore the magnitude of the impedance of the Warburg components, $Zw = \sqrt{R_w^2 + X_w^2}$, decreases with increasing frequency.

For the high current density used in defibrillation, the Warburg resistance (R_w) decreases and the Warburg capacitance (C_w) increases with increasing current density, as shown for sinusoidal alternating current in Fig. 4-10. Therefore the impedance of the Warburg components decreases with increasing current density, as shown in Fig. 4-10, C.

EQUIVALENT CIRCUIT FOR A PAIR OF ELECTRODES

It is now appropriate to examine the circuit appearing between the terminals of a pair of defibrillating electrodes. For simplicity, a 1 cm thick cylindrical column of low-resistivity electrode gel is placed between them. Fig. 4-11 illustrates the complete circuit consisting of R_{w1}, C_{w1}, R_{f1}, $E_{(1)1/2}$ and R_{w2}, C_{w2}, R_{f2}, $E_{(2)1/2}$ and the resistance R_e of the intervening electrolytic column.

With no current flowing through the electrodes, the potential E_{12} appearing between the electrode terminals (1,2) is $E_{(1)1/2} - E_{(2)1/2}$. If the two electrodes are identical and in contact with the same electrolyte at the same temperature, $E_{12} = 0$. If there is contamination on one electrode, or if the electrolytes are different, E_{12} will not be zero and the ECG will be faced with this offset potential, which may not be stable.[3]

During passage of the pulse of defibrillating current, the two half-cell potentials will change, but may not change by the same amount. Therefore after the current pulse when the defibrillating electrodes are connected to the ECG, it may take some time for the electrodes to recover to their preshock

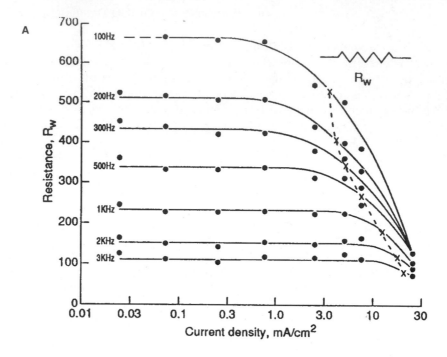

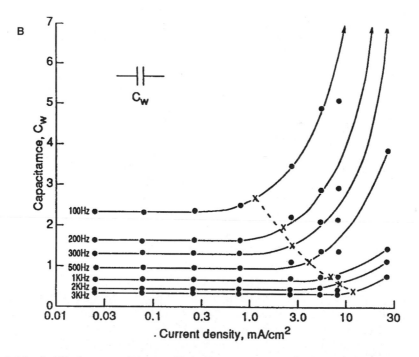

Fig. 4-10. A, Warburg resistance (R_w); **B**, capacitance (C_w); and **C**, impedance (Z_w) versus frequency for a 1 cm² stainless steel electrode in 0.9% saline operated at different current densities. (Redrawn from Geddes LA et al: The impedance of stainless steel electrodes, *Med Biol Eng Comput* 9:511, 1971.)

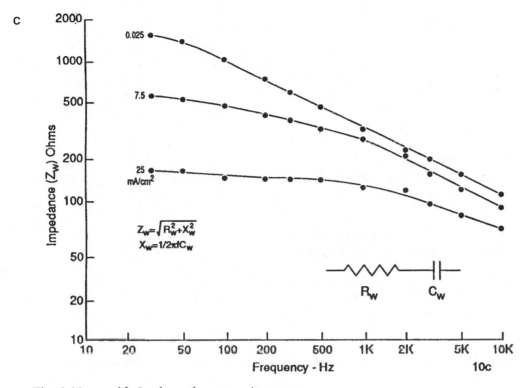

Fig. 4-10, cont'd. See legend on opposite page.

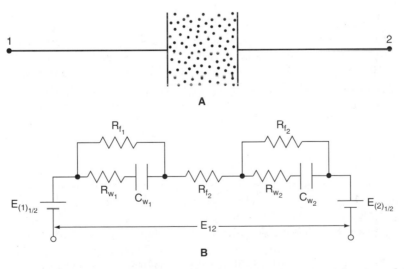

Fig. 4-11. Two defibrillating electrodes 8cm diameter in contact with a 1cm thick column of electrode gel (**A**) and the equivalent circuit (**B**).

potential. This is part of the reason why defibrillating electrodes may not permit recording the ECG immediately on cessation of the current pulse.

A second reason the voltage E_{12} is not zero immediately after the pulse of defibrillating current is because C_{w1} and C_{w2} become charged by the defibrillating current and must discharge through $R_w + R_f$. The recovery time also depends on how long the electrodes are connected to the defibrillator after the shock. The output impedance of a defibrillator is very low and can serve to bring E_{12} down quickly. If the electrodes are connected to the ECG quickly, E_{12} will decrease as C_{w1} discharges through R_{w1}, and R_{f1} and similarly C_{w2} discharges through R_{w2} and R_{f2}. The time taken for the amplifier to be able to display the ECG is called the recovery time. Obviously the recovery time will be shortest if separate ECG recording electrodes are used that carry no current.

PERFORMANCE STANDARD FOR RECORDING THE ECG FROM DEFIBRILLATION ELECTRODES

It is useful to recognize that defibrillating electrodes are required to deliver a substantial pulse of current to achieve defibrillation. Immediately thereafter, in many cases, the same electrodes are used to detect the electrical activity of the heart. This dual requirement places such electrodes in a special class because they must operate efficiently at a high current density to defibrillate, and then have little residual electrode potential after the shock so that the ECG amplifier will not be blocked and therefore can quickly detect cardiac electrical activity. There are established standards for defibrillating electrodes in their role as current-carrying and recording devices. These standards will be discussed later in this chapter.

Use of the defibrillating electrodes to record the ECG is very convenient because it allows both monitoring and defibrillation from only two electrodes. In emergency transchest defibrillation this saves time and reduces confusion. In the nonemergency case of transchest cardioversion or surgical defibrillation with hand-held electrodes, or for the ICD, separate recording electrodes are preferable. With this arrangement, artifacts in the ECG are less severe and, of course, in open-chest surgery the heart can be observed directly to identify defibrillation.

ECG STANDARD FOR ELECTRODES

For transchest emergency defibrillation there are standards of performance for defibrillating electrodes when used for ECG recording. The AAMI/ANSI Cardiac Defibrillator Devices standard states that the AAMI/ANSI Pregelled ECG Disposable Electrodes standard applies. In general this standard addresses two issues: (1) offset potential and (2) recovery from a defibrillator shock. The following will highlight these requirements, but the reader is strongly urged to access the original standard document.

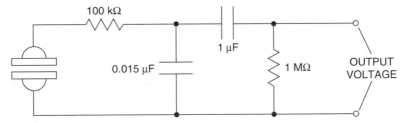

Fig. 4-12. Test circuit for offset instability/internal noise determination. (From AAMI/ANSI Disposable ECG Electrodes EC12, 1991. By permission from AAMI.)

OFFSET POTENTIAL

In essence, the ECG standard calls for the electrodes to be placed face-to-face (gel-to-gel) "and connected to the circuit shown in Fig. 4-12 to which is connected a DC voltmeter having a minimum input impedance of 10 megohms and a resolution of 1 mV or better. The measuring instrument shall apply less than 10 nA of bias current to the electrodes under test. The measurement shall be made after a 1-min stabilization period, but before 1.5 min have elapsed."

AAMI paragraph (3.2.2.3) defines the performance characteristics as follows:

> After a 1-min. stabilization period, the output voltage of the test circuit [Fig. 4-12] shall not exceed 150µV p-p over 5 minutes. Output voltage shall be measured with an instrument having a frequency-response range of 0.01 to 1000 Hz and a minimum input impedance of 10 Mω."

DEFIBRILLATOR OVERLOAD RECOVERY

The standard (3.2.2.4) provides a test circuit (Fig. 4-13) for assessing the recovery of a pair of ECG electrodes. The standard reads:

(1) A pair of electrodes shall be connected gel-to-gel and joined to the test circuit [Fig. 4-13] with switch SW1 closed and SW2 and SW3 open.
(2) At least 10 sec must be allowed for the capacitor to fully charge to 200 V; switch SW1 is then opened.
(3) The capacitor is immediately discharged through the electrode pair by holding switch SW2 closed long enough to discharge the capacitor to less than 2 V. (This time shall be no longer than 2 seconds.)
(4) Switch SW2 is opened and switch SW3 is closed immediately, thereby connecting the electrode pair to the offset measurement system.
(5) The electrode offset is recorded to the nearest 1 mV, 5 sec after the closing of switch SW3 and every 10 sec thereafter for the next 30 sec. The overload and measurement are repeated three times.

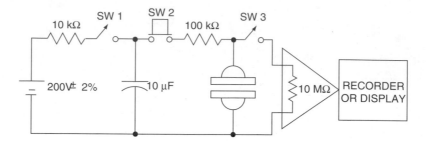

Fig. 4-13. Defibrillation overload test circuit. All capacitor and resistor values have a tolerance of ± 10 percent. (From AAMI/ANSI Disposable ECG Electrodes EC12, 1991. By permission from AAMI.)

(6) The test sequence above is repeated for n electrode pairs. For all electrode pairs tested, the 5-sec offset voltage after each of the four discharges of the capacitor shall not exceed 100mV, and any difference in adjacent 10-sec values (after the initial 5-sec period) shall not exceed ± 11mV (± 1 mV/sec).

As stated earlier, the foregoing is not a substitute for the information contained in the two standards. It is presented to indicate the type of test and performance required.

ELECTRODE IMPEDANCE

We will now focus on the impedance of the equivalent circuit shown in Fig. 4-10 and neglect the electrode potentials that have just been discussed because they are unimportant during defibrillation. By definition the term *impedance* refers to the opposition to the flow of sinusoidal alternating current and is defined as the ratio of rms voltage to rms current. However, in defibrillation studies many authors use the term *impedance* to mean the ratio of peak voltage to peak current for the defibrillating current pulse, regardless of waveform. Although this practice violates the strictest definition of impedance, the ratio so obtained informs about the quality of the conducting pathway.

SINUSOIDAL IMPEDANCE

It was shown earlier that the impedance of an electrode-electrolyte interface decreases with increasing frequency and with increasing current density. Fig. 4-14 shows the sinusoidal impedance for the two defibrillating electrodes in contact with a 1 cm thick cylindrical column of low-resistivity electrode gel. Note that (1) the decrease in impedance with increasing current density is more prominent in the low-frequency region as R_f, R_w, and X_w decrease, and (2) in the high-frequency region the asymptotic impedance is that of the resistance of the 1 cm thick intervening column of electrolyte.

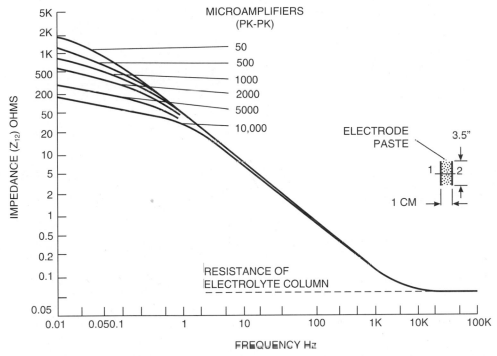

Fig. 4-14. Sinusoidal impedance-frequency relationship for 8 cm diameter electrodes in contact with a 1 cm column of electrode gel. Note the decrease in impedance with increasing current density in the low-frequency region. (Redrawn from Cardiac Defibrillation Conference, Oct 1-3, 1975, Purdue University, W Lafayette, IN 47907.)

IMPEDANCE OFFERED TO DEFIBRILLATING CURRENT PULSES

If a typical damped sine wave defibrillator is applied to the circuit shown in Fig. 4-11, the peak current that flows is not linearly related to the peak voltage in the low-voltage region, as shown in Fig. 4-15, *A*. Moreover the peak of the current and voltage waveforms are not quite coincident, there being a slight phase shift. Fig. 4-15, *B*, shows the ratio of the peak voltage to the peak current (apparent impedance) versus the peak current for the same electrodes. Observe that the apparent impedance decreases with increasing current, revealing that the Faradic and Warburg components of the electrode-electrolyte interface depend on current density. Parenthetically, electrolytes behave as almost pure resistances for defibrillating current pulses. However, the conductivity of a typical electrolyte increases by about 2% per degree Celsius increase in temperature.

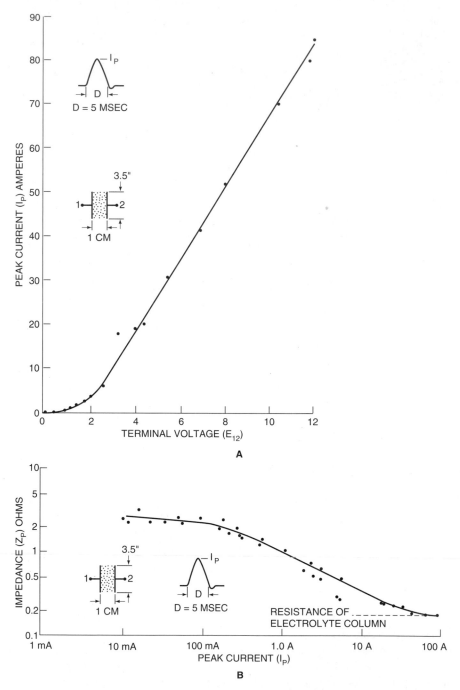

Fig. 4-15. Current-voltage (**A**) and impedance-current relationship (**B**) for two 8 cm diameter electrodes in contact with a 1 cm thick column of electrode gel. (Redrawn from Cardiac Defibrillation Conference, Oct 1-3, 1975, Purdue University, W Lafayette, IN 47907.)

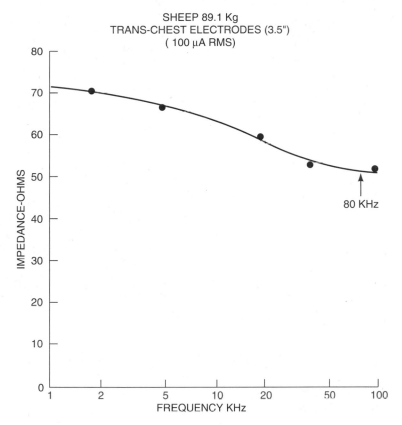

Fig. 4-16. Sinusoidal impedance-frequency relationship for defibrillating electrodes applied to the shaved chest of an 89.1 kg sheep. (Redrawn from Cardiac Defibrillation Conference, Oct 1-3, 1975, Purdue University, W Lafayette, IN 47907.)

IMPEDANCE OF ELECTRODES ON LIVING SUBJECTS

The foregoing discussion equated a 1 cm thick column of low-resistivity electrolytic gel to the subject. We will now examine the sine-wave impedance and the apparent impedance of a pair of 8 cm diameter defibrillating electrodes on living subjects. Data from a sheep with a shaved chest is used for illustration purposes. Fig. 4-16 shows the impedance offered to sinusoidal current in the frequency range extending from 1 kHz to 100 kHz. The impedance approaches an asymptote at about 100 kHz. For the same sheep, Fig. 4-17, *A*, shows the peak current versus the peak voltage for a typical damped sine wave applied to the same transchest electrodes. Fig. 4-17, *B* shows the apparent impedance versus peak current for this electrode pair on the sheep. Observe that the apparent impedance decreases with increasing current, as was found for the same electrodes applied to the 1 cm column of electrode gel.

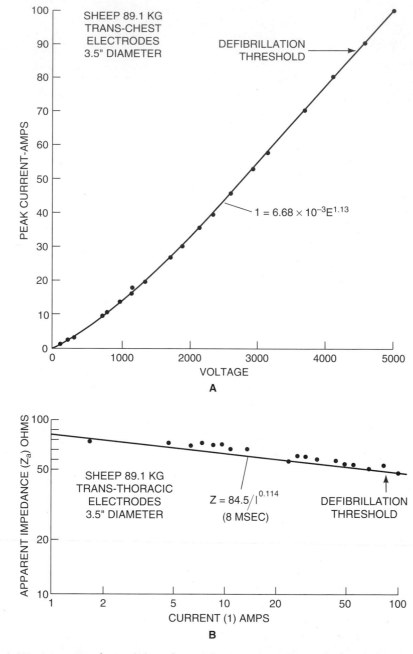

Fig. 4-17. Current-voltage (**A**) and impedance-current (**B**) relationships for damped sinusoidal current applied to transchest electrodes on an 89.1 kg sheep. (Redrawn from Cardiac Defibrillation Conference, Oct 1-3, 1975, Purdue University, W Lafayette, IN 47907.)

PREDICTION OF IMPEDANCE TO DEFIBRILLATING CURRENT

Before discussing a practical method for predicting the impedance presented to the defibrillating current with transchest electrodes, it is useful to review the data obtained in human defibrillation studies. Using standard defibrillating electrodes and a typical damped sine wave defibrillator, Machin[42] measured the voltage and current during defibrillation of adult male subjects. Fig. 4-18 is a histogram showing the number of subjects exhibiting impedances ranging from 24 to 105 ohms. Although the mean value was about 59 ohms, some subjects had much lower and others had higher impedances. Kerber et al.[38] reported a mean value of 79 +/− 15 ohms for handheld paddle electrodes and a mean value of 77.1 +/− 23.1 ohms for preapplied self-adhering electrodes on the human thorax. A damped sine wave defibrillator was used.

A typical defibrillator closely resembles a constant-voltage device, and the current that flows will depend on the energy setting and inversely on the impedance. Because it is current that accomplishes defibrillation for a given energy setting, the current will be less for a subject with high impedance and the chance of defibrillation will be less. Therefore it is necessary to establish a good contact between the electrodes and the subject. Modern defibrillators are calibrated to indicate the energy delivered into a 50 ohm resistive load.

Referring to the impedance-frequency curve for the sheep shown in Fig. 4-16, we see that by proper selection of a frequency the impedance corresponding to that offered to a selected defibrillation current can be identified. From Fig. 4-17, *B*, which relates the apparent impedance offered to defibrillating current at different current levels, it is possible to identify the impedance if the threshold defibrillating current is known. Therefore, if the impedance of the electrode-subject circuit is measured with the appropriate sinusoidal frequency, the impedance of the electrode-subject circuit will be known prior to application of the defibrillating current. In the example for the sheep shown in Fig. 4-17, *B*, the threshold current for defibrillation was 88 amps and from Fig. 4-15, the impedance offered to this current is 50 ohms. From Fig. 4-16, this impedance is offered to a sinusoidal current of 80kHz.

The principle just described was investigated by Geddes et al.,[27] who used the dog. It was found that a frequency of 20kHz provided a good estimate of thoracic impedance for threshold damped sinusoidal current. Kerber et al.[37,39] investigated the ability of a 31 kHz square wave to predict the thoracic impedance of human subjects to damped sinusoidal current using handheld paddles and preapplied electrodes. They found that the predicted (Z_p) impedance was related to the measured (Z_m) impedance as follows. For the handheld electrodes $Z_p = 0.90 Z_m + 12.1$, with a correlation coefficient of 0.90. For the preapplied electrodes $Z_p = 0.95 Z_m + 7.6$, with a correlation coefficient of 0.99.

One manufacturer (Hewlett-Packard) has incorporated the method just described into their defibrillator to provide a quality-of-electrode application indicator. On the paddle handle is a linear array of 10 colored bars that illu-

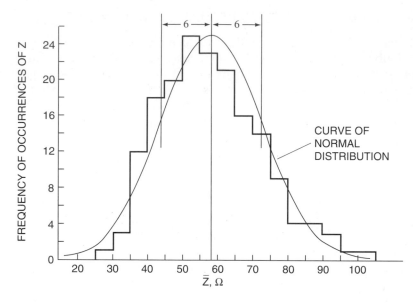

Fig. 4-18. Histogram showing the number of adult subjects exhibiting thoracic impedance (Z) in ohms for damped sine wave defibrillating current. (From Machin W: Thoracic impedance of human subjects, *Med Biol Eng Comput* 16:169, 1978. By permission.)

minate to identify the thoracic impedance. The green bars identify an impedance range of 40 to 90 ohms; the yellow bars identify 90 to 180 ohms; and the red bars cover the range from 180 to 230 ohms. Obviously the operator strives to apply the electrodes so that only the first few green bars are illuminated, indicating good electrical contact with the chest.

The ability to determine the transthoracic impedance prior to delivery of the shock leads to the possibility of automatic adjustment of defibrillator output. Kerber et al.[41] described a clinical study in which if the impedance to a 31 kHz square wave (predicted defibrillating-current impedance) exceeded 70 ohms, the defibrillator energy output was doubled automatically. They reported that the method was beneficial for both cardioversion and defibrillation and led to an increased percent of defibrillation success with the first shock.

IMPEDANCE CHANGES WITH SUCCESSIVE SHOCKS

Several investigators have reported that the (apparent) impedance offered to defibrillating shocks decreases with successive shocks. Using sheep, Geddes et al.[27] delivered successive 320 J shocks and noted an 18% decrease in impedance for the tenth shock. A similar result was obtained by Dahl et al.,[12] who delivered successive 245 J shocks to dogs. Using pigs, Geddes et al.[26] delivered successive 800 J shocks and noted a 28% decrease in impedance after the

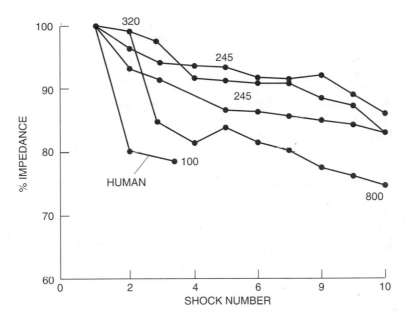

Fig. 4-19. Percent impedance versus shock number showing the decrease in impedance of the electrode-subject circuit with successive shocks. The numbers
on the curves represent the energy in joules. (Data from Geddes LA et al.
The prediction of the impedance of the thorax to defibrillation current, *Am
Heart J* 94: 67, 1976; Dahl CF et al: Transthoracic impedance to direct current discharge, *Med Instrum* 10:151, 1976; and Chambers W et al: Human
chest resistance during successive counter-shocks, *Circulation* 183 (suppl
III):1 1977.)

tenth shock. Chambers, et al.[9] delivered successive 100 J shocks and observed
a decrease in impedance of 21% with the third shock. The foregoing studies
are summarized in Fig. 4-19, which is a plot of percent impedance versus
shock number. The impedance for the first shock is 100% and in all cases the
electrode-subject impedance decreased with successive shocks.

The significance of the foregoing is that for a given energy setting, the peak
current will increase with each successive shock and may account, in part, for
some successful defibrillation with multiple, low-energy shocks. However, it
should be recognized that the use of multiple shocks to achieve defibrillation
increases the ischemic time for the myocardium, which in turn causes
myocardial depression, and the first postdefibrillation beat may be weak.

There are several factors that can account for the decrease in transthoracic
impedance with successive shocks; only a few have been investigated. Sirna et
al.,[46] in a 7-dog study using damped sinusoidal current and handheld paddle
electrodes, reported an increase in blood flow and edema at the electrode
sites. Both factors could decrease the impedance, but it was not proven that
they did so.

Other factors could contribute to the decrease in transthoracic impedance with successive shocks. For example, the dielectric properties of skin-cell membranes in the region of high current density could break down. There is a limited amount of information on the breakdown of cell membranes exposed to high-intensity field strengths. Coster and Zimmerman[10,11] used transmembrane electrodes to study the breakdown of membranes of valonia with 0.5–1 msec pulses. They found that the breakdown was local and recovery occurred in less than 4 sec. Gauger and Bentrup[19] investigated membrane breakdown in brown alga using pulses of 1–1760 μsec in duration and field strength of 50–400 V/cm. They too found that the breakdown was local and recovery occurred in less than 3 sec.

There is not much information available on the change in bulk resistivity of living tissue exposed to high current density. Tacker et al.[48] measured the resistivity of blood samples with single 30 msec rectangular-wave shocks with field strengths ranging from 30 to 403 V/cm. Packed-cell volumes ranging from 0% (plasma) to 98% were tested. Plasma exhibited virtually no change in resistivity; the higher packed-cell volume samples exhibited a decrease in resistivity with increasing field strength. The 90% packed-cell volume sample decreased from 2040 to 1509 ohm-cm for field strengths ranging from 30 to 403 V/cm. DeGaravilla et al.[13] studied the effect of 30 msec rectangular-wave shocks on the resistivity of cardiac muscle. Fifteen shocks, producing an electric field ranging from 33 to 405 V/cm, were delivered. In general, the bulk resistivity decreased with successive shocks, the decrease being slight for the 33 V/cm shocks and more for the shocks having higher field strengths. Tacker et al.[50] measured the decrease in bulk resistivity of skeletal muscle, skin, and fat exposed to 30 msec rectangular pulses with field strengths of 50 to 400 V/cm. The decrease in resistivity (ohm-cm) was most for skeletal muscle (1150 to 150), less for skin (2500 to 650) and least for fat (2300 to 1700). The current density is the electric field divided by the resistivity.

Another, but less prominent, factor contributing to the decrease in impedance with successive shocks is the very slight increase in temperature in the regions of tissue exposed to high current density. Electrolytes such as body fluids decrease their resistivity by about 2% for a 1°C rise in temperature. However, the temperature rise under defibrillating electrodes is very small for a single shock.

Although there is no complete explanation for the decrease in impedance with successive shocks, the phenomenon is real. The decrease depends on both the strength of each shock and the number of shocks delivered.

CURRENT-CARRYING LIMITS FOR DEFIBRILLATING ELECTRODES

All electrodes have a limited ability to carry current. Stated precisely, for a given electrode there is an inverse relationship between electrode current density (amps per square cm of electrode area) and the duration of the current pulse. Under high current density conditions, this limit can manifest itself by the evolution of gas bubbles in the electrolyte or an arc under an electrode. In fact, such a situation has led to surgical drapes catching fire in an operating room in the presence of oxygen. In our laboratories current-density limitations for defibrillating electrodes arose in the studies with catheter-borne electrodes in the right heart used for ventricular defibrillation. As defibrillating current was increased an audible thump was heard within the animal during current delivery, indicating the creation of a shock wave. The cause was shown by Bourland et al.[5] in a study in which a single electrode of the type used on the catheter was placed in an 0.9% saline volume conductor, and a second, large electrode distant from the active electrode was used to pass defibrillator shocks. The active electrode was observed carefully and photographed as the defibrillating current pulse was increased incrementally. With low current the electrode exhibited nothing. As the current was increased, small bubbles appeared. With higher current there were more and larger bubbles ejected from the electrode. Such gas bubbles are the result of electrolytic decomposition of the electrolyte. With higher current there occurred an intense blue-white flash and a loud sharp sound, indicating ionization of the gas bubbles and the creation of a shock wave. The same sequence occurred with either polarity for the active electrode. Fig. 4-20 shows a series of pictures of these events.

Having documented the nature of the events occurring at the surface of an active electrode operated at a high current density, Wessale et al.[55] quanti-

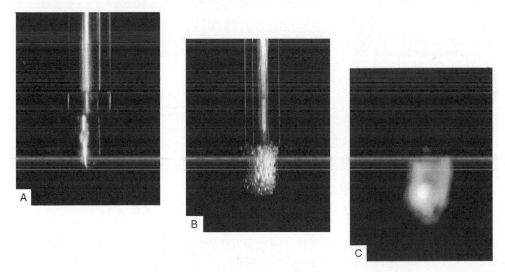

Fig. 4-20. A, Catheter-tip electrode (1.25cm^2) in 0.9% saline. **B**, The electrode (cathode) 11 msec after the application of a 500-V, 10.8-A current pulse. Note the gas bubbles. **C**, An underwater arc formed 17 msec after current application. The voltage source was removed at 20 msec. (From Geddes LA, Baker LE: *Principles of applied biomedical instrumentation*, ed 3, New York, 1989, Wiley Interscience. By permission.)

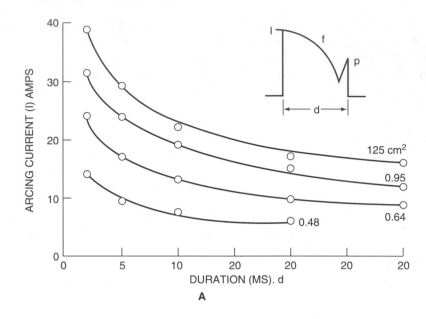

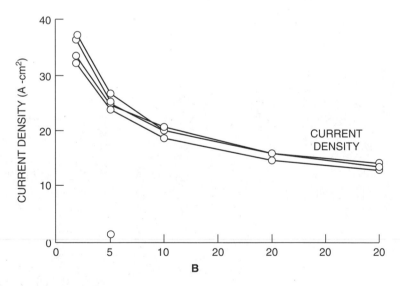

Fig. 4-21. Current pulse (*inset*) and strength-duration curves for arcing with electrodes of different areas. (Redrawn from Wessale JL et al: Arcing threshold and electrode surface area for catheter electrical ablation, *PACE* 10:487, 1987.

tated the factors underlying arc formation. Using a rectangular, constant-voltage, variable-duration pulse, they recorded the voltage and current for each pulse while incrementing the voltage applied to electrodes of different areas in an 0.9% saline volume conductor. A typical record of the current pulse is shown in the inset of Fig. 4-21, *A*. The fall (*f*) in current is likely due to the electrolytic formation of gas bubbles and the sudden peak (*p*) is due to ionization of the gas bubbles that give rise to the shock wave. The current pulse was terminated with the occurrence of the flash. Using the method just described, Wessale et al.[55] determined strength-duration curves for the production of arcs for electrodes of different areas. Fig. 4-21, *A*, shows the result. Fig. 4-21, *B*, presents the same data normalized for current density.

In summary, for a given electrode it is clear that there is an inverse relationship between the current-density limit and pulse duration. Although high-current density may not ordinarily be encountered with catheter-defibrillating electrodes, it can occur if the electrode area is small. The effect of a shock wave generated at a catheter electrode on the blood and myocardium are not known, but it is expected that the effects are deleterious.

Arcing at an electrode surface is not confined to small-area electrodes. Recall that the current density is highest under the perimeter of an electrode. On occasion arcs have been seen under the perimeter of a chest-surface electrode. This situation is exacerbated if the electrode-subject resistance is uneven or high. In animal studies conducted in a darkened room using preapplied electrodes, arcing has been seen with currents that are typical for human defibrillation.

THE UNIVERSAL ELECTRODE

At this time there are many efforts directed toward the creation of a preapplied body-surface electrode that can be used for ventricular defibrillation/cardioversion, pacing, and electrosurgery. It should be noted that the requirements for these three applications are very different. For defibrillation and cardioversion, a low-impedance contact is required to assure the delivery of adequate current. For closed-chest pacing it was shown by Zoll et al.[56] that the use of a thick film of a relatively high-resistivity gel (along with a pulse duration of about 40 msec) provides less skin sensation (that is, pain), which is an important requirement because the subject is conscious. Therefore the electrode-subject impedance can be high for this application. The thick film of high-resistivity gel reduces the high perimeter current density. For electrosurgery, which uses sinusoidal current with a frequency in the 0.5 to 2 MHz range, a low-impedance contact and a uniform current distribution are desirable. Gelled metal foil, conducting adhesive on metal foil, and adhering capacitive (insulated) electrodes are all used. Because of the relatively uniform current distribution with the capacitive electrode, there is increased use of this type for electrosurgery. It is definitely not useful for defibrillation because of its very high impedance to defibrillating current.

Whether a truly multipurpose electrode can be created is not known at present. Research is ongoing with conducting particles (for example, carbon or metal powder) in an adhesive to create such an electrode. At this point it is well to remember that for closed-chest defibrillation, the electrodes may carry 50 amps (pulse duration 5 to 10 msec). For closed-chest pacing, the electrodes carry 0.1 amp pulses (about 40 msec in duration), slightly more than once per second. For electrosurgery, intermittent radiofrequency currents (0.2 to 0.5 amps rms) are applied for a few seconds; these activations are repeated very often during surgery to coagulate bleeding vessels and to cut tissues. Ideally an electrode coupling agent that offers a high impedance to low current and a low impedance to high current would be desirable for defibrillation and pacing. Clearly the challenge is great—but so are the rewards.

REFERENCES

1. AAMI-ANSI National Standard for Cardiac Defibrillator Devices. May 26, 1989. Association for the Advancement of Medical Instrumentation (AAMI, 3330 Washington Blvd, Arlington, VA 22201-4598).
2. AAMI-ANSI Disposable ECG Electrodes EC12, 1991. Association for the Advancement of Medical Instrumentation (AAMI, 3330 Washington Blvd, Arlington, VA 22201-4598).
3. Aronson S, Geddes LA: Electrode potential stability, *IEEE Trans Biom Eng* 32:85, 1987.
4. Aylward PE et al: Defibrillator electrode chest-wall coupling agents, influence on transthoracic impedance and shock success, *J Am Coll Cardiol* 6:682, 1985.
5. Bourland JD et al: Bubble formation, arcing and waveform distortion produced in human blood by trapezoidal defibrillation current, *Proc AAMI 12th Ann Mtg*, p 409, March 13–17, 1977, San Francisco.
6. Bourland JD et al: Sequential pulse defibrillation for implantable defibrillators, *Med Instrum* 20:138, 1986.
7. Budde T et al: Bidirectional transvenous/subcutaneous defibrillation of ventricular fibrillation in dogs, *Eur Heart J* 9:92, 1988.
8. Caruso PM, Pearce JA, DeWitt DP: Temperature and current density distributions at electrosurgical dispersive electrode sites, *Proc 7th New Engl (NE) Bioeng Conf* 1979, Troy, NY, pp 373–376.
9. Chambers W, Miles R, Stratbucker R: Human chest resistance during successive countershocks, *Circulation* 183 (suppl III):1, 1977.
10. Coster HGL, Zimmerman U: The mechanism of electric breakdown in the membranes of valonia utricularis, *J Membr Biol* 22:73, 1975.
11. Coster HGL, Zimmerman U: Dielectric breakdown in the membranes of valonia utricularis, *Biochim Biophys Acta* 382:410, 1975.
12. Dahl CF, Ewy GA, Thomas ED: Transthoracic impedance to direct current discharge, *Med Instrum* 10:151, 1976.
13. DeGaravilla L et al: In vitro resistivity of canine heart to defibrillator shocks, *Proc 1981 AAMI 16th Ann Mtg*, p 28.
14. Dixon EG et al: Improved defibrillation thresholds with large contoured epicardial electrodes and biphasic waveforms, *Circulation* 76:1176, 1987.
15. ECRI/Emergency Care Research Institute, a non-profit agency that publishes Health Devices. 5200 Butler Pike, Plymouth Meeting, PA 19462.
16. Ewy GA, Taren D: Comparison of paddle electrode pastes used for defibrillation, *Heart and Lung* 6:817, 1977.
17. Ewy GA, Horan WJ, Ewy MD: Disposable defibrillator electrodes, *Heart and Lung* 6:127, 1977.
18. Furman S, Parker B, Escher D: Decreasing electrode size and increasing efficiency of cardiac stimulation, *J Surg Res* 11:105, 1971.
19. Gauger B, Bentrup FW: Study of dielectric breakdown, *Membr Biol* 48:249, 1979.

20. Geddes LA, de Costa C, Wise G: The impedance of stainless steel electrodes, *Med Biol Eng Comput* 9:511, 1971.

21. Geddes LA, Tacker WA: Engineering and physiological considerations of direct capacitor-discharge ventricular defibrillation, *Med Biol Eng Comput* 9:185, 1971.

22. Geddes LA: Characteristics of defibrillating electrodes and living tissue, Cardiac Defibrillation Conference, Purdue University, Oct 1–3, 1975.

23. Geddes LA et al: Electrical dose for ventricular defibrillation of large and small animals using precordial electrodes, *J Clin Invest* 53:310, 1974.

24. Geddes LA et al: The electrical dose for ventricular defibrillation with electrodes applied directly to the heart, *J Thor Cardiovasc Surg* 68:593, 1974.

25. Geddes LA et al: The decrease in transthoracic impedance during successive ventricular defibrillation trials, *Med Instrum* 9:177, 1975.

26. Geddes LA et al: The prediction of the impedance of the thorax to defibrillating current, *Med Instrum* 10:159, 1976.

27. Geddes LA et al: The thoracic windows for electrical ventricular defibrillation current, *Am Heart J* 94:67, 1977.

28. Geddes LA, Bourland JD, Terry RS: Method of and apparatus for automatically detecting and treating ventricular fibrillation: U.S. Patent 4,291,699, September 29, 1981. Canadian Patent 1,119,671, March 9, 1982. European Patent 0009255, June 1, 1983. Japanese Patent P-248-7.

29. Geddes LA, Baker LE: *Principles of applied biomedical instrumentation*, ed 3, New York, 1989, Wiley Interscience.

30. Guse PA et al: Defibrillation with low voltage using a left ventricular catheter and four cutaneous patch electrodes in dogs, *PACE* 14:443, 1991.

31. Health Devices, see ECRI.

32. Helmholtz H: Studien uber electrische Grenzschichten, *Ann Physik u Chemie* 7:337, 1879.

33. Heilman MS et al: Implantable electrodes for accomplishing ventricular defibrillation and pacing and method of electrode implantation and utilization. U.S. Patent 4,030,509. June 21, 1977.

34. Ideker RE et al: Current concepts for selecting the location, size and shape of defibrillation electrodes, *PACE* 14:227, 1991.

35. Jakobsson J, Odmansson I, Norlander R: Comparison of two different electrodes for the delivery of dc-shocks, *Resuscitation* 20:25, 1990.

36. Jones DL, Klein GJ, Kallok MJ: Improved internal defibrillation with twin pulse sequential energy delivery to different lead orientations in pigs, *Am J Cardiol* 55:821, 1985.

37. Kerber RE, Kouba C, Martins J: Advanced prediction of tissue impedance in human defibrillation and cardioversion: importance of impedance in determining the success of low-energy shocks, *Circulation* 70:303, 1984.

38. Kerber RE et al: Self adhesive preapplied electrode pads for defibrillation and cardioversion, *J Amer Coll Cardiol* 3:815, 1984.

39. Kerber RE et al: Experimental evaluation and initial clinical application of new self-adhesive defibrillating electrodes, *Int J Cardiol* 8:57, 1985.

40. Kerber RE, McPherson D, Charbonnier F: Automated impedance-based energy adjustment for defibrillation: experimental studies, *Circulation* 71:136, 1985.

41. Kerber RE et al: Energy, current and success in defibrillation and cardioversion: clinical studies using an automated impedance-based method of energy adjustment, *Circulation* 77:1038, 1988.

42. Machin W: Thoracic impedance of human subjects, *Med Biol Eng Comput* 16:169, 1978.

43. Mayer S et al: A new method for measuring the Faradic resistance of a single electrode-electrolyte interface, *Australasian Phys Eng Sci in Med* 15:38, 1992.

44. Ragheb T, Geddes LA: The polarization impedance of common electrode metals operated at low current density, *Ann Biomed Eng* 19:151, 1991.

45. Sirna SJ et al: Factors affecting transthoracic impedance during electrical cardioversion, *Am J Cardiol* 62:1048, 1988.

46. Sirna SJ et al: Mechanisms responsible for decline in transthoracic impedance after DC shocks, *Am J Physiol* 261:H1180, 1989.

47. Tacker WA, Geddes LA: *Electrical defibrillation*, Boca Raton, FL, 1980, CRC Press.

48. Tacker WA et al: Resistivity of blood to

defibrillator-strength shocks, *Proc 17th Ann Mtg* 1982, AAMI, p 121.

49. Tacker WA, Paris R: Transchest defibrillation effectiveness and electrical impedance using disposable conductive pads, *Heart and Lung* 12:510, 1983.

50. Tacker WA: Resistivity of skeletal muscle, skin, fat and lung to defibrillation shocks, *Proc AAMI 19th Ann Mtg*, Apr 14–18, 1984, p 81.

51. Troup OL et al: The implanted defibrillator *J Am Coll Cardiol* 6:1315, 1985.

52. Walcott GP et al: Defibrillation efficacy of consecutive versus single biphasic shocks, *PACE* 14:717, 1991 (abstract).

53. Warburg E: Ueber das Verhalten sorgenannter unpolarisbarer Elektroden gegen Wechselstrom, *Ann Physik Chem* 67:493, 1899.

54. Warburg E: Ueber die Polarisationscapacitat des Platins, *Ann Physik* 6:125, 1901.

55. Wessale JL et al: Arcing threshold and electrode surface area for catheter electrical ablation, North American Society Pacing Electrophysiology, 1987, Boston, MA, *PACE* 10:427, 1987.

56. Zoll PM, Zoll RM, Belgard H: External noninvasive electrical stimulation of the heart, *Crit Care Med* 9:393, 1981.

Chapter 5
Design of Transchest Defibrillators

W. A. Tacker

CLINICAL EXTERNAL DEFIBRILLATORS

External defibrillators are used for both emergency and elective treatment of cardiac arrhythmias. In this chapter defibrillator characteristics and design will be considered. Specific clinical uses are given in Chapters 6 to 9. Photographs of several currently available transchest defibrillators are shown in Fig. 5.1. Detailed descriptions of specific defibrillators with comparisons of features is beyond the scope of this book, but can be found in articles from *Health Devices*, a publication of ECRI, 5200 Butler Pike, Plymouth Meeting, PA, USA.

A defibrillator is a device that applies a strong electric shock (hundreds or thousands of volts) to a cardiac chamber in order to convert a tachyarrhythmia to a normal cardiac rhythm, preferably sinus rhythm.* Treatment of ventricular fibrillation is traditionally called defibrillation, whereas treatment of other tachyarrhythmias is called cardioversion.

Clinically popular defibrillators are of the damped sine wave type or the trapezoidal (truncated exponential decay) type, and both will be described. Other previously used waveforms have been shown to have serious safety and/or effectiveness problems and are no longer used. These include long-duration, or high-current and voltage alternating current (AC), untruncated capacitor discharge, and delay line designs.[3,4] Other waveforms, such as those described by Jones in Chapter 3, are considered experimental.

The typical defibrillator is characterized by the following functional components: power supply, energy storage capacitor, and discharge circuit, which includes controls, waveform shaping components, and electrodes. Fig. 5-2 presents a block diagram of the fundamental components of a typical defibrillator.[3] (Also seen in Fig. 5-2 is the optional synchronization capability of the defibrillator.) Electrodes are discussed elsewhere, in Chapters 4 and 8 and the section on features in this chapter.

---

*This is in contrast to a pacemaker, which generates weaker shocks (a few volts) in order to correct bradyarrhythmias, or which in some cases generates a burst of weak shocks to correct tachyarrhythmias. Most pacemakers are implanted, but transchest pacing is clinically feasible, and will be discussed later.

119

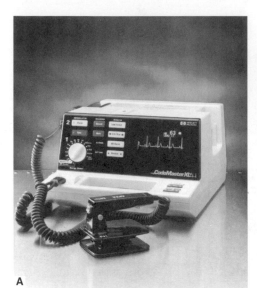

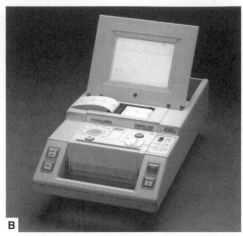

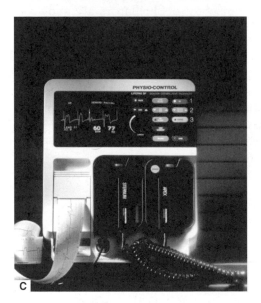

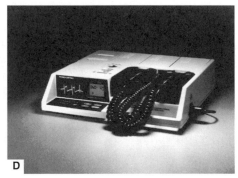

Fig. 5-1. Defibrillators for transchest use. **A,** HP Codemaster HL & defibrillator & external pacer. (From Hewlett-Packard Company. With permission.) **B,** Marquette series 1500 defibrillator (From Marquette Electronics. With permission.) **C,** Physio-Control Lifepak 9B. (From Physio-Control Corporation. With permission.) **D,** Physio-Control Lifepak 10. (From Physio-Control Corporation. With permission.)

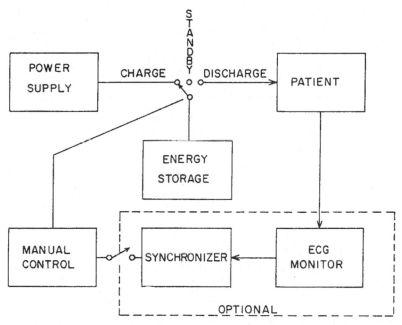

Fig. 5 2. Elements of a defibrillator. (From Feinberg B: *Handbook series in clinical laboratory science,* vol 2, Boca Raton, FL, 1980, CRC Press. With permission.)

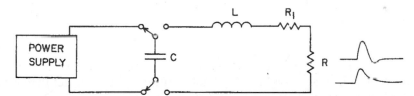

Fig. 5-3. Capacitor-inductor defibrillator. (From Feinberg B: *Handbook series in clinical laboratory science,* vol 2, Boca Raton, FL, 1980, CRC Press. With permission.)

DAMPED SINE WAVE

The defibrillators in most widespread use have the damped sine waveform. Typically they deliver a damped sinusoidal waveform and have a pulse duration of about 3 to 6 msec. A typical defibrillator stores a maximum of 440 J of energy and delivers about 80% of the stored energy into a 50 Ω resistive load. The waveform is generated by a resistor-inductor-capacitor (RLC) circuit, as shown in Fig. 5-3. The patient resistance forms part of the discharge circuit, and thus the duration and the damping characteristics of the waveform vary slightly because of the variation in resistance of different subjects. For most

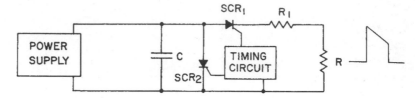

Fig. 5-4. Trapezoidal wave defibrillator. (From Feinberg B: *Handbook series in clinical laboratory science,* vol 2, Boca Raton, FL, CRC Press, 1980. With permis-

defibrillators the waveform is overdamped in high-resistance patients and underdamped in low-resistance patients. Electrodes may be either for precordial or chest-to-back placement and are more or less circular and 8 cm or larger in diameter.

TRUNCATED EXPONENTIAL DECAY (TRAPEZOIDAL WAVE) DEFIBRILLATORS

A typical circuit for truncated exponential decay (trapezoidal wave) defibrillators is shown in Fig. 5-4. The advent of the trapezoidal wave defibrillator was based on the premise that a lower voltage and hence lower-current defibrillation pulse would produce less cardiac damage. Trapezoidal waveform defibrillators with a servo-controlled pulse duration also have the presumed advantage of delivering exactly the energy selected.

BASIC ELEMENTS

POWER SUPPLY

The power supply may use alternating current from domestic power lines or batteries as the basic energy source. Older battery-powered defibrillators had longer charging times than line-powered units, but this is not a problem with state-of-the-art units. There is usually some form of battery testing mechanism on battery-powered defibrillators. This may be in the form of a push-to-test indicator, or there may be a low battery charge warning light that comes on when the battery has a marginal residual level of charge.

Several types of rechargable batteries have been used by different defibrillator manufacturers, including nickel-cadmium batteries and sealed lead-acid batteries. Jellied lead-acid batteries are not used in defibrillators because they have a high internal resistance. The sealed lead-acid battery is inexpensive and has a high energy density and low internal resistance. However, when totally discharged, it will be damaged and will not accept a recharge until its temperature is raised—for example, by being warmed in an oven. Hence, it is best to keep lead-acid batteries near full charge at all times and to avoid deep discharge. The nickel-cadmium (Nicad) battery has been popular in portable defibrillators. This battery is characterized by a moderately low internal resistance and fairly high power density. The Nicad battery is more expensive than the lead-acid battery. Also, proper use and maintenance are essential to obtain long life. The Nicad battery has a characteristic called "memory"—that is, if it is used on a limited basis for many cycles, the battery will not release more charge than has been used in the repeated partial cycles. This is a transient phenomenon and can be remedied by a "deep discharge" and recharge cycle, which will restore full function. Nickel-cadmium batteries also last longer if they are regularly exercised by the multiple discharge-charge cycles. Total discharge of a nickel-cadmium battery can cause permanent damage due to cell polarity reversal. The reverse polarity changes the chemical composition of the battery. Because these batteries lose 20% to 30% of their charge per month if not on a charging cycle, it is necessary to recharge the batteries periodically even when they are in storage.

Battery-operated defibrillators include a battery charger, which may be built into the defibrillator or may be separate. Some manufacturers provide either slow- or fast-charge capability. Most but not all defibrillators can operate from the 60 Hz AC power line when the batteries are depleted. A defibrillator with run-down batteries is useless if it cannot be operated from the power line in this condition. Many defibrillators are capable of working either from the batteries or domestic power line. Finally, some defibrillators will work even when the batteries are discharged and the defibrillator is in the charging mode.

CAPACITORS

All defibrillators in use today rely on capacitors for energy storage. Damped sine wave defibrillators in the United States generally contain either electrolytic or oil-filled capacitors. Trapezoidal wave defibrillators usually contain electrolytic capacitors. All capacitors have two problems in common, namely, that there are a limited number of charge-discharge cycles and that sustained charging to high voltages results in earlier failure. At one time the K-film capacitor was especially popular in portable defibrillators because of its light weight. However, this type of capacitor cannot be charged for long periods. The most common failure is due to internal shorting. K-film also has fairly high leakage characteristics, and leakage is much greater when the capacitor is first charged than after several seconds of charge-holding time. Recently developed thin film, self-healing oil-filled capacitors are protected from catastrophic failure (breakdown) and promise high-reliability defibrillators.

DISCHARGE CIRCUIT

Discharge circuits for all defibrillators are necessary to insure proper timing of the electric shock. Either mechanical relays or solid-state devices may be used. As with capacitors the high voltages across the relays accelerate failure rate. Some relays are of open-frame design, whereas others are encased or in a vacuum or inert gas environment. The typical open-frame relays exhibit a corona at 5 to 7 kV and so are used only below this voltage. Higher voltages require gas-filled enclosures, but in this latter design the arcing with each discharge ionizes the gas, and the enclosure medium deteriorates. After the concentration of ions becomes high, premature arcing occurs before contact closure. A very serious failure mode is welding of the contacts in the closed position, which can occur due to the high voltage arc. In such an event the defibrillator cannot be used. Limitations of solid-state switching are voltage limitations, high electrical leakage characteristics, and danger of failure in the closed mode. A potential advantage of solid-state switching would be for accurate production of multiple, closely spaced pulses.

An additional feature of the discharge circuit is waveform shaping. The damped sine wave is generated by inclusion of a series inductor to form an RCL circuit that damps the capacitor discharge spike to form the nominal 5 msec damped sine wave pulse, which is close to critical damping. Without the inductance (L), the waveform would have the faster rise time, higher amplitude, and much briefer duration typical of a capacitor discharge into a resistor.

The trapezoidal waveform defibrillator also has a waveform shaping function in the discharge circuit shown in Fig. 5-4 as SCR_2. This switches the capacitor to a low-resistance shunt, effectively truncating the pulse delivered to the patient before the capacitor has fully discharged. An advantage of solid-state switching is use in trapezoidal waveform defibrillation, because the solid-state switching has the capability to truncate at a preselected and accurate time.

Of course, controls for energy selection, charging, and discharging the defibrillator are necessary. Reliable control of the unit's performance is essential to both safety and effectiveness.

SAFETY AND EFFECTIVENESS

There are three categories of safety related to defibrillator use. The first is safety of the patient, the second is safety of the operator, and the third is safety of other equipment in the vicinity. A defibrillator is a potentially dangerous device. A shock applied to a nonfibrillating patient can precipitate ventricular fibrillation. Accidental shock may occur if the operator is not properly trained or if the defibrillator malfunctions. Accidental shock may be due to defibrillator discharge or to leakage currents from circuitry in the defibrillator. An important safety feature is the limitation of energy output for use with direct-heart electrodes. The AAMI standard limits internal defibrillation energy output to a maximum of 50 J. Modern defibrillators have automatic internal switching that accomplishes this objective, but some older units may be capable of delivering up to 300 J to direct-heart electrodes. Another patient safety feature is protection of the electrodes from 60 Hz leakage current. Also, defibrillators should not maintain a charge after they have been turned off or otherwise disabled. A defibrillator that has been turned off should not be capable of delivering any shock. Another patient safety feature, synchronization, will be discussed separately.

The second safety category relates to the operator of the defibrillator. Often the patient safety features are the same as those for the operator. Examples are the limitation of leakage currents and the automatic discharging feature. In addition, the provision of clear and simple instruction on proper use of the device is essential. Finally, if the defibrillator is not used with proper care, the operator may be inadvertently shocked.

The safety of other devices must also be considered; they include virtually all electronic equipment in the vicinity of a defibrillator and patient. Most commonly, this includes the ECG, which is attached to the patient for documentation of the rhythm disorder and may also include other monitoring equipment commonly found in the coronary-care unit, such as pressure transducers. Some manufacturers now provide special pressure transducers that are immune to defibrillation shocks encountered in high-voltage environments. Finally, implanted pacemakers or ICDs may be damaged by defibrillator shocks. The monopolar pacemakers are much more susceptible to damage since the potential that may be applied across the active and indifferent electrode may be high if the defibrillation electrodes are applied near to the pacemaker case, which is the indifferent electrode of the pacemaker.

Most defibrillators have the feature of automatically returning to the emergency defibrillation mode when the defibrillator is turned off and turned on again. This is valuable since the synchronized defibrillation procedure allows time for checking and preparation. On the other hand, in the emergency situation it is time-consuming and undesirable for the operator to have to check to be certain that the unit is in the emergency operating mode.

Some defibrillators have the feature of automatically switching to the defibrillation mode after a cardioversion shock, whereas others do not. This is a controversial issue, since unintentional ventricular fibrillation after cardioversion is uncommon and switching back to the synchronized mode is inconvenient. However, if ventricular fibrillation does follow a cardioversion attempt, some additional cardiac arrest time is added if the defibrillator must be switched to the defibrillation mode. Some users prefer automatic switching; others do not.

Defibrillators automatically discharge their energy into an internal resistor when the defibrillator is turned off. The AAMI standard specifies that defibrillators automatically disarm after 30 to 120 seconds if the unit is not discharged by the user. These safety features prevent accidental discharge due to retention of voltage on the capacitors that the operator may think has been discharged.

With optimized conditions, conventional defibrillators are very effective devices for defibrillation and cardioversion. The major limitation to defibrillation effectiveness seems to be delay after onset of fibrillation until applying the shock. When shocks are applied within seconds of the onset of fibrillation, the usual outcome is defibrillation. However, failure to defibrillate may occur if shock application is delayed or if the underlying problem (disease, drug toxicity, etc.) causes the ventricles to remain in fibrillation or to refibrillate immediately. Another cause of failure is application of excessively strong shocks to children who, because of their smaller size, require lower shock strength and are more susceptible to an overdose of the electric shock. The effectiveness of defibrillation has been greatly improved with widespread CPR training, inasmuch as the CPR maintains oxygenation and perfusion of the heart and other vital organs until a defibrillator shock is applied.

Cardioversion effectiveness for elective therapy is not very dependent on either CPR or time from diagnosis to treatment. The patient's medical status does not deteriorate rapidly, and passage of time is not rapidly deleterious, mostly because the progression of the medical problem is so slow. In the case of cardioversion, short-term success for conversion of atrial arrhythmias is limited by the fact that many patients revert to their arrhythmia because the underlying problem has not been corrected. For both defibrillation and cardioversion, proper concomitant medical therapy is essential to long-term success.

FEATURES

Defibrillator features include the specifications for output as well as the characteristics of various options, accessories, and capabilities. Since many of these are used with defibrillators, it is necessary for the user to determine which defibrillator features are of primary importance. For example, will the defibrillator be used for hospital application only or will it be used in ambulances or other situations where portability is essential? Will it be used for cardioversion or for emergency defibrillation? Will it be used in surgery for direct-heart defibrillation or is the unit intended for research purposes only? For those concerned with purchasing a defibrillator, appropriate selection follows identification of the primary use for the defibrillator.

MONITORS

Most defibrillation is performed only after the arrhythmia has been documented by display on a screen or graphic recorder. A monitor screen, such as an LCD flat display, has the advantage of not requiring paper. A disadvantage is that there is no permanent record. Most defibrillators are equipped with both options.

One of the considerations in choosing between these is that, in general, the monitor requires less energy and hence can operate on lighter-weight batteries than the graphic recorder, in which a thermal printer is heated and a motor is used to move the paper. Telemetry of the ECG is another possible option. Whether it is recorded on a monitor or on paper at the site of the event, the ECG may be transmitted to a central hospital facility. New solid-state recording systems have recently been incorporated into defibrillation monitors. These systems are very robust, convenient, and lightweight. They can record several minutes of ECG records.

There are a number of characteristics that are unique to the graphic recording and monitoring systems. When the ECG is recorded on paper, the defibrillator is usually supplied with a single-channel recorder, which may accept an input from either the defibrillation electrodes or from separate electrodes placed on the limbs or chest. With graphic recorders or monitors, a number of characteristics must be considered. These include the frequency response, capability for calibrating the record, recovery time of the trace following application of the shock, and the sensitivity for recording the ECG signal. Considerations for monitors also include trace intensity (brightness), whether or not the monitor has a "memory" for freezing the ECG for careful inspection, and whether or not there is a variable time base (sweep speed). A variable time base may be available so that the defibrillator operator can examine recordings at high speed to make a diagnosis. The size of the monitor screen is also important. Small screens are usually associated with light weight and small size but have the disadvantage of being harder to see.

There is a wide variety of ECG lead selection among defibrillators. In most cases monitoring through the defibrillation electrodes is highly desirable because the ECG can be obtained almost immediately after a shock is applied. However, it is usually desirable to have an accessory input to the ECG section in order that the ECG can be monitored for long periods without having to hold the defibrillation electrodes in place. There is a developing trend for defibrillators to have capability for multiple lead selection in order to provide for taking a standard 12 lead ECG. However, this can be a disadvantage because of additional switches and controls on the defibrillator, which may confuse the operator. Desirable accessories for defibrillators may be auxiliary input terminals from another ECG so that it can be used in conjunction with the defibrillator. An auxiliary output from monitors is desirable so that hard-copy records can be made of the electrocardiogram.

Heart-rate counters and/or alarm systems are available on most defibrillators for long-term monitoring of the electrocardiogram. An additional feature is a tone modulation system, which allows transmission of the electrocardiogram over domestic telephone lines.

Some systems provide two-way voice communication with a central monitoring station. The advantage of this system is that a single physician can monitor a large geographic area and be responsible for several mobile units simultaneously. Telemetry is more commonly included in new mobile care programs that have defibrillators operated by paramedic (nonphysician) rescuers. Defibrillators used in the vicinity of a telemetry system should have adequate radio frequency shielding to prevent stray signals from being recorded on the oscilloscope or graphic record.

Some defibrillators permit tape recording the ECG and voice as events occur. Tape recording has advantages for research and educational purposes as well as utility with regard to accurate documentation of the events at the emergency site. It may have value in cases of litigation.

SYNCHRONIZATION

Most defibrillators have synchronized shock capability. Synchronization is described in more detail in Chapter 7. However, two characteristics of synchronization systems will be emphasized here. The first is that modern defibrillators have a fixed maximum time delay between sensing of the QRS wave of the ECG and application of the shock. This feature has been provided because incorrect adjustment of the defibrillators during treatment of ventricular tachycardia or junctional tachycardia causes delivery of a shock during the vulnerable period of the atria, and this sometimes results in undesirable precipitation of atrial fibrillation.

Second, a spike or bright dot on the CRT screen (Fig. 5-5) indicates timing of the shock. Personal preference is the only determinant of which of these is desirable. Synchronization capability is truly a built-in safety feature that is intended for atrial defibrillation or the termination of ventricular tachyarrhythmias other than fibrillation.

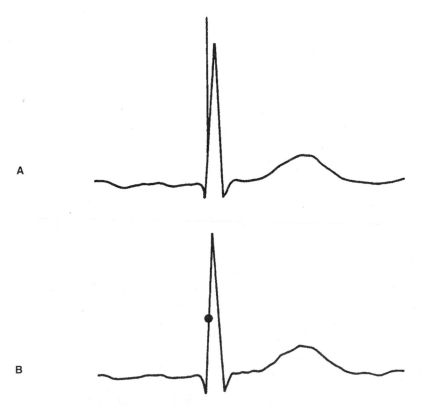

Fig. 5-5. Spike (**A**) and dot (**B**) type markers for synchronization.

SIZE, WEIGHT, AND RUGGEDNESS

The introduction of defibrillators for out-of-hospital use brought attention to the benefits of small size and light weight for many defibrillator uses. A portable defibrillator is lightweight and has a built-in energy source in the form of batteries. A defibrillator weighing about 10 kg is fairly easy to carry in the field. However, the advantages of the small, lightweight, portable defibrillator in ambulances or for other out-of-hospital use do not always carry over to defibrillators intended for hospital use. For example, very small defibrillators necessarily have a small ECG display. This is a disadvantage if the unit is used in an environment such as the coronary care unit, where a larger screen is needed for easy observation from a distance.

Some defibrillators are modular in construction—that is, the defibrillator may be separated from the ECG monitor. Such an arrangement may be convenient because it will allow use of the monitoring separately if such need arises. Also, the defibrillator can be carried more easily if it is broken down into two separate lightweight sections.

Because a charger is required with battery-operated defibrillators and because a battery-check circuit must be included, these units are generally more expensive than line-operated defibrillators. Because battery function is dependent on temperature and other environmental variables, a defibrillator that uses batteries requires careful attention to battery condition.

In general, the defibrillator must be built of rugged material with attention given to how and where it will be used. For example, portable defibrillators will have more stringent environmental requirements, such as use at temperature extremes, high altitude, high humidity, and tolerance to vibration in transport. Of course, the unit should be made of durable materials that can withstand the abuse frequently given in clinical use. The case should be rugged and capable of withstanding exposure to impact. The electrodes should be capable of withstanding abuse such as being dropped or stepped on. Obviously, the defibrillator should be electrically insulated so that accidental shock is not applied to the subject or to any other instruments or people in the environment.

SHOCK STRENGTH SELECTION AND CONTROLS

The method for displaying the energy setting on a defibrillator has been standardized. Modern defibrillators show the energy delivered either into a 50 Ω load or into the patient. Some defibrillator manufacturers use meters; others use displays to indicate the charge; and still other manufacturers use labeled pushbuttons. With most models, when the selected energy has been achieved, a light blinks or a buzzer sounds to indicate that the unit is charged to the desired setting. An additional method for displaying the energy is that a defibrillator with a display for monitoring the ECG may show a bar of light that moves along a vertical or horizontal line that is calibrated in energy units. All these energy selecting and indicating methods are satisfactory. The personal preference of the operator determines which of these various configurations is desirable. It should be pointed out that when stepped controls or pushbuttons are used for defibrillation, several energy levels should be provided. Typically 8 to 14 choices are provided from 1 to 2 J (minimum) up to 360 J (maximum).

There also may be an indicator that displays the energy that has been actually delivered following application of each shock. Patient transthoracic impedance and/or peak current may also be displayed. This feature allows the user to evaluate the shock strength that was actually delivered to a patient. The operator can take corrective action for such conditions as high patient resistance due to poor electrode contact. Some defibrillators measure patient impedance before discharge and indicate on a display whether impedance is high, low, or intermediate.

The controls that appear on various defibrillators are limited only by the ingenuity of the designer. The AAMI standard requires functional grouping of all controls for defibrillation into a single clearly defined area. Obviously, controls should be arranged so that the average medical person can use the defibrillator without delay. There should be few controls, and they should be clearly labeled, visible, and placed so that the defibrillation procedure is relatively self-evident. When instructions are printed on the defibrillator, they should be brief and in large print. Controls for most defibrillators are located entirely on the front panel, except for the discharge buttons, which are often on the electrode handles. Some defibrillators have controls on the electrode handles so that the defibrillator can be recharged and discharged without releasing the electrodes.

ELECTRODES

Electrodes for defibrillation are covered in Chapter 4. It is emphasized here, however, that electrodes should be of adequate surface area (probably 70 to 100 square cm) and must be in good contact with the skin. Also, use of a low-resistivity coupling material between the metal conductor and the skin is essential. Either handheld metal plates with a liquid or solid conductive gel or self-adhesive "hands-off" electrodes can be used. Both precordial and anterior-to-posterior electrode positions are effective.

It is appropriate to point out that connectors for electrodes to the defibrillator have not been standardized by the defibrillator industry. For this reason no defibrillation electrodes can be, or should be, used with a defibrillator of a different manufacturer. In fact, different models of defibrillators made by the same manufacturer often cannot be interchanged. In most cases the connectors will not mate and such interchanging of electrodes and defibrillators is not possible. Since manufacturers have used different connector pins for different uses, it would be very dangerous to use an electrode with a defibrillator for which the electrode has not been designed. For this reason it is usually desirable to order at least two pairs of electrodes for each defibrillator. Otherwise, failure of the electrodes because of conductor breakage, switch malfunction, and so forth will result in the defibrillator being inoperable. Obviously the electrode handles, cables, and connectors must be adequately insulated to protect the patient and operator.

BUILT-IN TESTING

Most defibrillators have a built-in testing capability, and some will automatically self-test when switched on. The functions being tested vary from one unit to another. Some tests deliver energy into a resistor that is built into the defibrillator; others provide for testing the built-in synchronizer, whereas other testing procedures may only document that the discharge control circuitry is functional. Some others do major functional tests.

TRANSCHEST PACING

Transchest pacing, also called noninvasive or external pacing, is not new, having been introduced several decades ago by Zoll.[2] However, it has increased in popularity during the past decade, and the feature now appears as an available option in many defibrillators. Detailed consideration of transchest pacing[2] is beyond the scope of this book, but a few comments are in order to point out some of the issues related to defibrillators with transchest pacing capability.

Transchest pacing is used for emergency treatment of Adams-Stokes bradycardia or cardiac arrest. A problem associated with this use is the pain caused by the strong (40 to 250 ma), long-duration (up to 40 msec), electric pulses. Successful treatment may bring the patient to consciousness and to recognition of the pain. The transchest pacer is also useful as a prophylactic device for patients at risk of asystole or bradycardia. These patients can have a transchest pacer applied for "demand" pacing if needed. If no pacing is ever needed, the risks and morbidity of transvenous pacer implant are avoided. If bradycardia does occur, the patient will be safely paced until a transvenous electrode is inserted, thus reducing the urgency of the clinical situation. There are certain clinical situations in which this is particularly important, for instance in a patient who is taking anticoagulants and therefore is a poor venotomy risk. Advantages include low cost, ease and speed of patient preparation, and absence of complications including bleeding, infection, arrhythmias produced by mechanical stimulation of the heart, thrombosis and embolism, pneumothorax, and cardiac tamponade.[1]

Since diagnosis of the underlying cause of cardiac arrest requires ECG monitoring and treatment may require either pacing, defibrillation, or both, there is a logical case to be made for devices with all these capabilities. There are, of course, a number of special considerations associated with this combination. First, sensing of the ECG during pacing poses special challenges in device design since automated and controlled sensing and stimulation are required. Second, there is a low risk that pacing may cause ventricular fibrillation, especially if pacing is asynchronous. Third, more training of personnel may be required due to the complexity of these devices. Fourth, if separate electrodes are used for all three functions, the profusion of cables, the limited space on the chest, and the time required to apply and maintain electrodes become problems. Some manufacturers provide a single pair of large self-adhesive electrodes for all three purposes. However, it is generally held that the lower-impedance electrodes required for defibrillation produce more pain if used for pacing than do higher-impedance electrodes. Improved electrode design may obviate this issue in the future, as discussed in Chapter 4. Although adding a transchest pacer to a defibrillator provides added capability to treat cardiac arrest, adding a pacer to a defibrillator also adds complexity, size, and weight as well as cost. The overall benefit-to-liability remains to be determined.

The majority of the features listed above add somewhat to the size, weight, and cost of the defibrillator. Therefore the user can often save money if the situation in which the defibrillator will be used is evaluated, and only the needed features are purchased.

The author would like to express his appreciation to Clif Alferness, Francis Charbonnier, and Carl Morgan for their review of and helpful suggestions for this chapter.

REFERENCES

1. Austin JL et al: Analysis of pacemaker malfunction and complications of temporary pacing in the coronary care unit, *Am J Cardio*, 49:301, 1982.
2. Emergency Cardiac Care Committee and Subcommittees, American Heart Association. Guidelines for cardiopulmonary resuscitation and emergency cardiac care, III: Adult Advanced Cardiac Life Support, *JAMA* 268:2199, 1992.
3. Tacker WA: Defibrillators. In Feinberg BN, editor: *Handbook of clinical engineering*, vol 1, Boca Raton, FL, 1980, CRC Press, pp 151-176.
4. Tacker WA, Geddes LA: *Electrical defibrillation*, Boca Raton, FL, 1980, CRC Press.

Chapter 6
Clinical Defibrillation: Optimal Transthoracic and Open Chest Techniques

Karl B. Kern
Gordon A. Ewy

Cardiac arrest continues to occur at an alarming rate in the United States, affecting over 500,000 individuals each year.[8] Fortunately, more than 70% of out-of-hospital cardiac arrests are secondary to ventricular tachycardia or ventricular fibrillation, dysrhythmias amenable to electroshock therapy. Effective electroshock treatment for patients with cardiac arrest from ventricular arrhythmias may be life saving. Defibrillation is the nonsynchronized application of electrical energy to interrupt hemodynamically compromising ventricular arrhythmias, thereby allowing the spontaneous restoration of a potentially perfusing rhythm. It is well recognized that the most important determinant of survival from sudden cardiac arrest is early intervention; that is, the early application of basic cardiopulmonary resuscitation (bystander CPR) and the early use of defibrillation.[26] Timely defibrillation is the only curative therapy currently available for cardiac arrest caused by ventricular fibrillation. Basic life support, including chest compressions and ventilation, merely temporizes and slows myocardial and cerebral death. Though important, such therapy does not restore the cardiac rhythm needed for survival. While other methods of defibrillation are of interest, the application of a direct current shock is the only reliable method to achieve ventricular defibrillation.

Who, then, should receive defibrillation therapy? Certainly anyone suffering unexpected hemodynamic collapse secondary to ventricular tachyarrhythmias is a potential candidate. Noncandidates are patients who have previ-

133

ously designated that they prefer not to undergo such resuscitative measures secondary to chronic illnesses, poor prognoses, or unacceptable life-styles. If such wishes are documented or well known, defibrillation therapy is inappropriate. However, in most circumstances where such information is not available, early defibrillation should be considered in the treatment of cardiopulmonary arrest.

The ability to defibrillate should be readily available in hospitals, not only in intensive care units but also throughout the facility. Emergency departments should be prepared to defibrillate by either external or internal techniques. The ability to defibrillate is frequently needed in out-of-the-hospital emergency services. Previously, only paramedic units have been equipped with a defibrillator, but the development of automatic and semiautomatic external defibrillators has allowed many communities to staff all first-responding units ("EMT-D") with the equipment necessary to defibrillate. Interest has grown in equipping large community functions such as sporting or entertainment events with equipment to automatically or semi-automatically externally defibrillate. Recently a call has been made for more widespread use of such automatic defibrillators by persons other than emergency medical technicians or paramedics.[22]

THE IMPORTANCE OF RAPID DEFIBRILLATION

The rapidity with which defibrillation is delivered is a major determinant of survival from cardiac arrest secondary to ventricular fibrillation.* The importance of early basic life support and defibrillation has been documented by several studies. Time is the most important variable for survival from cardiac arrest. Seattle investigators have shown that when a victim of cardiac arrest secondary to ventricular fibrillation receives basic life support within 4 minutes and defibrillation within 8 minutes, survival is greater than 40%.[61] If either of these factors is unduly delayed, survival rapidly declines. Even with the institution of basic life support (that is, early CPR) if definitive treatment with defibrillation does not occur before 16 minutes, survival declines to 10%. If CPR and defibrillation are each delayed greater than 12 minutes, survival does not occur.[61] Table 6-1 illustrates this data. Not only is survival improved with early defibrillation, but neurologic outcome is also improved where early defibrillation is accomplished.[120]

Cardiac rehabilitation programs have provided further evidence of the importance and success of early defibrillation. Though cardiac arrest is rare during supervised cardiac rehabilitation programs, it has occurred. A number of reports have shown that when cardiac arrest is immediately treated with basic life support and early defibrillation in the cardiac rehabilitation setting, the overall survival of such cardiac arrest victims approaches 90%.[26,44,56,58,113]

A significant advance in promoting early defibrillation has been the devel-

*References 34-37, 61, 71, 92, 117, 119-120.

Table 6-1
Cardiac Arrest: Time to Initiation of Therapy and Subsequent Survival

	Defibrillation		
	<8 Min	8–16 Min	>16 Min
CPR <4 min	43%	19%	10%
CPR 4-8 min	27%	19%	6%
CPR > 8 min	—	7%	0%

Reproduced with permission from Eisenberg MS, Bergner L, Hallstrom A: Cardiac resuscitation in the community: importance of rapid provision and implications for program planning, *JAMA* 241:1905, 1979.

opment of automatic and semiautomatic external defibrillators. Such devices are reliable and simple to operate. In both urban and rural environments studies have shown that emergency medical technicians given a relatively short training course can learn and use these devices in a lifesaving manner. The devices are operated by placing the electrodes on the cardiac arrest victim and then activating the computer program for diagnosis. Algorithms have been developed that are both specific and sensitive for the identification of ventricular fibrillation.[32,104] The semiautomatic external defibrillators require a second interaction, with the operator pushing a button once the diagnosis has been made. After placed and activated, the automatic device will deliver a shock without any further input once ventricular fibrillation is positively identified and the absence of respiration is noted by the lack of impedance changes. Numerous studies have shown improvement in survival rates for out-of-hospital cardiac arrest with the use of external defibrillators.[25,38,59,105,121] Table 6-2 outlines a number of such studies, showing the success rate before and after the use of automatic or semiautomatic external defibrillators by first responders. Enthusiasm has grown more widespread for the use of the devices, particularly where there is a large public gathering.[21,24,39,54,118] Such devices will allow early defibrillation before paramedic arrival. Weaver et al. trained security personnel at the 1986 World Expedition in Vancouver, British Columbia, to use these automatic defibrillators in the event of cardiac arrest. Five such arrests occurred. Two of the victims were in ventricular fibrillation, and both were successfully resuscitated by early defibrillation through the use of automatic external defibrillators.[118] Currently, enthusiasm is mounting to place these devices in public places such as large airports and skyscrapers or in remote locations such as cruise ships or airplanes.

The evidence supporting the importance of early defibrillation is so compelling that the American Heart Association and the American College of Cardiology endorsed a position statement on early defibrillation, calling for training of all emergency personnel to operate a defibrillator. This training should include "all first-responding emergency personnel, both hospital and nonhos-

Table 6-2
Effectiveness of Early Defibrillation Programs: Survival from Ventricular Fibrillation

Location	Before Early Defibrillation	After Early Defibrillation	Odds Ratio for Improved Survival*
King County[88]	7% (4/56)	26% (10/38)	4.6
Iowa[90]	3% (1/31)	19% (12/64)	6.9
Southeastern Minnesota[119]	4% (1/27)	17% (6/36)	5.2
Northeastern Minnesota[77]	3% (3/118)	10% (8/81)	4.2
Wisconsin[122]	4% (32/893)	11% (33/304)	3.3

Reproduced with permission from Cummins RO et al: Improving survival from sudden cardiac arrest: the "chain of survival concept," *Circulation* 83:1838, 1991.

pital (for example, emergency medical technicians [EMTs], non-EMT first responders, firefighters, volunteer emergency personnel, physicians, nurses, and paramedics)."[60]

A study by Martin et al.[73] in the mid-1980s examined physician-directed paramedic treatment of cardiac arrest in the field utilizing either immediate defibrillation shock or a period of CPR and drug therapy prior to defibrillation. Early defibrillation resulted in a significant improvement in survival, 12% vs 4%. In view of this and other evidence supporting the effectiveness of early defibrillation in improving cardiac arrest survival, the American Heart Association has recommended in its standards and guidelines for cardiopulmonary resuscitation that cardiac arrest victims in ventricular fibrillation undergo three attempts at external defibrillation as the initial step to resuscitation.[100] The current recommendations suggest an initial shock of 200 J followed by a second immediate shock of 200 to 300 J if the victim remains in ventricular fibrillation. A third attempt using 360 J is immediately applied if the first two lower-energy attempts fail. These recommendations for immediate defibrillation are not without some controversy. Yakaitis and Ewy found that when defibrillation was performed within minutes of the onset of cardiac arrest, no CPR or drug therapy was needed. However, if cardiac arrest continued for more than 5 minutes before defibrillation was attempted, administration of epinephrine and then external chest compressions were helpful prior to defibrillation in restoring a perfusion rhythm.[125] More recently Neimann et al., using an animal model of ventricular fibrillation cardiac arrest, found that following $7\frac{1}{2}$ minutes of untreated ventricular fibrillation animals initially given high-dose epinephrine and manual closed-chest CPR for approximately 5 minutes prior to defibrillation attempts had a higher resuscitation rate (9 of 14) than those treated with initial countershock (3 of 14).[81] Their findings suggested that following prolonged ventricular fibrillation a brief period of myocardial perfusion before countershock may improve successful resuscitation. Since the duration of arrest is most often unknown, the recommendations of the American Heart Association Emergency Cardiac Care Conference guidelines for CPR are as follows: (1) three initial defibrillation shocks; and if (2) shocks prove unsuccessful, then intravenous epinephrine, chest compressions, and ventilation followed by another series of defibrillation shocks.

CONVENTIONAL TECHNIQUES

PRECORDIAL THUMP

The precordial thump is the easiest, though least effective, form of defibrillation. First reported in the early 1960s as capable of defibrillating ventricular fibrillation,[55] it became apparent that precordial thumps could also convert ventricular tachycardia to ventricular fibrillation.[4] Because of that concern, the American Heart Association recommended in 1986 that a precordial thump be utilized only in patients with "monitored ventricular fibrillation or in witnessed cardiac arrest if a defibrillator is unavailable."[73] Precordial thumps defibrillate only 2% of patients with very recent onset of ventricular fibrillation. However, attempts utilizing precordial thump appear justified because of the rapidity and ease of delivery, particularly in patients with witnessed hemodynamic collapse.[19] Nevertheless, a defibrillator should be available before application of precordial thump in patients with ventricular tachycardia who have a pulse since the mechanical stimulus can induce ventricular fibrillation.[73]

TRANSTHORACIC DEFIBRILLATION

Successful transthoracic external defibrillation requires several steps (box). An important determinant of successful defibrillation is transthoracic impedance. Transthoracic impedance varies widely among victims of cardiac arrest.

Procedure for External Defibrillation

1. Ensure that the patient is in cardiac arrest.
2. Power the defibrillator on.
3. Use "quick look" paddles for rhythm diagnosis.
4. Select the energy level desired.
5. Apply electrode paste or conductive pads.
6. Position electrodes.
7. Ensure all personnel are clear of patient and bed.
8. Discharge defibrillator.
9. Reassess for cardiac arrest and "quick look" at the rhythm.
10. Repeat steps as necessary.

A study by Kerber et al.[64] showed that transthoracic impedance could range from 15 to 143 ohms, thereby varying by a factor of nearly 10. In our experience another factor that affects transthoracic impedance is the diameter of the electrode.* Work performed in our experimental laboratory indicates that as one increases the diameter of such external electrodes, the impedance decreases. With lower impedance defibrillation effectiveness should improve, and in a canine cardiac arrest model this proved to be true. Standard 8-cm diameter electrodes applied within the first minutes of ventricular fibrillation successfully defibrillated 38 of 53 animals (71%). A larger electrode with a 12.8-cm diameter successfully defibrillated within the same time period 66 of 75 animals (88%).[110] Kerber et al.[64] showed lower impedance with larger (13 cm) electrodes in human defibrillation and, when coupled with firm pressure to the chest, better current delivery.

If very large electrodes are used, the impedance is even lower, but defibrillation effectiveness is lower, showing that current density through the heart is the major factor in defibrillation. In our animal studies the optimal electrode size is the same as the heart size cross-sectional area in the animal. Optimal paddle size in human defibrillation remains uncertain.

A second factor known to affect transthoracic impedance and thus defibrillation success is the interface between the chest wall and the electrode.[23] Impedance can be very high if the electrodes are applied directly to the skin without some form of conductive medium. The impedance will drop by adding appropriate gels, pastes, or saline-soaked gauze pads.

In our laboratory we found a wide discrepancy in the ability of commercially available creams, pastes, and gels to decrease the impedance. Of the 26 products tested, we found the American Writer, Cor-gel, GE gel, and Redux paste as having the lowest impedance scores.[42] One should avoid high-impedance gels, for example the gels used for echocardiography.

An alternative to paste and gels is disposable electrode pads. Ewy and Taren[41] compared two such disposable pads (SAF-D-FIB and DEFIB-PADS) with Redux paste as the interface between the defibrillator electrode and the chest wall. One hundred watt-second and 400 watt-second defibrillation shocks were given, and impedance was measured. In all cases the paste electrode resulted in significantly lower impedance levels than the disposable defibrillation pads. Kerber et al., using a more recently developed defibrillation and cardioversion pad (R2 Corporation), found that in 80 patients receiving 267 shocks all but two patients achieved defibrillation or cardioversion at least once. The measured transthoracic impedance with such pads was 75 ± 21 ohms, similar to previous results by these investigators with standard hand-held electrodes (67 ± 36 ohms).[63] In our studies of cardioversion in humans, the impedance with hand-held electrodes in the anterior (8 cm)-posterior (12.8 cm) position was a mean of 50 ± 12 ohms in those successfully cardioverted and 59 ± 10 ohms in those not cardioverted. These values from

---

*Numerous reports refer to "paddles" in reference to defibrillation. "Electrodes" has been the term used throughout this chapter for hand-held transthoracic defibrillation electrodes.

Hewlett-Packard Redux paste and metal electrodes are much lower than that from the disposable R-2 electrodes. Though some have concluded that the self-adhesive disposable electrode pads are effective for routine defibrillation and cardioversion and that they provide an advantage in certain circumstances (such as in the electrophysiologic laboratory and in the transportation of the high-risk patient with cardiac disease),[63] we believe that because of their high impedance they are *not* optimal for cardioversion or defibrillation.

In a report from 1985 Aylward and colleagues detailed tests of three different electrode-chest wall coupling agents: Harcow pads (Hewlett-Packard), Littman pads (3M), and Redux paste (Hewlett-Packard). In a canine model of ventricular fibrillation cardiac arrest, defibrillation attempted 15 seconds following arrest at three different energy levels (50, 100, 150 J) showed that the Redux paste provided significantly lower impedance resulting in higher current delivery than the two disposable preformed pads; however, there was no significant difference in defibrillation success among the three agents. The investigators concluded that in the experimental cardiac arrest model disposable coupling pads were as effective as electrode paste for successful defibrillation, in spite of the fact that there was slightly higher impedance with the pads.[9]

Another determinant of transthoracic impedance to DC shock is the phase of respiration. Our laboratory has demonstrated higher impedance and decreased defibrillation effectiveness when shocks are delivered at full inspiration (from artificial inspiration) rather than during expiration. Likewise, defibrillation is rarely possible if there is a left-sided pneumothorax, an indication for open-chest defibrillation.

Correct positioning of the external defibrillation electrodes is crucial in optimizing successful defibrillation. The most common mistake in conventional transthoracic defibrillation is probably the incorrect placement of the electrodes. Though it is not necessary to defibrillate every myofibril, it does appear that a critical myocardial mass must be defibrillated. If the electrodes are placed too close together, the current that passes through the myocardium may be inadequate to successfully defibrillate. With proper spacing and placement of the electrodes, the current is more uniformly transmitted through the ventricular mass providing a better chance of defibrillation. An excellent example was seen by the senior author several years ago. In consultation he examined a patient who the night before required defibrillation but who was successfully defibrillated only after numerous attempts. It was obvious by inspection of the patient's chest that the electrodes had been placed too close together, as indicated by faint skin burns on the precordium (Fig. 6-1). Adequate distance must be maintained between the electrodes to ensure adequate current distribution to the fibrillating myocardium (Fig. 6-2).

There are several possible positions that will allow adequate current delivery to the fibrillating myocardium. The standard precordial position (or anterior apical) consists of one electrode placed at the right upper sternal border with another electrode at the left ventricular apex, lateral to the 5th intercostal space in the anterior axillary line (Fig. 6-3). This is the most commonly

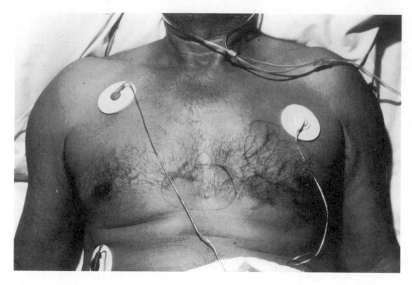

Fig. 6-1. Defibrillation burns indicating inappropriate paddle placement with electrode paddles too close together.

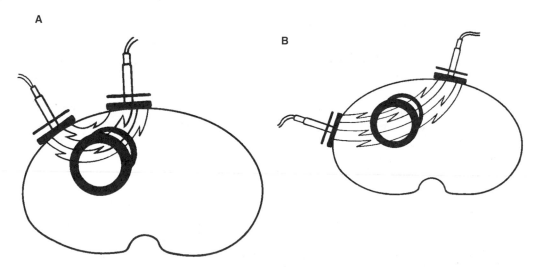

Fig. 6-2. A, The schematic showing the current pathway when the paddles are placed too closely together. **B,** A more optimal current pathway when the paddles are placed in the standard position. (Reproduced with permission from Ewy GA, Bressler R, editors: *Cardiovascular drugs and the management of heart disease,* New York, 1982, Raven Press.)

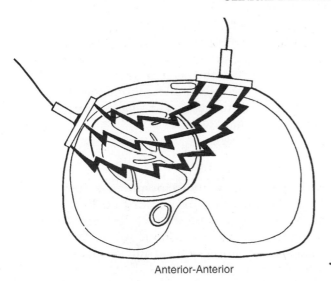

Anterior-Anterior

Fig. 6-3. The correct positioning for the standard anterior apical electrode placement.

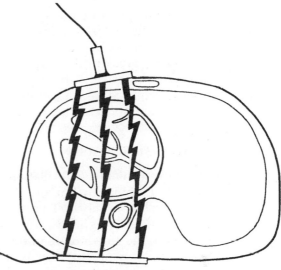

L-Anterior-Posterior

Fig. 6-4. The standard anterior-posterior positioning of the defibrillation electrodes.

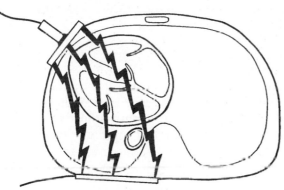

Apical-posterior

Fig. 6-5. An alternative anterior-posterior positioning also called the apex posterior position.

used electrode positioning and is easy and quick to employ. There are certain cases, however, where other positions may be desirable. For example, many permanent pacemaker pockets are placed in the right infra-clavicular area, which would be very close to the right parasternal anterior electrode position when using the standard position. In such a case an anterior-posterior positioning is less likely to cause the loss of pacemaker function after direct current shock. In the left anterior-posterior position one electrode is placed at the anterior apex just left of the palpable cardiac apex with the posterior electrode placed in the left infrascapular area (Fig. 6-4). In the apical posterior position one electrode is placed at the left ventricular apex while the posterior electrode is placed just inferior to the left scapula (Fig. 6-5).

Adequate pressure must be applied to the hand-held electrodes to ensure a low-impedance electrode-thoracic interface. Typical recommendations are for application of at least a 25-pound pressure. Self-adhesive electrode pads are said to have an advantage when applied prior to the need of defibrillation in high-risk patients, thereby ensuring correct positioning should defibrillation be required at a later time.[9,41] Their disadvantages are the lack of firm pressure and the less than optimal impedance characteristics.

BLIND DEFIBRILLATION

Currently available defibrillation devices have the ability to monitor the electrocardiographic rhythm and thereby confirm the diagnosis prior to delivery of defibrillation shock. This is done using the electrodes as electrocardiographic monitoring leads. The machine is turned on, a conductive paste is applied to the electrode to optimize the chest wall-to-electrode interface, and with firm pressure the electrodes are placed in the standard defibrillation positions. The electrocardiographic lead can be altered by changing the position of the electrodes. The ability to monitor patients in such a fashion has precluded the previously common use of "blind defibrillation." In rare circumstances when "quick look" monitoring is not possible, blind defibrillation can be attempted. Blind defibrillation is essentially the delivery of a defibrillation shock to a cardiac arrest victim without prior knowledge of the exact cardiac rhythm. Such an approach is acceptable with the knowledge that ventricular fibrillation is common among cardiac arrest victims and that it is the cause most amenable to therapy. Indeed, most survivors of cardiac arrest are those individuals whose arrest was caused by ventricular fibrillation. Delivering a defibrillation shock to a patient in asystole or electromechanical dissociation generally will not be successful, but there is no evidence that such an attempt will be detrimental. In cases where the patient is in ventricular fibrillation, such blind attempts can be life saving.[50]

DEFIBRILLATOR OPERATIONS

The actual operation of a conventional external defibrillator requires several steps (box, p. 137 and Fig. 6-6). The device must first be operational, and power must be turned on. A separate switch is used to charge the capacitor with the necessary energy to deliver the defibrillation shock. Typically, a button must be pushed to charge the device. All the devices have some method of measuring the energy. The desired energy must be selected, usually by the use of a dial indicating the desired joules from 0 to 360. Once fully charged and ready to deliver the selected energy shock, the electrodes should be firmly (we strongly favor hand-held electrodes) placed in an appropriate defibrillation position, and a warning should be given for all associated personnel to avoid contact with the victim prior to the delivery of the shock. Applying firm pressure to each electrode, the shock should then be delivered. As a safety mea-

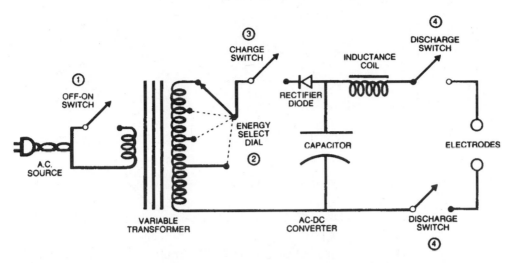

Fig. 6-6. Defibrillation steps illustrated as a function of the defibrillator. (Reproduced with permission. *Textbook of Advanced Cardiac Life Support*, 1987, 1990. Copyright American Heart Association.)

sure most devices have switch buttons on each electrode that must be simultaneously depressed to deliver the shock.

If a shock is not delivered, several troubleshooting steps should be taken. First, ensure that the device has power. Second, check that the device was adequately charged and ready to deliver the shock. Third, be certain that the device is in the asynchronous mode. Most defibrillators with ECG monitors now come with the capacity not only for defibrillation but for synchronized cardioversion as well. When the synchronized circuit is activated, the unit will monitor the electrocardiogram, specifically the QRS complex, and then deliver the countershock on or immediately after the R wave. In the presence of ventricular fibrillation the device will appropriately not recognize a QRS complex and will continue to monitor the electrocardiogram, but will not discharge. Defibrillation shocks can only be delivered in the asynchronous mode. Following application of a defibrillation shock, the cardiac arrest victim should be reassessed, both clinically and with the monitoring electrode. The electrocardiogram can be reassessed through the electrodes, and the presence or absence of the pulse should be determined. If the patient remains in ventricular fibrillation, repeated shocks can be performed.

ENERGY FOR DEFIBRILLATION

Energy requirements for successful defibrillation have been studied carefully in both experimental models and in clinical trials. Most experimental work has corroborated that a defibrillation threshold exists, and therefore shocks of inadequate strength will not defibrillate.[45,127] However, excessive defibrillation

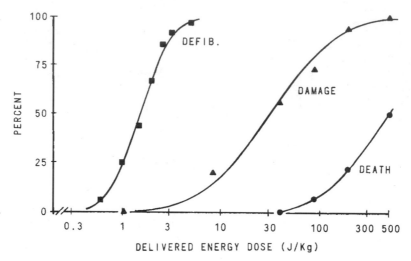

Fig. 6-7. Dose response curves showing the potential for morbidity and mortality with excessive strength shocks.

energy shocks are known to produce both dysrthymias and myocardial damage (Fig. 6-7).[27,33,116] Initial work within the experimental model of cardiac arrest indicates that body size and the strength of defibrillation shock required for successful defibrillation correlate quite well.[48] It is also known that smaller defibrillation shocks are needed for defibrillation in small children than those needed for adults.[52] However, among the size range of adulthood, it has been difficult to correlate energy requirement with body size.[3,85,107]

Classic clinical trials have shown in both outpatients and inpatients that initial shocks with 200 J are usually adequate.[61,122] In an out-of-the-hospital study Weaver and associates compared low- and high-energy shocks in 249 patients with ventricular fibrillation. Two 175-J delivered energy shocks and, if ineffective, a third shock at 320 J delivered energy were compared with three consecutive high-energy (320 J) shocks. Defibrillation rates were not different, and the proportion of patients successfully resuscitated and discharged from the hospital was also similar (Fig. 6-8).[122] Since the average transthoracic impedance is 50 ohms (see below), 200 J stored energy delivers 175 J, and 360 J stored energy delivers 320 J. Kerber and colleagues conducted a prospective in-hospital study of 183 patients requiring defibrillation. Patients received initial countershocks of either 200 J or 300 to 400 J. This study also showed no difference in first shock or accumulative success rates at the two energy levels.[61]

The rationale for a lower-energy shock (200 J) is that less myocardial damage occurs. Weaver found a higher incidence of atrioventricular block in the patients receiving the higher-dose shocks compared to those receiving lower-

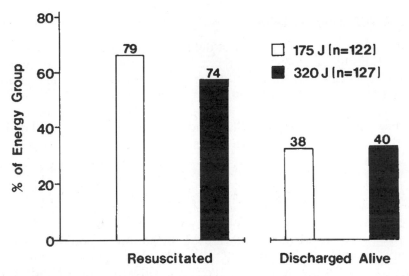

Fig. 6-8. Defibrillation results comparing 175 J and 320 J. (Reprinted, by permission of *The New England Journal of Medicine*, 307:1104, 1982.)

energy defibrillation. These data have resulted in the American Heart Association's present guidelines for defibrillation that recommend an initial shock at 200 J. If successful defibrillation has not occurred after one or two shocks at the lower level, then a high-energy shock at 360 J should be attempted.[73] The recommendation for the energy level of the second shock is either 200 or 300 J. Several studies have shown that transthoracic impedance declines with repeated shocks.[28,47] Such a decline in transthoracic impedence results in greater current delivery to the myocardium using the same shock energy and should enhance the possibility of achieving successful defibrillation. This is the rationale for delivering a second shock of the same energy. However, in humans Kerber found little or no decrease in transthoracic impedance with a rapidly delivered second shock and advocated the shock strength be 300 J. If ventricular fibrillation continues after the second attempt of 200 or 300 J, a higher energy level (360 J) should be used for the third and subsequent shocks.

Recurrent ventricular fibrillation may occur even after successful defibrillation. In such circumstances it is reasonable to use energy levels similar to those that were previously effective. Energy levels should be kept as low as possible to minimize myocardial damage, particularly in the cases where ventricular fibrillation reoccurs frequently. Myocardial injury associated with defibrillation corresponds not only with total energy (joules) used but also with the frequency of the defibrillation shocks.[27] Electrode size is a third factor, with the most damage occurring when high energy is delivered repeatedly at short intervals via small electrodes.[27]

OPEN-CHEST DEFIBRILLATION

The most common use of open-chest defibrillation is during cardiac surgery. Current cardiothoracic surgery practice rarely uses deliberate ventricular fibrillation; cold cardioplegia and full cardiac arrest are now the usual methods. Nonetheless, ventricular fibrillation can result under a variety of circumstances in the operating room. During induction of anesthesia, cardiac surgery patients occasionally fibrillate and are treated with external defibrillation in the usual fashion. Once the chest has been opened, it is possible to defibrillate by external means,[16,17,91] but internal defibrillation is usually utilized if ventricular fibrillation occurs. The most common scenario for ventricular fibrillation requiring internal defibrillation is at the conclusion of the surgical procedure. On rewarming and unclamping of the aorta, approximately 40% to 50% of the patients will experience ventricular fibrillation.[30]

The equipment needed for internal defibrillation is somewhat different than that needed for external defibrillation. The electrodes are usually 8 cm in diameter (or smaller for children) and cup-shaped with longer handles so that they can be inserted into the chest cavity. The heart is cradled between the two electrodes, typically with one over the right ventricle and the other at the left ventricular apex. Adequate force is used to apply the electrode firmly to the myocardial surface, and an electrical shock is delivered. This position seems to be optimal for accomplishing defibrillation with the lowest current.[127] It was recommended formerly that a gauze sponge soaked in normal saline be used to decrease the likelihood of shock producing cardiac damage.[89] However, that is not the current standard of care. It is important that all operating-room personnel stand back at the time of shock delivery and that they not be in contact with the patient or the operating-room table. In most cases discharge of the internal defibrillator shock is performed by a button on the front panel of the defibrillator rather than from the electrodes themselves.

Several studies have examined the optimal dose for internal defibrillation. Tacker et al. published a series of 100 patients undergoing cardiothoracic surgery who required defibrillation. Ninety-three of these 100 patients required 10 Js or less for successful defibrillation.[108] Forty-eight or almost 50% required 5 J or less. The authors concluded that most human hearts can be defibrillated directly with 10 J of energy or less. They suggested that this may be preferable to the standard 20 to 50 Js often used in hospitals because of decreased risk of electrical damage. In a separate study, Lake and colleagues found that approximately 90% of 150 cardiac surgical patients could be defibrillated successfully with 10 or less J.[69] These authors also suggested starting at low levels of energy and increasing only if the lower levels failed to successfully defibrillate, thereby avoiding possible myocardial damage from high-dose defibrillation. Pugsley et al.[87] found similar results in a study of 168 patients showing that 98% could be defibrillated internally with less than 10 J of energy.

PLATE 1

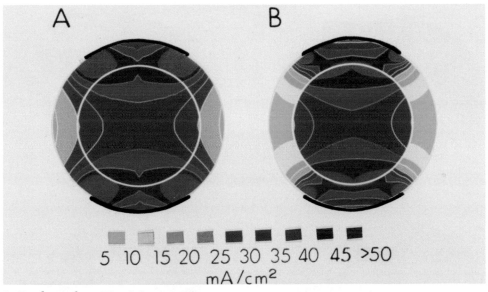

A, For legend see Fig. 2-2, page 18.

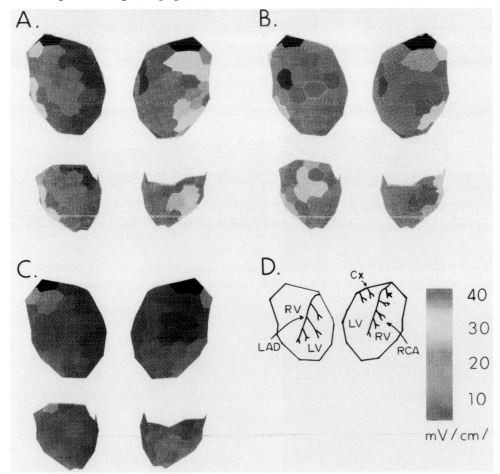

B, For legend see Fig. 2-12, page 30.

PLATE 2

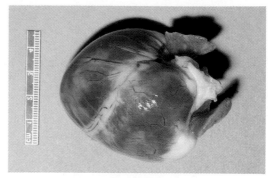

A, For legend see Fig. 12-1, page 261.

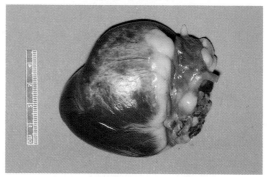

B For legend see Fig. 12-2, page 261.

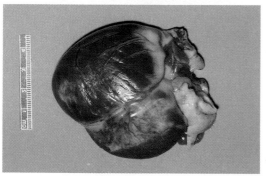

C, For legend see Fig. 12-3, *A*, page 262.

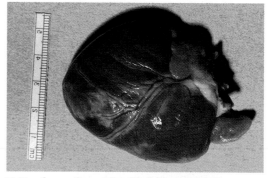

D, For legend see Fig. 12-3, *B*, page 262.

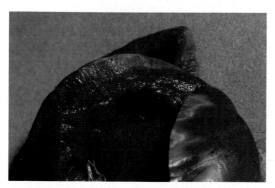

E, For legend see Fig. 12-4, page 263.

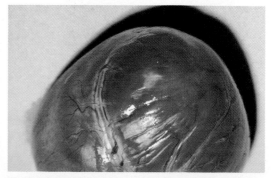

F, For legend see Fig. 12-5, *A*, page 263.

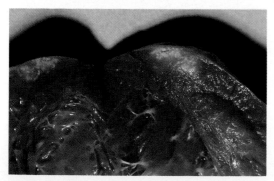

G, For legend see Fig. 12-5, *B*, page 264.

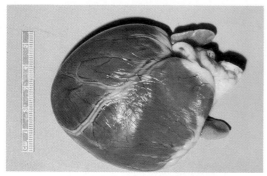

H, For legend see Fig. 12-6, page 264.

Another less common use for open-chest defibrillation occurs during emergency circumstances where closed-chest resuscitation efforts have failed and more aggressive open-chest measures have been employed. Open-chest cardiopulmonary resuscitation and subsequent internal defibrillation have been shown to be more effective than closed-chest techniques in a number of circumstances.[29,123] Myocardial and cerebral perfusion with open-chest CPR techniques are clearly superior to those with closed-chest efforts,[10,14-15] and subsequent short- and long-term survival in animal models have been substantially better.[13,67,96-97] The most difficult decision in using open-chest techniques is *when* to employ such invasive techniques (emergent thoracotomy and open-chest resuscitation). The American Heart Association recommendations concerning the use of invasive techniques are shown in the accompanying box.[101]

We studied the time-course feasibility of instituting open-chest cardiopulmonary resuscitation and direct defibrillation after various periods of unsuccessful closed-chest efforts and found that after a period of 25 or 30 minutes of ineffective closed-chest efforts, the institution of open-chest invasive resuscitation did not result in long-term benefits.[96] Hence, the decision to use invasive techniques must be made relatively early, probably within 15 minutes of cardiac arrest and failed closed-chest efforts.

One of the questions in using emergent open-chest efforts and internal defibrillation is "Who should perform such techniques?" In the early 1980s, McNulty from the University of Pittsburgh interviewed groups of physicians who in the 1950s had routinely performed open-chest cardiac cardiopul-

---

American Heart Association's Recommendatons for Open-Chest Cardiopulmonary Resuscitation and Internal Defibrillation

1. Cardiac arrest associated with penetrating chest trauma.
2. Anatomical chest wall deformities precluding effective external chest compressions (including severe emphysema).
3. Cardiac arrest associated with hypothermia.
4. Cardiac arrest secondary to a ruptured aortic aneurysm, where cardiopulmonary bypass is immediately available.
5. Cardiac tamponade.
6. Cardiac arrest in the operating suite, where the chest is already open.
7. Cardiac arrest associated with a "crushed chest" injury.
8. "Rarely, where there is failure of adequately applied closed-chest compressions and ventricular fibrillation refractory to external defibrillation."

Adapted from American Medical Association: *JAMA* 255:2937, 1986.

monary resuscitation. Four decades ago physicians of various disciplines had become skilled in the performance of invasive resuscitation, including its use in the emergency room and on regular hospital wards.[94] Concern about overwhelming morbidity and infection following the emergent thoracotomy has not been realized.[6] Whether this technique should be further espoused among nonphysicians (i.e., paramedics) has not been addressed.

The thorax can be emergently opened by a 4th or 5th left intercostal space incision. Bleeding can be minimized by cutting through only the skin and outer fascia and then inserting a finger or blunt instrument and tearing a rend into the thoracic cavity. Such a technique causes spasm of the arterioles and capillaries, thereby markedly reducing the amount of postresuscitation bleeding at the entrance site.

DETERMINANTS OF SUCCESSFUL DEFIBRILLATION

A number of variables have been shown to affect defibrillation success, such as concurrent disease or patient condition. The accompanying box lists a number of such variables. The duration of ventricular fibrillation prior to attempts at defibrillation appears to be one of the more powerful predictors of failure to defibrillate. Yakaitis and Ewy[125] found that the duration of ventricular fibrillation is inversely proportional to successful defibrillation (Fig. 6-9). They also found that the energy requirement for defibrillation was directly proportional to the duration of fibrillation in an experimental canine model.[125] Kerber and Sarnat,[65] in a review of patients undergoing defibrillation attempts, found that a prolonged delay in defibrillation efforts was a significant factor in defibrillation failure. Not all investigators have agreed with these conclusions. Gascho and coworkers,[46] in studying 88 adult patients undergoing cardiac resuscitation, did not find duration of ventricular fibrillation to be important in predicting success. The vast majority of patients in this study were treated quickly and defibrillation attempted early, usually within 2 to 3 minutes, with a mean time to defibrillation attempt of 2.9 ± 5.4 minutes. The investigators found the patient's underlying diagnosis and the

Variables Affecting Defibrillation Success
1. Duration of ventricular fibrillation.
2. Automatic internal defibrillator patches.

Variable Having No Effect on Defibrillation Success
1. Acid-base status.
2. Left ventricular hypertrophy.
3. Hypoxia.
4. Ischemia.
5. Epinephrine usage.

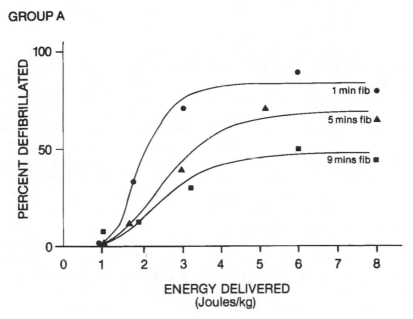

GROUP A

Fig. 6-9. Influence on successful outcome of cardiac arrest time prior to defibrillation attempts. (Reproduced from RW Yakaitis, GA Ewy, CW Otto et al: Influence of time and therapy on ventricular defibrillation in dogs, *Crit Care Med* 8:157-163, © by Williams and Wilkins [1982].)

setting in which ventricular fibrillation occurred influenced the success of defibrillation more than the duration of ventricular fibrillation. The difference among these studies appears to be the length of fibrillation. If the duration of ventricular fibrillation is short, then it may not be an important factor; when the duration approaches 5 to 10 minutes or greater, it becomes extremely important.

Other evidence indicating that the duration of ventricular fibrillation is important in determining defibrillation success comes from evaluating adenosine triphosphate energy stores in the myocardium during ventricular fibrillation. We found that with increasing time of ventricular fibrillation, myocardium energy stores of adenosine triphosphate (ATP) decline in a non-linear fashion, and that below a certain level successful defibrillation could not be achieved.[66] Brown and colleagues have found similar results examining high-energy phosphate levels in the fibrillating myocardium.[82] These investigators have also reported the use of ventricular fibrillation frequency analysis using fast fourier transformation to estimate the duration of ventricular fibrillation. The goal is to select the best therapeutic options during cardiopulmonary resuscitation.[72] The duration of ventricular fibrillation is clearly a major factor in defibrillation success. Since ventricular fibrillation is an energy-consuming rhythm, the longer the patient remains in ventricular fibrillation without circulatory support, the lower the myocardial energy stores and the greater the myocardial damage.

A number of factors have been found not to have any effect on either defibrillation threshold or defibrillation success. These include left ventricular hypertrophy, acidosis, hypoxia, ischemia, and ischemic load.[62,126] The use of epinephrine to improve defibrillation has also been evaluated in an experimental model by Otto and colleagues at the University of Arizona. It was found to have little effect. Though epinephrine can be helpful during cardiopulmonary resuscitation by improving myocardial blood flow and perfusion, there does not appear to be any advantage to epinephrine use in countershock therapy during resuscitation of animals with myocardial ischemia.[84]

In the present era of automatic internal defibrillators, it is important to note that there are several reports showing that epicardial patch electrodes used for internal defibrillators have a negative impact on transthoracic defibrillation. In such circumstances if external defibrillation fails, it is suggested that the orientation of the thoracic electrodes be varied from the standard positions to attempt a more favorable defibrillation pathway.[70,115]

Patient conditions during internal cardiac defibrillation are less well described, but several are elucidated. Hypothermia often results in refibrillation even after successful defibrillation. The effect of ischemia during internal defibrillation is somewhat less defined. Tacker found that with an open-chest preparation the defibrillation threshold for direct cardiac defibrillation increased with ischemia.[109] However, Ruffy et al.,[93] also using an open-chest experimental preparation, found no effect of ischemia on defibrillation threshold.[93]

COMMON PROBLEMS IN CONVENTIONAL DEFIBRILLATION

An initial problem to successful defibrillation can be the accurate determination of the diagnosis. Ventricular fibrillation is a well-recognized arrhythmia and has been classified generally as "coarse" or "fine." "Fine" ventricular fibrillation is most likely the result of a coarse ventricular fibrillation degenerating over time. When evaluating a victim of cardiac arrest, it is important to determine whether ventricular fibrillation or asystole is present. Ventricular fibrillation can be successfully treated by electrical defibrillation. Asystole generally is not successfully defibrillated. However, it has been shown that ventricular fibrillation (much like atrial fibrillation) may have an electrical vector, and depending on the leads monitored, a null vector may be produced mimicking a straight-line asystolic rhythm (Fig. 6-10). Ewy et al.[43] reported finding such "straight-line" ventricular fibrillation by monitoring leads AVL or AVR in five of the 11 animals electrically fibrillated. McDonald published a case report on a human cardiac arrest showing a similar phenomenon. On arrival at the emergency department the patient's electrocardiogram revealed asystole or very fine ventricular fibrillation, but with a lead change, coarse ventricular fibrillation became apparent.[74]

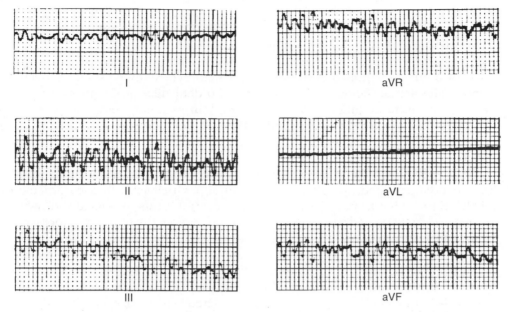

Fig. 6-10. Coarse ventricular fibrillation seen in an experimental model with a null electrical vector apparent in lead AVL. Note that this lead is the sum of AVR and AVF. When these two leads are the exact mirror image, a straight line is produced. (Reproduced from GA Ewy, DF Dahl, M Zimmerman et al: Ventricular fibrillation masquerading as ventricular stand still, *Crit Care Med* 9;841-844, © by Williams and Wilkins [1981].)

In cases of recurrent ventricular fibrillation it is recommended that to limit myocardial damage the previously successful or even lower energy level be employed. Repetitive shocks may result in myocardial damage. Ewy et al. have shown that repeat shocks at 15-second intervals resulted in myocardial damage.[127] Such damage may manifest itself as ST segment elevation on the electrocardiogram; the appearance of other arrhythmias, including premature beats or heart block; the elevation of myocardial enzymes; and the development of left ventricular failure.[1,57,77,78,83]

Defibrillation shocks may produce nonperfusing rhythms, such as electromechanical disassociation or postshock asystole. The most appropriate therapy for these rhythms appears to be aggressive cardiopulmonary resuscitation producing the maximal achievable myocardial perfusion, with either the return of a perfusing rhythm or the reversion to ventricular fibrillation and then further defibrillation attempts.

RISK OF DEFIBRILLATION TO RESCUER

The safety of defibrillation must be considered. For the patient requiring defibrillation, risks are described in Chapter 5. For the individual delivering the defibrillation shock, precautions must also be taken to limit any inherent dangers. Gibbs reported on the severity of injuries to prehospital emergency personnel in King County, Washington. Questionnaires mailed to the paramedics in the King County emergency medical system documented only eight cases of injury to paramedics or emergency medical technicians over a 9-year period. The actual incidence was one in 1700 defibrillation attempts among paramedics and one in 1000 defibrillation attempts among emergency medical technicians trained to defibrillate. Most of the incidences resulted from contact with the cardiac arrest victim during the defibrillation shock, producing localized transmission of a portion of electrical current culminating in extremity tingling or soreness. One equipment failure, a crack in the defibrillator paddle, resulted in a more significant shock delivered to a paramedic, resulting in frequent premature ventricular ectopic beats and localized muscle spasms requiring admission to the hospital. No deaths have been reported from accidental injury to the administrators of the defibrillation shock. The incidence of defibrillator-associated injuries to prehospital emergency personnel appears to be low and the nature of the injuries minimal. However, safety must continue to be stressed and efforts made to eliminate all such injuries.[49] Case reports of defibrillation hazards associated with nitroglycerin patches are of interest. Ren reported a case of a small explosion in a nitroglycerin patch during the defibrillation attempt when an electrode was placed directly on such a patch. Though no adverse effects occurred in this patient, the dangers of "arcing" during defibrillation and ineffective delivery of current in reference to patches or ointments, particularly nitroglycerin, should be considered.[124]

It should be emphasized that there is essentially no danger to CPR providers from the discharge of automatic implantable cardioverter defibrillators (ICDs).

WHEN TO STOP RESUSCITATION AND DEFIBRILLATION EFFORTS

Both in-hospital and out-of-hospital studies have shown that successful resuscitation and defibrillation are functions of time. The longer the patient remains in a nonperfusing cardiac rhythm, the greater the likelihood of a poor outcome. The decision to stop resuscitation efforts is difficult. Each patient and circumstance must be carefully evaluated to avoid premature termination of potentially successful efforts. However, there are data indicating that beyond a certain point in time further efforts at resuscitation and defibrillation are probably futile. Bedell et al. found that in an in-hospital setting cardiopulmonary resuscitation efforts, including defibrillation, did not result in long-term survival if the duration of arrest and resuscitation effort was greater than 30 minutes.[12] Among 241 inpatients whose arrest continued for more than 15 minutes, only 5% survived. Tortolani and colleagues found similar data during the 1990s. Among 470 adults suffering cardiac arrest in the hospital setting, independent correlates of 24-hour survival included CPR durations of less than 15 minutes.[111] Therefore, it seems reasonable to conclude that in an in-hospital setting if resuscitation efforts, including defibrillation, have not resulted in a perfusing cardiac rhythm by 30 minutes, further efforts are rarely successful. Obviously, there are certain circumstances where this may not be true, such as in profound hypothermia, and individual specifics must always be considered.

We have found monitoring end-tidal carbon dioxide to be a valuable tool during resuscitation efforts. In a study of adults suffering nontraumatic cardiac arrest in whom expired end-tidal carbon dioxide was measured during CPR, we found that levels below 10 torr were associated with a poor outcome. Only one of 51 patients had an average end-tidal carbon dioxide level of less the 10 torr and survived.[98] Monitoring for expired end-tidal carbon dioxide levels may be another way to objectively assess the possibilities for successful resuscitation and in some cases provide information on when to stop resuscitation efforts.

Out-of-hospital cardiac arrest resuscitation success is also time dependent. Gray et al. found that of 185 patients presenting to the emergency department after initially suffering cardiac arrest and unsuccessful resuscitation efforts in the prehospital setting, only 16 were resuscitated (9%) and none survived to hospital discharge.[51] They concluded that to continue resuscitation efforts in the emergency department for victims of cardiac arrest who were initially unsuccessfully treated in a prehospital setting was not worthwhile. Though no one has specifically determined the maximum time limit for out-of-hospital cardiac arrest efforts, as has been done for in-hospital arrests, it seems reasonable to conclude that a similar time frame is applicable. Hence, after 25 or 30 minutes of efforts if defibrillation and CPR have not resulted in a successful resuscitation, it seems legitimate to consider stopping further efforts. Exceptions to this guideline include young individuals and patients with hypothermia.

THERAPY AFTER SUCCESSFUL DEFIBRILLATION

The care of the successfully defibrillated patient can be divided into three major categories: the immediate postresuscitation period, the management of the postresuscitation syndrome, and the long-term follow-up care to prevent recurrence. Following cardiac arrest and subsequent restoration of spontaneous perfusion, the patient who was immediately defibrillated is restored to his or her pre-ventricular fibrillation state. With more prolonged arrest the the patient will suffer varying degrees of multiple organ failure, which may be temporary or permanent. Negovsky[80] was the first to describe this condition in the 1950s, which he later labeled "postresuscitation disease." Much of the previous work with postresuscitation illness has centered on the central nervous system. Ames[7] has shown that individual cerebral neurons can tolerate up to 20 minutes of cardiac arrest before irreversible damage occurs. Safar and coworkers have subsequently determined the limits of global total ischemia tolerated by the *in vivo* central nervous system also to be 20 minutes before functional recovery is markedly limited.[76,88,95] They have also investigated multiple therapeutic interventions to combat postresuscitation central nervous system damage. A large clinical trial of barbiturate therapy following resuscitation failed to show any benefit,[2] but some encouraging results from experimental work[102,103,112] and some clinical trials[90] have suggested that calcium entry blockers may be somewhat helpful.

Less is known about postresuscitation myocardial dysfunction. Regional myocardial stunning from various periods of coronary occlusion and reperfusion is well described. Myocardial function, including both systolic contraction and diastolic relaxation, may remain impaired long after reperfusion and myocardial blood flow are restored.[18,86] Global stunning of the myocardium from cardiac arrest has not been studied as thoroughly. Investigators at the University of Pittsburgh have reported the only evaluation of myocardial function following prolonged cardiac arrest and successful resuscitation in dogs.[20] Cerchiari found that following cardiac arrest of 71/2 to 10 minutes, cardiac index had fallen by 30% at 2 to 4 hours following resuscitation. Full recovery to prearrest levels was seen by 12 hours; however, if the cardiac arrest was longer than 121/2 minutes, cardiac index declined again by 30% but did not return to normal within 24 hours. Pulmonary capillary wedge pressure rose in all groups and remained elevated in those animals resuscitated after 121/2 minutes of untreated cardiac arrest. Postresuscitation myocardial dysfunction continues to be a major limitation for long-term survival after resuscitation. Little is understood about its prevention or treatment. Elucidation of postresuscitation systolic and diastolic myocardial dysfunction with examination of potential therapeutic options is needed.

The myocardium may also show electrical instability after defibrillation, particularly where high-level energy was required for successful defibrillation. Liberthson and colleagues found that initially rapid post-defibrillation heart rates, including sinus tachycardia or atrial fibrillation, were associated with a better outcome than were slow heart rates of any origin after defibrillation.[71]

The long-term management of victims of cardiac arrest who are successfully defibrillated focuses on preventing recurrence of their ventricular fibrillation. Data from the Seattle Heart Watch Program indicated that patients with primary ventricular fibrillation (ventricular fibrillation not associated with an acute myocardial infarction) had a high recurrence rate of 47% at 2 years. Those whose cardiac arrest was associated with an acute transmural Q wave infarction had a mortality rate of only 14% during the 2-year follow-up.[11] Liberthson studied 301 subjects with prehospital ventricular fibrillation. Defibrillation was successful in 199. Ninety-eight died prior to admission, while 101 were successfully hospitalized. Fifty-nine of those died in the hospital. Forty-two patients survived and were eventually discharged from the hospital. Ventricular fibrillation or rapid ventricular tachycardia reoccurred in

57% of the hospitalized patients within the first day. Of the 42 patients eventually discharged from the hospital, 28% died suddenly after discharge.[71] Hence, the recurrence rate for sudden cardiac death secondary to ventricular fibrillation in initial defibrillation survivors appears to be quite high, somewhere between 28% and 47% over a 2-year period. Schaffer and Cobb[99] followed 234 successfully resuscitated patients over 50 months and found a 38% recurrence during that period. Reports from a decade later continued to show a high recurrence rate, though somewhat less than the initial reports. Myerberg found a 25% recurrence during a 5-year follow-up ending in 1984. Two thirds of the deaths in his group were from recurrent sudden cardiac death during that 5-year period.[79]

Several risk factors have been identified in the survivors of ventricular fibrillation that predispose them to further events. Left ventricular dysfunction is a powerful predictor. Smoking has been reported as a primary risk factor for recurrence of sudden cardiac arrest; the cessation of smoking decreased the incidence of ventricular fibrillation.[53] In a group of 310 survivors of out-of-hospital cardiac arrest, those who stopped smoking had a lower incidence of recurrent cardiac arrest than those patients who continued to smoke (19% vs 27% at 3 years). Recently, Cobb and associates[40] have shown that coronary bypass surgery may also reduce the incidence of recurrent sudden cardiac death in suitable patients resuscitated from an episode of ventricular fibrillation.

The current evaluation of out-of-hospital sudden cardiac death survivors should include both noninvasive and invasive testing. Waldo and colleagues[114] have outlined an extensive and complete evaluation for such patients. They suggest that it include not only a detailed history, routine chest x ray, and 12 lead electrocardiogram but also a number of laboratory tests such as electrolytes, cardiac enzymes, and plasma drug levels. Continuous monitoring of the electrocardiogram by Holter monitor or telemetry is also deemed important in assessing risk of recurrence. A measurement of left ventricular function is indicated and can be accomplished either by nuclear techniques or by echocardiography. Assessment of coronary anatomy is essential. Waldo et al.[114] suggest that cardiac catheterization should be considered in all instances of sudden cardiac death survival and should be performed in most cases. Finally, invasive electrophysiologic testing is indicated in virtually all cases except where out-of-hospital sudden cardiac death can be attributed to a cause that does not require further elucidation, such as drug intoxication, or complete heart block.[114]

Treatment of recurrent ventricular fibrillation by empiric drug therapy has not proven efficacious.[68] Some experts believe that such an approach will have little impact on the community incidence of sudden cardiac death.[22] However, the use of the internal automatic defibrillator and semiautomatic and fully automatic external defibrillators may have a strong impact on improving survival for sudden cardiac arrest victims.[5,31,75]

SUMMARY

Conventional defibrillation, both transthoracic and open-chest, can be a life-saving treatment for patients in ventricular fibrillation. The importance of early defibrillation cannot be overemphasized, and great efforts are currently under way to provide for early defibrillation by the more extensive use of semiautomatic and fully automatic external defibrillators. The patient population at greatest risk for ventricular fibrillation sudden cardiac death is comprised of the survivors of an initial such episode. These patients deserve a careful evaluation and follow-up and, in many instances, the placement of an internal automatic defibrillator device.

REFERENCES

1. Aberg H, Cullhed I: Direct current countershock complications, *Acta Med Scand* 183:415, 1968.
2. Abramson NS et al: Randomized clinical study of cardiopulmonary-cerebral resuscitation: thiopental loading in comatose cardiac arrest survivors, *N Engl J Med* 314:397, 1986.
3. Adgey AAJ et al: Ventricular defibrillation: appropriate energy levels, *Circulation* 60:219, 1979.
4. Adgey AAJ, Webb SW: The treatment of ventricular arrhythmias in acute myocardial infarction, *Br J Hosp Med* 21:356, 1979.
5. Akhtar M et al: Role of implantable cardioverter defibrillator therapy in the management of high-risk patients, *Circulation* 85(Suppl 1):I-131, 1992.
6. Altemeier WA, Todd J: Studies on the incidence of infection following open-chest cardiac massage for cardiac arrest, *Ann Surg* 158:596, 1963.
7. Ames A III, Nesbett FB: Pathophysiology of ischemic cell death. I. Time of onset of irreversible damage: importance of the different components of the ischemic insult, *Stroke* 14:219, 1983.
8. 1992 Heart Facts, American Heart Association, Dallas, Texas.
9. Aylward PE et al: Defibrillator electrode-chest wall coupling agents: influence on transthoracic impedance and shock success, *J Am Coll Cardiol* 6:682, 1985.
10. Bartlett RL et al: Comparative study of three methods of resuscitation: closed-chest, open-chest manual and direct mechanical ventricular system, *Ann Emerg Med* 13:773, 1984.
11. Baum RS, Alvalrez H III, Cobb LA: Survival after resuscitation from out-of-hospital ventricular fibrillation, *Circulation* 50:1231, 1974.
12. Bedell SE et al: Survival after cardiopulmonary resuscitation in the hospital, *N Engl J Med* 309:569, 1983.
13. Bircher N, Safar P: Cerebral preservation during cardiopulmonary resuscitation, *Crit Care Med* 13:185, 1985.
14. Bircher N, Safar P: Comparison of standard "new" closed-chest CPR and open-chest CPR in dogs, *Crit Care Med* 9:384, 1981.
15. Bircher N, Safar P, Stewart R: A comparison of standard, "mast"-augmented and open-chest CPR in dogs, *Crit Care Med* 8:147, 1980.
16. Bojar RM et al: Use of self-adhesive external defibrillator pads for complex cardiac surgical procedures, *Ann Thorac Surg* 46:587, 1988.
17. Borman JB et al: External-internal defibrillation, an experimental and clinical appraisal, *J Thorac Cardiovasc Surg* 62:98, 1971.
18. Braunwald E, Kloner RA: The stunned myocardium: prolonged, post-ischemic ventricular dysfunction, *Circulation* 66:1146, 1982.
19. Caldwell G et al: Simple mechanical methods for cardioversion: defense of the precordial thump and cough version, *Br Med J* 291:627, 1985.
20. Cerchiari E et al: Cardiovascular post

resuscitation syndrome (PRS) after ventricular fibrillation cardiac arrest (VFCA) in dogs, *Crit Care Med* 16:445, 1988 (abstract).

21. Chadda KD, Kammerer R: Early experiences with the portable automatic external defibrillator in the home and public places, *Am J Cardiol* 60:732, 1987.

22. Cobb LA et al: Community-based interventions for sudden cardiac death, *Circulation* 85(Suppl I):I-98, 1992.

23. Connell PN et al: Transthoracic impedance to defibrillator discharge. Effect of electrode size and electrode-chest wall interface, *J Electrocardiol* 6:313, 1973.

24. Cummins RO et al: Automatic external defibrillation: evaluations of its role in the home and in emergency medical services, *Ann Emerg Med* 13:789, 1984.

25. Cummins RO et al: Automatic external defibrillators used by emergency medical technicians. A controlled clinical trial, *JAMA* 257:1605, 1987.

26. Cummins RO et al: Improving survival from sudden cardiac arrest: the "chain of survival" concept, *Circulation* 83:1832, 1991.

27. Dahl CF et al: Myocardial necrosis from direct current countershock, *Circulation* 50:956, 1974.

28. Dahl CF, Ewy GA, Thomas ED: Transthoracic impedance to direct current discharge: effect of repeated countershocks, *Med Instrum* 10:151, 1976.

29. Del Guercio LRM et al: Comparison of blood flow during external and internal cardiac massage in man, *Circulation* 31(Suppl I):I-171, 1965.

30. DiNardo J: Management of cardiopulmonary bypass. In DiNardo J, Schwartz MJ, editors: *Anesthesia for cardiac surgery*, Norwalk, Conn, 1990, Appleton & Lange.

31. Echt DS et al: Clinical experience, complications, and survival in 70 patients with the automatic implantable cardioverter/defibrillator, *Circulation* 71:289, 1985.

32. Edwards DG: Development of a decision algorithm for a semiautomatic defibrillator, *Ann Emerg Med* 18:1276, 1989.

33. Ehsani A, Ewy GA, Sobel BE: Effects of electrical countershock on serum crea-

tine phosphokinase (CPK) isoenzyme activity, *Am J Cardiol* 37:12, 1976.

34. Eisenberg MS, Bergner L, Hallstrom A: Cardiac resuscitation in the community: importance of rapid provision and implications for program planning, *JAMA* 241:1905, 1979.

35. Eisenberg M, Bergner L, Hallstrom A: Paramedic programs and out-of-hospital cardiac arrest. I. Factors associated with successful resuscitation, *Am J Public Health* 69:30, 1979.

36. Eisenberg MS et al: Management of out-of-hospital cardiac arrest. Failure of basic emergency medical technician services, *JAMA* 243:1049, 1980.

37. Eisenberg MS et al: Treatment of out-of-hospital cardiac arrest with rapid defibrillation by emergency medical technicians, *N Engl J Med* 302:1379, 1980.

38. Eisenberg MS et al: Treatment of ventricular fibrillation: emergency medical technician defibrillation and paramedic services, *JAMA* 251:1723, 1984.

39. Eisenberg MS et al: Use of the automatic external defibrillator in home of survivors of out-of-hospital ventricular fibrillation, *Am J Cardiol* 63:443, 1989.

40. Every NR et al: Influence of coronary bypass surgery on subsequent outcome of patients resuscitated from out-of-hospital cardiac arrest, *J Am Coll Cardiol* 19:1435, 1992.

41. Ewy GA, Taren D: Comparison of paddle electrode paste used for defibrillation, *Heart Lung* 6:847, 1977.

42. Ewy GA, Taren D: Relative impedance of gels to defibrillator discharge, *Med Instrum* 13:295, 1979.

43. Ewy GA et al: Ventricular fibrillation masquerading as ventricular standstill, *Crit Care Med* 9:841, 1981.

44. Fletcher GF, Cantwell JD: Ventricular fibrillation in a medically supervised cardiac exercise program: clinical, angiographic, and surgical correlations, *JAMA* 238:2627, 1977.

45. Garrey WE: The nature of fibrillatory contractions of the heart and its relation to tissue mass and form, *Am J Physiol* 33:397, 1914.

46. Gascho JA et al: Determinants of ventric-

ular defibrillation in adults, *Circulation* 60:231, 1979.

47. Geddes LA et al: Decrease in transthoracic resistance during successive ventricular defibrillation trials, *Med Instrum* 9:179, 1975.

48. Geddes LA et al: Electrical dose for ventricular defibrillation of large and small animals using precordial electrodes, *J Clin Invest* 53:310, 1974.

49. Gibbs W, Eisenberg M, Daman KD: Dangers of defibrillation: injuries to emergency personnel during patient resuscitation, *Am J Emerg Med* 8:101, 1990.

50. Grace WJ, Kennedy RJ, Nolte CT: Blind defibrillation, *Am J Cardiol* 34:115, 1974.

51. Gray WA, Capone RJ, Most AS: Unsuccessful emergency medical resuscitation. Are continued efforts in the emergency department justified? *N Engl J Med* 325:1393, 1991.

52. Gutgesell HP et al: Energy dose for defibrillation in children, *Pediatrics* 58:898, 1976.

53. Hallstrom AP, Cobb LA, Ray R: Smoking as a risk factor for recurrence of sudden cardiac arrest, *N Engl J Med* 314:271, 1986.

54. Hallstrom AP, Eisenberg MS, Bergner L: The potential use of automatic defibrillators in the home for management of cardiac arrest, *Med Care* 22:1083, 1984.

55. Harwood-Nash DCF: Thumping of the precordium in ventricular fibrillation, *S Afr Med J* 36:280, 1962.

56. Haskell WL: Cardiovascular complications during exercise training of cardiac patients, *Circulation* 57:920, 1978.

57. Honey M, Nicholls TT, Towers MK: Pulmonary edema following direct current defibrillation, *Lancet* 1:765, 1965.

58. Hossack KF, Hartwig R: Cardiac arrest associated with supervised cardiac rehabilitation, *J Cardiac Rehab* 2:402, 1982.

59. Jaggarao NS et al: Use of an automated external defibrillator-pacemaker by ambulance staff, *Lancet* 2:73, 1982.

60. Kerber RE: AHA medical/scientific statement: statement on early defibrillation, *Circulation* 83:2233, 1991.

61. Kerber RE et al: Determinants of defibrillation: prospective analysis of 183 patients, *Am J Cardiol* 52:739, 1983.

62. Kerber RE et al: Effect of ischemia, hypertrophy, hypoxia, acidosis, and alkalosis on canine defibrillation, *Am J Physiol* 244:H825, 1983.

63. Kerber RE et al: Self-adhesive preapplied electrode pads for defibrillation and cardioversion, *J Am Coll Cardiol* 3:815, 1984.

64. Kerber RE et al: Transthoracic resistance in human defibrillation, *Circulation* 63:676, 1981.

65. Kerber RE, Sarnat W: Factors influencing the success of ventricular defibrillation in man, *Circulation* 60:226, 1979.

66. Kern KB et al: Depletion of myocardial adenosine triphosphate during prolonged untreated ventricular fibrillation: effect on defibrillation success, *Resuscitation* 20:221, 1990.

67. Kern KB et al: Long-term survival with open-chest cardiac massage after ineffective closed-chest compression in a canine preparation, *Circulation* 75:498, 1987.

68. Knilans TK, Prystowsky EN: Antiarrhythmic drug therapy in the management of cardiac arrest survivors, *Circulation* 85(Suppl1):I-118, 1992.

69. Lake CL et al: Energy dose and other variables possibly affecting ventricular defibrillation during cardiac surgery, *Anesth Analg* 63:743, 1984.

70. Lerman BB, Deale OC: Effect of epicardial patch electrodes on transthoracic defibrillation, *Circulation* 81:1409, 1990.

71. Liberthson RR et al: Prehospital ventricular defibrillation. Prognosis and follow-up course, *N Engl J Med* 291:317, 1974.

72. Martin DR, Brown CG, Dzwonczk R: Frequency analysis of the human and swine electrocardiogram during ventricular fibrillation, *Resuscitation* 22:85, 1991.

73. Martin TG et al: Initial treatment of ventricular fibrillation: defibrillation or drug therapy, *Am J Emerg Med* 6:113, 1986.

74. McDonald JL: Coarse ventricular fibrillation presenting as asystole or very low amplitude ventricular fibrillation, *Crit Care Med* 10:790, 1982.

75. Mirowski M et al: Termination of malignant ventricular arrhythmias with an implanted automatic defibrillator in human beings, *N Engl J Med* 303:322, 1980.

76. Moosy J et al: Pathophysiologic limits to the reversibility of clinical death, *Crit Care Med* 16:1077, 1988.

77. Morris JJ Jr et al: The changes in cardiac output with reversion of atrial fibrillation to sinus rhythm, *Circulation* 31:670, 1965.

78. Morris JJ Jr, Peter RH, McIntosh HD: Electrical conversion of atrial fibrillation. Immediate and long-term results and selection of patients, *Ann Intern Med* 65:216, 1966.

79. Myerburg RJ et al: Long-term survival after pre-hospital cardiac arrest: analysis of outcome during an 8 year study, *Circulation* 70:538, 1984.

80. Negovsky VA: Post-resuscitation disease, *Crit Care Med* 16:942, 1988.

81. Neimann JT et al: Treatment of prolonged ventricular fibrillation: immediate countershock versus high dose epinephrine and CPR preceding countershock, *Circulation* 85:281, 1992.

82. Neumar RW et al: Myocardial high energy phosphate metabolism during ventricular fibrillation with total circulatory arrest, *Resuscitation* 19:199, 1990.

83. Oram S, Davies JPH: Further experience of electrical conversion of atrial fibrillation to sinus rhythm: analysis of 100 patients, *Lancet* 1:1294, 1964.

84. Otto CW, Yakaitis RW, Ewy GA: Effect of epinephrine on defibrillation in ischemic ventricular fibrillation, *Am J Emerg Med* 3:285, 1985.

85. Pantridge JR et al: Electrical requirements for ventricular defibrillation, *Br Med J* 2:313, 1975.

86. Przyklenk K, Patel B, Kloner RA: Diastolic abnormalities of post-ischemic "stunned" myocardium, *Am J Cardiol* 60:1211, 1987.

87. Pugsley WB et al: Low energy level internal defibrillation during cardiopulmonary bypass, *Eur J Cardiothorac Surg* 3:273, 1989.

88. Reich H et al: Reversibility limits for heart and brain of ventricular fibrillation cardiac arrest in dogs, *Crit Care Med* 16:390, 1988.

89. Rifkin LM: The defibrillator and cardiac burns, *J Thorac Cardiovasc Surg* 46:755, 1963.

90. Roine RO et al: Nimodipine after resuscitation from out-of-hospital ventricular fibrillation, *JAMA* 264:3171, 1990.

91. Rostelli CC et al: Experimental study and clinical appraisal of external defibrillation with the thorax open, *J Thorac Cardiovasc Surg* 55:116, 1968.

92. Roth R et al: Out-of-hospital cardiac arrest: factors associated with survival, *Ann Emerg Med* 13:237, 1984.

93. Ruffy R, Schwartz DJ, Hieb BR: Influence of acute coronary artery occlusion on direct ventricular defibrillation in dogs, *Med Instrum* 14:23, 1980.

94. Safar P, Bircher N: *Cardiopulmonary cerebral resuscitation*, ed 3, Philadelphia, 1988, Saunders.

95. Safar P et al: Recommendations for future research on the reversibility of clinical death, *Crit Care Med* 16:1077, 1988.

96. Sanders AB et al: Importance of the duration of inadequate coronary perfusion pressure on resuscitation from cardiac arrest, *J Am Coll Cardiol* 6:113, 1985.

97. Sanders AB et al: Improved resuscitation from cardiac arrest with open-chest massage, *Ann Emerg Med* 13:672, 1984.

98. Sanders A et al: Negative predictive value of end-tidal carbon dioxide for the resuscitation of patients in cardiac arrest, *J Am Coll Cardiol* 17:180, 1991 (abstract).

99. Schaffer WA, Cobb LA: Recurrent ventricular fibrillation and modes of death in survivors of out-of-hospital ventricular fibrillation, *N Engl J Med* 293:259, 1975.

100. Guidelines for cardiopulmonary resuscitation and emergency cardiac care, *JAMA* 268:2171, 1992.

101. Standards and guidelines for cardiopulmonary resuscitation and emergency cardiac care, *JAMA* 255:2937, 1986.

102. Steen PA et al: Cerebral blood flow and neurologic outcome when nimodipine is given after complete cerebral ischemia in the dog, *J Cereb Blood Flow Metab* 4:82, 1984.

103. Steen PA et al: Nimodipine improves outcome when given after complete ischemia in primates, *Anesthesiology* 62:406, 1985.

104. Stults KR, Brown DD, Kerber RE: Efficacy of an automated external defibrillator in the management of out-

of-hospital cardiac arrest: validation of the diagnostic algorithm and initial experience in a rural environment, *Circulation* 73:701, 1986.

105. Stults KR et al: Pre-hospital defibrillation performed by emergency medical technicians in rural communities, *N Engl J Med* 310:219, 1984.

106. Stults KR et al: Self-adhesive monitor/defibrillation pads improve pre-hospital defibrillation success, *Ann Emerg Med* 16:872, 1987.

107. Tacker WA, Ewy GA: Emergency defibrillation dose: recommendation and rationale, *Circulation* 60:223, 1979.

108. Tacker WA et al: The electrical dose for direct ventricular defibrillation in man, *J Thorac Cardiovasc Surg* 75:224, 1978.

109. Tacker WA et al: Electrical threshold for defibrillation of canine ventricles following myocardial infarction, *Am Heart J* 88:476, 1974.

110. Thomas ED et al: Effectiveness of direct current defibrillation: role of paddle electrode size, *Am Heart J* 93:463, 1977.

111. Tortolani AJ et al: In-hospital cardiopulmonary resuscitation: patient, arrest, and resuscitation factors associated with survival, *Resuscitation* 20:115, 1990.

112. Vaagenes P et al: Amelioration of brain damage by lidoflazine after prolonged ventricular fibrillation cardiac arrest in dogs, *Crit Care Med* 12:846, 1984.

113. Van Camp SP, Peterson RA: Cardiovascular complications of outpatient cardiac rehabilitation programs, *JAMA* 256:1160, 1986.

114. Waldo AL, Biblo LA, Carlson MD: General evaluation of out-of-hospital sudden cardiac death survivors, *Circulation* 85(Suppl 1):103, 1992.

115. Walls JT et al: Adverse effects of permanent cardiac internal defibrillator patches on external defibrillation, *Am J Cardiol* 64:1144, 1989.

116. Warner ED, Dahl CF, Ewy GA: Myocardial injury from transthoracic defibrillator countershock, *Arch Pathol* 99:55, 1975.

117. Weaver WD et al: Considerations for improving survival from out-of-hospital cardiac arrest, *Ann Emerg Med* 15:1181, 1986.

118. Weaver WD et al: Emergency medical care requirements for large public assemblies and a new strategy for managing cardiac arrest in this setting, *Ann Emerg Med* 18:155, 1989.

119. Weaver WD et al: Factors influencing survival after out-of-hospital cardiac arrest, *J Am Coll Cardiol* 7:752, 1986.

120. Weaver WD et al: Improved neurologic recovery and survival after early defibrillation, *Circulation* 69:943, 1984.

121. Weaver WD et al: Use of the automatic external defibrillator in the management of out-of-hospital cardiac arrest, *N Engl J Med* 319:661, 1988.

122. Weaver et al: Ventricular defibrillation— a comparative trial using 175-J and 320-J shocks, *N Engl J Med* 307:1101, 1982.

123. Weisner FM, Adler LN, Kuhn LA: Hemodynamic effects of closed and open-chest cardiac resuscitation in normal dogs and those with acute myocardial infarction, *Am J Cardiol* 10:555, 1962.

124. Wrenn K: The hazards of defibrillation through nitroglycerin patches, *Ann Emerg Med* 19:1327, 1990.

125. Yakaitis RW et al: Influence of time and therapy on ventricular defibrillation in dogs, *Crit Care Med* 8:157, 1980.

126. Yakaitis RW, Thomas JD, Mahaffey JE: Influence of pH and hypoxia on the success of defibrillation, *Crit Care Med* 3:139, 1975.

127. Zipes DP et al: Termination of ventricular fibrillation in dogs by depolarizing a critical amount of myocardium, *Am J*

Chapter 7
Transchest Cardioversion: Optimal Techniques

Richard E. Kerber

Electrical therapy of cardiac arrhythmias was introduced for ventricular fibrillation,[24,35] but it is also effective for the termination of atrial arrhythmias.[27] The exact mechanism of termination of atrial fibrillation by direct current electric shock is not known; concepts of *ventricular* fibrillation termination (critical mass, critical current density)[30,34] may apply to the *atria* as well. Arrhythmias such as atrial flutter and supraventricular tachycardia are more electrically organized and probably are terminated by depolarization of the myocardial segments that lie in the immediate path of the advancing wavefront. This concept is also thought to apply to the organized rhythm of monomorphic ventricular tachycardia. All of the more organized cardiac arrhythmias require relatively low energy and current to terminate.[21,23]

INDICATIONS AND PATIENT SELECTION

Cardiac performance is optimized by the presence of sinus rhythm, especially in patients with mitral stenosis, left ventricular hypertrophy (aortic stenosis, hypertension, idiopathic hypertrophic subaortic stenosis), and/or diminished myocardial reserve (congestive heart failure, myocardial ischemia). The coordinated atrial contraction of sinus rhythm improves ventricular filling, and cardiac rate is usually slower. Thus patients with the above conditions are candidates for *elective* cardioversion.

Urgent cardioversion may be required for patients with atrial or ventricular arrhythmias who are hypotensive and/or in pulmonary edema.

The etiology of any of the arrhythmias treatable by cardioversion should be sought because in some cases treatment of the underlying condition may restore sinus rhythm without the necessity of electric cardioversion. Common causes of atrial arrhythmias include hyperthyroidism, pulmonary embolism, congestive heart failure, and mitral stenosis. Postoperative cardiac patients frequently experience transient rhythm disturbances.

Interrelated factors that determine the immediate and long-term success of electric cardioversion of atrial fibrillation include the duration of the arrhythmia, the extent of atrial fibrosis, and the size of the left atrium. Early success rates of 75% to 80% have been reported for cardioversion of atrial fibrillation and atrial flutter; monomorphic ventricular tachycardia may yield similar high success rates.[21,23] However, a large fibrotic atrium that has been fibrillating for months to years has a low probability of achieving and maintaining sinus rhythm after electric shock.[13,29]

In elective cardioversion systemic anticoagulation is generally undertaken for 3 weeks prior to the electric shock to reduce the risk of systemic thromboembolism. A large left atrium, mitral stenosis, and previous thromboembolic events mandate anticoagulation, but anticoagulation may be omitted in patients who have a very short duration of arrhythmia and/or a small left atrium and no mitral valve disease. Thromboembolism is less likely to occur after cardioversion of atrial flutter than atrial fibrillation.[2]

Transesophageal echocardiography is an excellent technique for imaging the left atrium, including the left atrial appendage, which is the most common site of left atrial thrombus formation. Whether the absence of a left atrial appendage thrombus by transesophageal echocardiography allows omission of precardioversion anticoagulation has yet to be determined. In any case, since *mechanical* atrial contraction may not resume for some time after resumption of sinus rhythm, and since a large noncontractile left atrium is a likely source of thromboembolism even when sinus rhythm has been reestablished, *post*cardioversion anticoagulation is generally employed. If intermittent or permanent atrial fibrillation is likely to recur (for example, mitral stenosis), permanent anticoagulation may be appropriate.

Cardiac automaticity is increased by digitalis, and the inadvertent complication of ventricular tachycardia or ventricular fibrillation may occur if electric shocks are delivered to the digitalis-toxic patient.[28] Digitalis toxicity is therefore a contraindication to cardioversion. Although it is customary to withhold digitalis on the day of elective cardioversion, therapeutic levels of digitalis are rarely associated with postcardioversion arrhythmias.

PREPARATION FOR CARDIOVERSION

As discussed previously, most patients undergoing elective cardioversion for atrial fibrillation are treated with anticoagulant; this may not be necessary for atrial flutter.[2] Quinidine is frequently begun before the cardioversion attempt in order to maintain sinus rhythm after cardioversion, and pharmacologic cardioversion frequently occurs even before the shock.

Anesthesia is necessary to avoid the pain of the tetanic muscular contraction induced by the electric current through the thorax. It should also be sufficient to induce amnesia; mere sedation is generally inadequate. Endotracheal intubation may be necessary.

EQUIPMENT AND TECHNIQUE

A direct current defibrillator with the capability of delivering synchronized shocks is required for cardioversion. Handheld electrodes have traditionally been used, but more recently self-adhesive monitor-defibrillator pad electrodes have been shown to be effective.[18]

Placement of the electrodes must maximize transmyocardial current flow, and incorrect electrode placement may result in failure to terminate the arrhythmia.[7] However, a number of electrode placements and current pathways are effective. The most commonly used pathway is the apex-anterior one, but other pathways used successfully are anterior-posterior, apex-posterior, and even vertical pathways using tongue-epigastric electrodes.[17,20] Three of these are illustrated in Fig. 7-1. There is little evidence to suggest that any one of these pathways is generally preferred over the others. However, in individual patients shocks given through an alternative pathway may succeed even after previous shocks using another pathway have failed. Thus if shocks up to maximal energy levels have failed using one electrode placement, the operator may choose another placement and rearrange the electrodes while the patient is still anesthetized in order to administer additional shocks.

Electrodes should be placed to avoid permanent pacemaker generators lest damage occur to the generators, and/or myocardial injury occur from current transmitted along the low-impedance pathway of the pacemaker wire.[4]

Standard electrode sizes vary from 8 to 12 cm diameter. Use of smaller electrodes may be associated with high transthoracic impedance and inadequate current flow, while use of very large electrodes may result in more current following extracardiac pathways through the thorax, thereby "missing" the heart. In experimental canine studies we found that intracardiac voltage gradients (current density) were maximal using an intermediate external electrode size.[14] Small "pediatric" electrodes are available for use in children. However, their use in children larger than 10 kg (about 1 year old) is associated with high transthoracic impedance.[3] Standard "adult" electrodes should be used in such children.

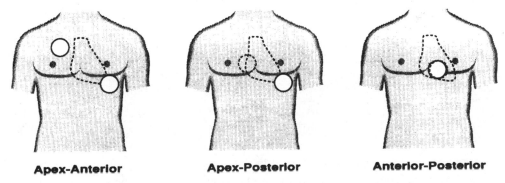

Apex-Anterior   **Apex-Posterior**   **Anterior-Posterior**

Fig. 7-1. Various electrode positions that can be used for cardioversion. All are effective.

Proper synchronization of shock delivery is critical during elective cardioversion. If the shock is administered during the "vulnerable" portion of the cardiac cycle (which roughly approximates the T-wave) ventricular fibrillation may be induced. To avoid this, synchronization circuitry identifies the QRS complex and restricts shock delivery to within a few milliseconds of this "safe" portion of the cardiac cycle. Most defibrillators identify the putative QRS complex by a mark displayed on both the oscilloscopic screen and also on the hard-copy electrocardiographic printout. The operator should verify that the ECG waveform identified as the QRS is in fact correct, since occasionally an unusually large or peaked T-wave or P-wave can be misidentified as the QRS complex.

Failure of the operator to enable the synchronization device is, in the author's experience, the most common cause of ventricular fibrillation (VF) being induced by elective cardioversion. An example is shown in Fig. 7-2. Should ventricular fibrillation be inadvertently induced, an immediate additional shock should terminate the arrhythmia. Some defibrillators require that the synchronization device be reenabled before each shock—the rationale being that if VF were to be accidentally induced, a subsequent rescue shock could not be delivered because there would be no QRS complex for the synchronizer to sense. The disadvantage of this approach is that if a first (synchronized) shock fails to convert an arrhythmia and a subsequent shock is required, the operator must remember to resynchronize—or the second shock will unintentionally be delivered at some random point within the cardiac cycle and may induce VF. Obviously, the operator must be intimately familiar with the details of the particular defibrillator being used.

Supraventricular arrhythmias such as atrial fibrillation, atrial flutter, and supraventricular tachycardia pose no problem for synchronization. Ventricular tachycardia may be more difficult due to the wide-complex morphology of the arrhythmia and the associated heterogeneity of ventricular depolarization and repolarization. When justified by clinical urgency (shock, pulmonary edema, angina), rapid ventricular arrhythmias should be cardioverted without attempts to synchronize.

Energy selection in cardioversion is arrhythmia-dependent.[21] Atrial fibrilla-

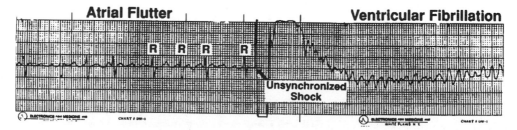

Fig. 7-2. An unsynchronized shock (*arrow*) induces ventricular fibrillation (VF). This complication of cardioversion can be avoided by using the synchronization device so the shock is given on the R wave of the QRS complex rather than, as here, on the "vulnerable" T wave.

Table 7-1
Energy Requirements for Various Arrhythmias

Arrhythmia Energies	Initial Shock Energy	Subsequent Shock
Atrial fibrillation	100 J	200, 300, 360 J
Atrial flutter	50 J	100, 200, 300, 360 J
Supraventricular tachycardia	50 J	100, 200, 300, 360 J
Monomorphic ventricular tachycardia	100 J	200, 300, 360 J
Polymorphic ventricular tachycardia	200 J	300, 360 J
Ventricular fibrillation	200 J	300, 360 J

tion and monomorphic ventricular tachycardia usually respond to initial shocks of 100 J. Atrial flutter and supraventricular tachycardia require lower energies—50 J is an appropriate initial shock. Polymorphic venricular tachycardia, a disorganized arrhythmia, behaves like VF and requires 200 J for the initial shock.[23] In all cases, if the initial shock fails, subsequent shocks are usually delivered at increasing energy levels. These shock recommendations are summarized in Table 7-1.

COMPLICATIONS AND FOLLOW-UP OF CARDIOVERSION

Elective cardioversion is a relatively safe procedure when properly performed. The most serious potential complications—induction of ventricular fibrillation and systemic embolization—have already been discussed. Both are largely preventable by use of appropriate synchronization and by anticoagulation. Myocardial damage can occur from excessive energy and current; although this is demonstrable in animals,[5,15,33] its occurrence in humans appears infrequent.[17] Use of the energy selection protocols discussed above should minimize the risk of myocardial damage.

Erythema at the sites of elective placement are common after cardioversion; but these usually reflect local hyperemia in the current pathway and are not "burns."[32] Skin sloughing rarely occurs.

Follow-up therapy of the cardioversion patient depends on the clinical circumstances and arrhythmia etiology. Long-term antiarrhythmic and anticoagulation therapy is appropriate in patients who have chronic cardiac disorders that predispose them to arrhythmia recurrences (for example, mitral stenosis, dilated or ischemic cardiomyopathy). Patients who experience postoperative atrial arrhythmias rarely have recurrences after the perioperative period and require little follow-up.

NEW DEVELOPMENTS: CURRENT-BASED CARDIOVERSION

In order to achieve cardioversion an adequate current flow and/or current density must traverse the atrial or ventricular myocardium. The two principal determinants of current flow are the operator-selected energy (traditionally denominated in Joules or watt-seconds) and the transthoracic impedance (in ohms). Multiple determinants of transthoracic impedance have been described: chest size (interelectrode distance), electrode size, electrode-chest wall couplant, electrode-chest wall contact pressure, phase of respiration, and previous shocks.* A wide range of transthoracic impedance has been found in adults, 28 to 150 ohms (average about 75 ohms).[21]

Since the range of impedance varies fivefold, shocks administered according to the energy protocols given earlier will actually produce wide ranges of current, which may be inadequate (if transthoracic impedance is high) or excessive (if impedance is low).[19,25] An appealing approach to circumventing this problem would be to employ a *current*-based cardioversion technique. Technology now exists to instantaneously determine impedance without having to actually administer a shock.[1,12,19] We have also determined the current requirements for termination of common atrial and ventricular arrhythmias.[21] Optimal current for termination of ventricular and atrial fibrillation is 30 to 41 amps; 14 to 25 amps are needed for atrial flutter.[21] Monomorphic ventricular tachycardia requires 18 amps; polymorphic ventricular tachycardia is similar to VF and requires 25 to 30 amps.[23] These requirements are illustrated in Figs. 7-3 and 7-4.

*References 6, 9, 11, 16, 31, 32.

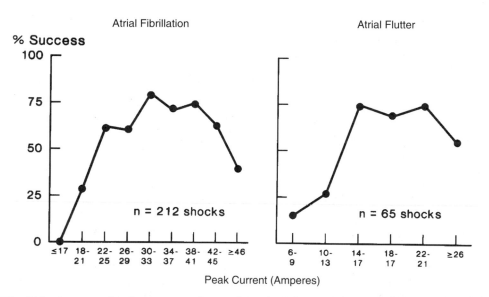

Fig. 7-3. Current-shock success relationships for the cardioversion of atrial fibrillation and atrial flutter. The optimal current for atrial flutter should be 14 to 25 amps; for atrial fibrillation 30 to 41 amps. (Reproduced by permission of the American Heart Association, Inc., from Kerber RE et al: Energy, current, and success in defibrillation and cardioversion: clinical studies using an automated impedance based method of energy adjustment, *Circulation* 77:1038, 1988.)

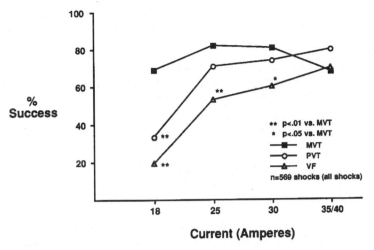

Fig. 7-4. Current-shock success relationships for the cardioversion of monomorphic and polymorphic ventricular tachycardia and ventricular fibrillation. Monomorphic VT is relatively easy to cardiovert, often requiring only 18 amps. Polymorphic VT requires more current, 25 to 30 amps, similar to VF. (Reproduced by permission of the American Heart Assoc., Inc., from Kerber RE et al: Ventricular tachycardia rate and morphology determine energy and current requirements for transthoracic cardioversion, *Circulation* 85:158, 1992.)

A feasible system would allow the operator to select the desired current, based on the arrhythmia being treated and the above recommendations. Then a microprocessor in the defibrillator would determine the transthoracic impedance, and the capacitor would be charged to generate the operator-selected current. Several initial studies have suggested that the approach is feasible and is particularly effective for high- or low-impedance patients.[8,22,26] Further experience with current-based defibrillation and cardioversion will define its role in the clinical treatment of cardiac arrhythmias.

REFERENCES

1. Armayor MR et al: Ventricular defibrillation threshold with capacitor discharge, *Med Biol Eng Comp* 17:435, 1979.
2. Arnold AZ et al: Role of prophylactic anticoagulation for direct current cardioversion in patients with atrial fibrillation or atrial flutter, *J Am Coll Cardiol* 19:851, 1992.
3. Atkins DL et al: Pediatric defibrillation: importance of paddle size in determining transthoracic impedance, *Pediatrics* 82:914, 1988.
4. Aylward P, Blood R, Tonkin A: Complications with defibrillation with permanent pacemakers in situ, *PACE* 2:462, 1988.
5. Babbs CF et al: Therapeutic indices for transchest defibrillator shocks: effective, damaging and lethal electrical doses, *Am Heart J* 99:734, 1980.
6. Connell PN et al: Transthoracic impedance to defibrillator discharge. Effect of electrode size and electrode-chest wall interface, *J Electrocardiol* 6:313, 1973.
7. Crampton RA: Accepted, controversial and speculative aspects of ventricular defibrillation, *Prog Cardiovasc Dis* 23:167, 1980.
8. Dalzell GWN et al: Initial experience with a microprocessor-controlled current-based defibrillator, *Br Heart J* 61:502, 1989.

9. Ewy GA et al: Influence of ventilation phase on transthoracic impedance and defibrillation effectiveness, *Crit Care Med* 8:164, 1980.

10. Geddes LA et al: Electrical dose for ventricular defibrillation of large and small animals using precordial electrodes, *J Clin Invest* 53:310, 1980.

11. Geddes LA et al: Decrease in transthoracic resistance during successive ventricular defibrillation trials, *Med Instrum* 9:179, 1975.

12. Geddes LA et al: The prediction of the impedance of the thorax to a defibrillating current, *Med Instrum* 10:159, 1976.

13. Henry WL et al: Relation between echocardiographically determined left atrial size and atrial fibrillation, *Circulation* 53:273, 1976.

14. Hoyt R, Grayzel J, Kerber RE: Determinants of intracardiac current and defibrillation: experimental studies in dogs, *Circulation* 64:818, 1981.

15. Kerber RE et al: Effect of direct current countershocks on regional myocardial contractility and perfusion: experimental studies, *Circulation* 63:323, 1981.

16. Kerber RE et al: Transthoracic resistance in human defibrillation: influence of body weight, chest size, serial shocks, paddle size and paddle contact pressure, *Circulation* 63:676, 1981.

17. Kerber RE et al: Elective cardioversion: influence of paddle electrode location and size on success rates and energy requirements, *N Engl J Med* 305:658, 1981.

18. Kerber RE et al: Self-adhesive, pre-applied electrode pads for defibrillation and cardioversion, *J Am Coll Cardiol* 3:815, 1984.

19. Kerber RE et al: Advance prediction of transthoracic impedance in human defibrillation and cardioversion: importance of impedance in determining the success of low energy shocks, *Circulation* 70:303, 1984.

20. Kerber RE et al: Evaluation of a new defibrillation pathway: tongue-epigastric/tongue-apex. II. Impedance characteristics in human subjects, *J Am Coll Cardiol* 4:253, 1984.

21. Kerber RE et al: Energy, current, and success in defibrillation and cardioversion: clinical studies using an automated impedance based method of energy adjustment, *Circulation* 77:1038, 1988.

22. Kerber RE et al: Current-based transthoracic defibrillation and cardioversion: initial report of a prospective multi-center study, *Circulation* (Suppl II) 78:II-46, 1988.

23. Kerber RE et al: Ventricular tachycardia rate and morphology determine energy and current requirements for transthoracic cardioversion, *Circulation* 85:158, 1992.

24. Kowenhowen WB et al: Closed-chest defibrillation of the heart, *Surgery* 42:550, 1954.

25. Lerman B et al: Relationship between canine transthoracic impedance and defibrillation threshold. Evidence for current-based defibrillation, *J Clin Invest* 80:7017, 1987.

26. Lerman B, DiMarco JP, Haines DE: Current-based vs. energy-based ventricular defibrillation: a prospective study, *J Am Coll Cardiol* 12:1259, 1988.

27. Lown BR, Amarasingham R, Newman J: New method for terminating cardiac arrhythmias: use of synchronized capacity discharge, *JAMA* 182:548, 1962.

28. Lown B, Krieger R, Williams J: Cardioversion and digitalis drugs: changed threshold to electric shock in digitalized animals, *Circ Res* 17:519, 1965.

29. Resnekov L, McDonald L: Appraisal of electroconversion and treatment of cardiac dysrhythmias, *Br Heart J* 30:786, 1968.

30. Shibata N et al: Epicardial activation after unsuccessful defibrillation shocks in dogs, *Am J Physiol* 255:H902, 1988.

31. Sirna SJ et al: Electrical cardioversion in humans: factors affecting transthoracic impedance, *Am J Cardiol* 62:1048, 1988.

32. Sirna SJ et al: What is the mechanism of the decline in transthoracic impedance after direct current shock? *Am J Physiol* 26:1180, 1989.

33. Warner ED, Dahl C, Ewy GA: Myocardial injury from transthoracic defibrillator countershock, *Arch Pathol* 99:55, 1975.

34. Zipes DP et al: Termination of ventricular fibrillation in dogs by depolarizing a critical amount of myocardium, *Am J Cardiol* 36:37, 1975.

35. Zoll PM, Linenthal AJ, Gibson W: Termination of ventricular fibrillation in man by externally applied electric countershock, *N Engl J Med* 274:727, 1956.

Chapter 8
Pediatric Defibrillation: Optimal Techniques

Dianne L. Atkins

Life-threatening dysrhythmias are less common in the pediatric age group than in the adult population. In children congenital heart disease or myocarditis is a more likely cause than coronary artery disease. Children also suffer from supraventricular arrhythmias, which occasionally require urgent or elective cardioversion. Thus the need for defibrillation or cardioversion exists, and an understanding of the differences between defibrillation in children and defibrillation in adults is a requirement of all personnel who participate in the critical care of children. Unfortunately, there is a marked paucity of experimental data concerning the optimal equipment and energy dose for pediatric defibrillation or cardioversion, which is in contrast to the extensive studies documenting efficacy, safety, and proper technique in adult patients.* Lack of data and relative infrequency of use has led to a fear of defibrillation of children that is great enough for some to recommend withholding defibrillation unless "specifically authorized by . . . medical authorities."[12]

This chapter will discuss differences between adults and children, the special considerations and equipment necessary to provide safe and effective treatment, and patient selection. My goal is to ease the apprehension of defibrillating or cardioverting a child while focusing on areas of inadequate information to heighten interest in answering these questions.

DIFFERENCES BETWEEN CHILDREN AND ADULTS

The most obvious difference between children and adults is the difference in body mass. This necessitates smaller electrode size and a delivered energy dose related to body weight. Other dissimilarities include differing frequencies and etiologies of rhythm disturbances, which may have an impact on shock success. Less apparent distinctions include variations in body composi-

*References 3, 6, 18, 38-41, 63.

tion and chest configuration. Infants and small children have a much higher percentage of body water than do adults and a fat distribution differing from adults, which could affect transthoracic impedance and current flow, the major determinants of shock success. In the child the length of the chest in relation to total length is shorter and the heart is positioned higher in the chest so that the electrode position needs to be adjusted accordingly.

SPECIAL CONSIDERATIONS FOR CHILDREN

TRANSTHORACIC IMPEDANCE

Transthoracic impedance is the major determinant of current flow during defibrillation. Studies performed *in vitro* or with adult subjects identified several variables that influence transthoracic impedance.[6,14,27,38] Kerber and colleagues[38] documented that oversized electrodes (13 cm, 132 cm^2) reduced transthoracic impedance by 21% when compared with standard adult electrodes (8 cm, 50 cm^2). A direct relationship between transthoracic impedance and chest width indicated that larger patients have high impedance.[38,54] Based on the hypothesis that children would have lower impedance because of small body mass, we measured transthoracic impedance in an outpatient pediatric population[5] using both "pediatric" (21 cm^2) and "adult" (83 cm^2) electrodes. We were able to capitalize on the test-pulse technique,[41] which permits measurement of transthoracic impedance without actually delivering a shock. Body weight and body surface area were significantly correlated with transthoracic impedance, but the correlations were not sufficiently great to be clinically useful (Table 8-1). Rather, electrode size was the major determinant

Table 8-1
Transthoracic Impedance and Its Determinants

Determinant and Paddle Size	r Value	P Value
Weight		
Pediatric	.52	<.01
Adult	.47	<.05
Body surface area		
Pediatric	.49	<.01
Adult	.44	<.05
Age		
Pediatric	.44	<.05
Adult	.36	NS
Interelectrode distance		
Pediatric	.39	<.05
Adult	.23	NS

From Atkins DL et al: Pediatric defibrillation: importance of paddle size in determining transthoracic impedance, *Pediatrics* 82:914, 1988. Reprinted with permission from *Pediatrics*.

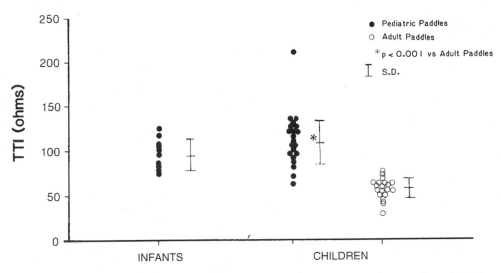

Fig. 8-1. Effect of paddle electrode size on transthoracic impedance. *Closed circles,* Pediatric paddles (21 cm²); *open circles,* adult paddles (83 cm²); *p < .001 vs. adult paddles; bars indicate mean ± standard deviation. (From Atkins DL, Sirna S, Kieso R: Pediatric defibrillation: importance of paddle size in determining transthoracic impedance, *Pediatrics* 82:914, 1988. Reprinted with permission from *Pediatrics*.)

of transthoracic impedance (Fig. 8-1). Standard adult electrodes halved transthoracic impedance (compared with pediatric electrodes) in infants and children when the chest was large enough to accommodate the larger surface area. We have since demonstrated that this relationship was present during actual shock delivery.[4] We recommended that the larger electrodes be used when the child's thorax is large enough to permit electrode-to-chest contact over the entire surface. This transition occurred at an approximate weight of 10 kg, the average weight of a 1-year-old child.

ENERGY DOSE

Currently, there are no human experimental data to identify the appropriate energy dose for defibrillation or cardioversion in children based on weight or rhythm. Animal studies have shown that the energy threshold for defibrillation ranged from 0.5 to 10 J/kg, with the energy requirement per kilogram increasing with body weight.[32] Gutgesell et al.[33] reviewed 71 defibrillation attempts in 27 children and found that 91% of shocks delivered within 10 J above or below 2 J/kg were effective (Fig. 8-2). However, only two patients received significantly less than 2 J/kg. Although they were not successfully defibrillated, there are so many other factors contributing to success or failure (that is, duration of ventricular fibrillation, hypoxia, and acid-base imbalance) that to say the minimum dose is 2 J/kg may not be justified. There did

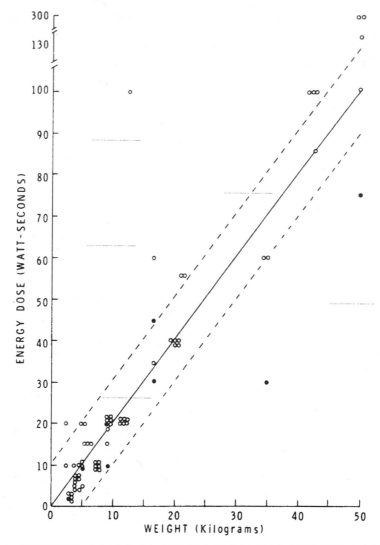

Fig. 8-2. Relationship of energy dose versus body weight during pediatric defibrillation. *Open circles,* successful shocks; *closed circles,* unsuccessful shocks. Solid line represents energy dose 2 J/kg; area between dotted lines represents 10 J above and below this dose. (From Gutgesell HP et al: Energy dose for ventricular defibrillation of children, *Pediatrics* 58:898, 1976. Reprinted with permission from *Pediatrics*.)

not appear to be any increase in energy requirements (based on a per kilogram measure) as patient size increased (Fig. 8-2).

The current recommendation of 0.5 to 1 J/kg for cardioversion of supraventricular tachyarrhythmias is derived by consensus and experience of pediatric cardiologists[1,2] and is supported by adult data, indicating energy requirements less than defibrillation doses[1] to terminate SVT or atrial flutter.

Indeed, cardioversion of supraventricular rhythms is easily achieved in children and is difficult only in the presence of significant structural heart disease.

ELECTRODES

Standard electrode size for adults is 8 to 10 cm in diameter. Small infants require smaller electrodes so that there is complete contact between the electrode surface and skin to reduce current density. There are no human studies to suggest ideal size for infants and children. Patel and Galysh[51] suggested that 5-cm electrodes were appropriate for pediatric use based on their study in dogs weighing less than 9 kg. Transthoracic impedance, delivered energy, and peak voltage were inversely proportional to diameter, with excessive energy and voltage delivered using sizes less than 5 cm. In fact, delivered energy was 35% above selected energy with the 3-cm electrodes. The American Heart Association recommends that pediatric electrodes be 4.5 cm, the size mostly readily available on commercial defibrillators.[1]

The self-adhesive electrodes have not been studied in children, although they are commercially available in "pediatric" sizes and are widely used during electrophysiologic testing. Kerber et al. have shown in adults that the transthoracic impedance is similar to standard electrodes and success rates are similar to those observed with standard electrodes.[42]

ELECTRODE POSITION

The most commonly used position is the anterolateral position, although the anterior posterior position may improve current flow at lower energy levels.[21,47] The anterior-posterior position has not received wide clinical acceptance because of the difficulty of placing the posterior electrode. However, an infant or young child can be supported on his side with the electrodes, making this a more realistic option. The advantage of this position is that the larger electrodes could be used with very small infants.

DEFIBRILLATOR DESIGN

All defibrillators currently marketed are equipped to provide the full range of needs for emergency treatment of adults. Not all units are suited for pediatric use. It is the author's opinion that the flexibility to care for all patients should be available on every defibrillator. The primary requirements for pediatric use are a broad range of accurately delivered energy levels and easily accessible pediatric electrodes. There should be the capability of selecting a very low energy dose (no greater than 2 J) with small increments of 1 to 10 J. Available energies of 2, 3, 5, 10, 20, 30, 40, 50, 70, and 100 J provide a reasonable range for patients who weigh 1 to 50 kg. Additionally, adaptation for using pediatric electrodes should be simple. Many units provide pediatric adaptors that clip on over adult electrodes, or electrodes that are entirely separate, requiring the operator to unplug the adult electrodes and plug in the pediatric ones. Both systems require additional storage space on or around the defibrillator and risk loss of the pediatric accessories. Removable adult electrodes, with pediatric ones directly beneath, provide easy accessibility and storage. Design features such as monitors, synchronizing switches, and recorders are standard.

COMPLICATIONS

Application of direct current countershock is known to produce mitochondrial disruption,[17,24,36] contraction-band necrosis,[22] and subepicardial coagulation and necrosis.[17] The extent and distribution of the damage depends on energy dose,[35] electrode size,[16] and number of shocks.[22] Analysis of the effects of direct current countershock in young animals and humans is limited. Gaba and Talner[30] demonstrated that myocardial damage, as measured by technetium-99m pyrophosphate uptake, was not apparent until shocks of 150 J/kg were given. In contrast, Karch[35] analyzed autopsied specimens from children who had received defibrillation during resuscitation. Contraction-band necrosis was present in all patients who received countershocks, while focal hemorrhages and epicardial coagulation were observed in a majority of the patients. These findings were accentuated if catecholamines had also been administered during the resuscitation efforts. The significance of these data are unclear, although arrhythmias and hemodynamic dysfunction are observed in children who are successfully resuscitated.

The potential exists for serious complications if excessive energy doses are given to children, particularly in the prehospital situation. If the defibrillator unit is not equipped to deliver low-energy shocks (2 to 50 J), then children may receive inappropriately high doses. Children have received 10 to 30 J/kg shocks, with cumulative doses reaching 700 J. None of these children survived (personal observation, personal communication from Dr. W.A. Tacker, Jr.).

Skin burns may occur after defibrillation and are more apparent with smaller electrodes or incomplete contact with the skin, situations which increase current density. Burns also occur if the conductive interface (gel or cream) is too sparingly applied to the surface. Conversely, if excessive medium is used, there is the possibility that the medium can smear across the patient's chest, resulting in formation of an electrical bridge. This will cause electrical arcing between the electrodes and inadequate current delivery to the myocardium.

Immediately after cardioversion in adults a more malignant arrhythmia such as ventricular fibrillation may emerge.[1,20] This is an extremely rare event in pediatrics, but the treatment is immediate defibrillation. Most pediatric cardiologists administer lidocaine, 1 mg/kg, prior to cardioversion or defibrillation if the patient is known to be taking digoxin.

There is one report of spinal cord damage after defibrillation with anterior-posterior paddles,[50] but the paddle size, number of shocks, and delivered energy dose were not recorded, and a true cause-and-effect relationship cannot be established.[37]

PATIENT SELECTION AND INDICATIONS

All rhythm disorders of adults are observed in children, the only differences being the relative frequency of individual rhythms and ventricular rate. A supraventricular origin is far more common than ventricular origin, and ventricular rates are more rapid since the atrioventricular node of a child is able to conduct more frequent impulses. Prior to treatment for any rhythm disturbance in children, a 12-lead electrocardiogram should be obtained to accurately diagnose the dysrhythmia and to avoid potentially lethal complications from inappropriate treatment. The only exceptions to this rule are the presence of ventricular fibrillation or pulseless tachycardia as detected on a monitor.

SUPRAVENTRICULAR TACHYCARDIA

Supraventricular tachycardia is the most common rhythm disturbance identified in infants and children. Despite tachycardia rates greater than 230 beats per minute, many children suffer only mild to moderate hemodynamic compromise, allowing time for vagal maneuvers, esophageal pacing, or pharmacologic treatment to be used safely. However, a small proportion of young patients, for example newborns or those with congenital heart disease, tolerate the tachycardia less well because of a greater dependence on heart rate to maintain adequate cardiac output. Multiple treatment options for SVT exist,[8,9,49,60,61] but in practice the appropriate treatment depends on the experience of the physician and the available facilities. Vagal maneuvers, especially ice water to the face, are rapid and extremely effective.[11] Adenosine has been used safely and successfully in children,[49,60] and despite a limited experience in this age group, is quickly becoming the drug of choice.[61] Verapamil has been recommended for use in children,[52,55,56] but there are multiple reports of catastrophic bradycardia and hypotension in infants less than 1 year old, thus limiting its usefulness in the population.[23,53] Esophageal pacing[8,9] is preferred by physicians who have the appropriate equipment and training. Of the many other antiarrhythmic agents available, most have significant toxicity and should not be administered to a child without additional physician familiarity or specific recommendations of a pediatric cardiologist.

Electrocardioversion is the indicated therapy if significant hemodynamic compromise is present or other maneuvers have failed. It is safe, easily administered, and highly effective. If the physician has any reluctance to treat pharmacologically, cardioversion is always an acceptable alternative. The appropriate dose for cardioversion in children has never been scientifically tested. By consensus and experience the recommended dose is 0.5 to 1 J/kg.[1,2]

If this does not terminate the tachycardia, the same dose may be repeated or doubled to 2 J/kg.[2] Normal sinus rhythm will be restored in virtually all patients with reentrant SVT.[58]

Unless life-threatening cardiogenic shock is present, all patients, including infants, should receive sedation prior to application of the shock. Morphine 0.1 mg/kg IV provides analgesia, and when combined with a benzodiazepine, adequate sedation and amnesia are achieved. Ketamine, 1 mg/kg IM or IV, is useful for children less than 10 years old and has the advantage of minimal respiratory depression. Ketamine, however, can increase the tachycardia rate, so care must be taken to prevent further hemodynamic deterioration. If the personnel and facilities are available, short-acting barbiturates are highly effective.

ATRIAL FLUTTER AND FIBRILLATION

Atrial flutter and fibrillation are increasingly seen in the pediatric population as a long-term consequence of extensive atrial surgery for congenital heart disease. Patients with myopathies, both primary cardiac and systemic, are at risk of developing atrial flutter or fibrillation. In the absence of heart disease, atrial flutter occurs in 14% of infants and children with narrow-complex tachycardia.[43] The indications for cardioversion are the same as for supraventricular tachycardia; however, medically refractory tachycardia is much more common in this group. Most patients can be cardioverted with low-energy dosing, the one exception being those with significant atrial pathology.

Anticoagulation prior to cardioversion is generally recommended in patients with poor ventricular function or if the duration of atrial fibrillation is greater than 1 week. Children who have undergone the atrial switch operation for D-transposition of the great vessels or a Fontan-type procedure frequently have underlying sinus node dysfunction and are at higher risk for profound bradycardia after cardioversion. Diminished sinus node function may be accentuated by concurrent antiarrhythmic drugs. Cardiac pacing might be required after cardioversion, and a route for doing this must be anticipated.

WIDE-COMPLEX TACHYCARDIA

Wide-complex tachycardias occur much less frequently in children than in adults, although the mechanisms of the tachycardias are the same. Ventricular tachycardia is the most common etiology of a wide-complex tachycardia followed by the rhythms associated with antegrade connection over an accessory pathway.[10] The hemodynamic condition of the patient is not a reliable discriminator among the various etiologies. A frequent mistake is to assume that a conscious, young patient with wide-complex tachycardia has SVT with aberrancy. In fact, SVT with aberrancy is very rare in the pediatric population.[31] Of 217 pediatric patients with SVT only 10 had a wide complex, including seven with known preexisting bundle branch block. This becomes an important issue because the drug treatment of SVT (that is, digoxin or verapamil) can have devastating effects when used to treat ventricular tachycardia.[13] Thus extreme caution should be used when treating a hemodynamically stable wide-complex tachycardia. If it is deemed necessary to treat, cardioversion with sedation is the safest option. If hemodynamic compromise is present, defibrillation should be performed immediately.

The optimal energy level to terminate ventricular tachycardia in children has not been tested, and the recommended doses are those based on experience in treatment of ventricular fibrillation.[33] The AHA recommends 1 to 2 J/kg, repeating the same dose or doubling it if necessary.[2] If more than three shocks are required, reassessment of the clinical status is appropriate.

VENTRICULAR FIBRILLATION

Ventricular fibrillation is an uncommon event in pediatric patients[62] but can be observed after electrocution, open-heart surgery, or in the presence of myocardial disease such as hypertrophic cardiomyopathy, which predisposes to ventricular arrhythmias. Explanations for the low incidence include the dominance of parasympathetic over sympathetic innervation in infants[29] and the low frequency of primary myocardial disease in children. The hypothesis that a "critical mass" is necessary to support ventricular fibrillation may also explain the low incidence of ventricular fibrillation in this population.[15,65] This may be the explanation for spontaneous termination of ventricular fibrillation, observed occasionally in children but rare enough that it is not a justification to postpone defibrillation. The energy dose is 2 J/kg, repeating it immediately if a stable rhythm is not present. Again, the operator has the option of doubling the dose to 4 J/kg with the second or third shock. If a sinus or other stable rhythm is not present after three shocks, the clinical status of the patient should be addressed prior to further shocks.[1,2]

ASYSTOLE

Ventricular fibrillation can mimic asystole in adults,[25,26] and anecdotal reports of successful electro-countershock conversion of asystole to an organized rhythm has provided the impetus to consider this as initial therapy.[59] Losek et al.[46] reviewed prehospital defibrillation of pediatric asystole and found it to be an ineffective treatment while prolonging the time at the scene. The increased time was related to the time required to apply and check three EKG leads instead of one. Intubation was delayed in 88% of the patients. Since respiratory support has first priority in pediatric patients, based on known etiologies of cardiopulmonary arrest, immediate countershock of asystole will likely have a deleterious effect on resuscitation success and is not recommended in the pediatric population.[2,46]

IMPLANTED CARDIOVERTER DEFIBRILLATOR IN PEDIATRICS

Young patients with malignant ventricular arrhythmias have a dismally poor prognosis despite medical therapy.[7,19,48,57] Although cardiomyopathy or congenital heart disease is usually known to be present, sudden cardiac death may be the first indication of cardiac disease.[7,48] The development of the automatic cardioverter defibrillator has contributed to improved survival in the adult population with similar arrhythmias.[64] However, its size and initial lack of programmability limited its use in children. Several reports have documented successful implantation and follow-up in patients less than 20 years old.[34,44,45] Patients' ages ranged from 8 to 19 years, and their weights ranged from 30 to 86 kg. Surgical implantation was not unduly complicated by the presence of congenital heart disease, and the epicardial electrodes were placed without difficulty. Although some patients may require transvenous sensing or defibrillation electrodes, this is best avoided in growing patients. The major limiting factor has been the size of the defibrillator (235 grams), but careful surgical technique can overcome this problem.[34] During a 29-month follow-up period, 43% of the patients sustained appropriate shocks, 27% spurious or indeterminate shocks, and 30% received no discharges.[45] Actuarial survival analysis disclosed survival rates, free of sudden cardiac death, to be 0.94 and 0.88 at 12 and 33 months, respectively.

Of major concern to this population is the psychologic acceptance of the device and resumption of normal activities. Most patients and families adjust well to the device, primarily because of the severity and progressive nature of the underlying disease process if left untreated. Life-style restrictions, such as limited athletic activities, are usually a consequence of the primary disease, and few additional constraints are imposed solely because of the device. The major limitation involves driving privileges. Although there are no consistent recommendations, most physicians discourage driving and may forbid it altogether.[45] As with the adult population,[28] these patients and their families benefit from ongoing counseling and psychologic support. Continued improvement in design and function should broaden the usefulness of this therapy in pediatrics.

SUMMARY

Pediatric defibrillation is a useful and underutilized treatment for pediatric dysrhythmias. Although energy doses have not been as thoroughly tested for children as for adults, the guidelines published by the American Heart Association have stood the test of time. Physicians and medical personnel need to be aware of the appropriate indications and techniques with respect to the age and size of the patient to use defibrillation safely, effectively, and wisely.

REFERENCES

1. Guidelines for cardiopulmonary resuscitation and emergency cardiac care, *JAMA* 268:2171, 1992.

2. *Textbook of pediatric advanced life support*, 1988, American Heart Association.

3. Alexander S: The new era of cardioversion, *JAMA* 256:628, 1986.

4. Atkins DL, Kerber RE: Relationship of selected and delivered energy in pediatric defibrillation, *Clin Res* 38:877A, 1990 (abstract).

5. Atkins DL et al: Pediatric defibrillation: importance of paddle size in determining transthoracic impedance, *Pediatrics* 82:914, 1988.

6. Aylward PE, et al: Defibrillator electrode-chest wall coupling agents: influence on transthoracic impedance and shock success, *J Am Coll Cardiol* 6:682, 1985.

7. Benson DW Jr et al: Cardiac arrest in young, ostensibly healthy patients: clinical, hemodynamic, and electrophysiologic findings, *Am J Cardiol* 52:65, 1983.

8. Benson DW Jr et al: Transesophageal study of infant supraventricular tachycardia: electrophysiologic characteristics, *Am J Cardiol* 52:1002, 1983.

9. Benson DW Jr et al: Transesophageal cardiac pacing: history, application, technique, *Clin Prog Pacing Electrophysiol* 2:360, 1984.

10. Benson DW Jr et al: Mechanisms of regular, wide QRS tachycardia in infants and children, *Am J Cardiol* 49:1778, 1982.

11. Bisset GS III, Gaum W, Kaplan S: The ice bag: a new technique for interruption of supraventricular tachycardia, *J Pediatr* 97:593, 1980.

12. Bunting-Blake L, Parker J, Weigel A: Defibrillation procedures. In *Defibrillation. A manual for the EMT*, Philadelphia, 1985, JB Lippincott.

13. Buxton AE et al: Hazards of intravenous verapamil for sustained ventricular tachycardia, *Am J Cardiol* 59:1107, 1987.

14. Connell PN et al: Transthoracic impedance to defibrillator discharge: effect of electrode size and electrode chest wall interface, *J Electrocardiol* 6:313, 1973.

15. Crampton R: Accepted, controversial, and speculative aspects of ventricular defibrillation, *Prog Cardiovasc Dis* 23:167, 1980.

16. Dahl CF, Ewy GA, Warner ED: Myocardial necrosis from direct current countershock: effect of paddle electrode size and time interval between discharges, *Circulation* 50:956, 1974.

17. Dahl CF et al: Myocardial necrosis from direct current countershock, *Circulation* 50:956, 1974.

18. Dalzell GWN, Adgey AAJ: Determinants of successful transthoracic defibrillation and outcome in ventricular fibrillation, *Br Heart J* 65:311, 1991.

19. Deal BJ et al: Ventricular tachycardia in a young population without overt heart disease, *Circulation* 73:1111, 1986.

20. DeSilva RA et al: Cardioversion and defibrillation, *Am Heart J* 100:881, 1980.

21. DeSilva RA, Lown B: Energy requirement for cardioversion for atrial fibrillation as a function of body weight and chest size. In *Third Purdue Conference on Cardiac Defibrillation and Cardiopulmonary Resuscitation*, West Lafayette, Ind., 1979.

22. Doherty PW et al: Cardiac damage produced by direct current countershock applied to the heart, *Am J Cardiol* 43:225, 1979.

23. Epstein ML, Kiel EA, Victorica BE: Cardiac decompensation following verapamil therapy in infants with supraventricular tachycardia, *Pediatrics* 75:737, 1985.

24. Ewy GA: Cardiac arrest and resuscitation: defibrillators and defibrillation, *Curr Probl Cardiol* 2:45, 1978.

25. Ewy GA: Ventricular fibrillation masquerading as asystole, *Ann Emerg Med* 13(Part 2):811, 1984.

26. Ewy GA et al: Ventricular fibrillation masquerading as ventricular standstill, *Crit Care Med* 9:841, 1981.

27. Ewy GA, Taren D: Impedance to transthoracic direct current discharge: a model for testing interface material, *Med Instrum* 12:47, 1978.

28. Fricchione GL, Olson LC, Vlay SC: Psychiatric syndromes in patients with the auto-

matic internal cardioverter defibrillator: anxiety, psychological dependence, abuse, and withdrawal, *Am Heart J* 117:1411, 1989.

29. Friedman WF: The intrinsic physiologic properties of the developing heart, *Prog Cardiovasc Dis* 15:87, 1972.

30. Gaba DM, Talner NS: Myocardial damage following transthoracic direct current countershock in newborn piglets, *Pediatr Cardiol* 2:281, 1982.

31. Garson A Jr, Gillette PC, McNamara DG: Supraventricular tachycardia in children: clinical features, response to treatment, and long-term follow-up in 217 patients, *J Pediatr* 98:875, 1981.

32. Geddes LA et al: Electrical dose for ventricular defibrillation of large and small subjects using precordial electrodes, *J Clin Invest* 53:310, 1974.

33. Gutgesell HP et al: Energy dose for ventricular defibrillation of children, *Pediatrics* 58:898, 1976.

34. Kaminer SJ et al: Cardiomyopathy and the use of implanted cardio-defibrillators in children, *PACE* 13:593, 1990.

35. Karch SB: Resuscitation-induced myocardial necrosis. Catecholamines and defibrillation, *Am J Forensic Med Pathol* 8:3, 1987.

36. Karch SB, Billingham ME: Myocardial contraction bands revisited, *Hum Pathol* 17:9, 1986.

37. Kerber RE: Infantile hematomyelia complicating electrocardioversion, *Arch Pathol Lab Med* 109:974, 1985.

38. Kerber RE et al: Transthoracic resistance in human defibrillation. Influence of body weight, chest size, serial shocks, paddle size and paddle contact pressure, *Circulation* 63:676, 1981.

39. Kerber RE et al: Determinants of defibrillation: prospective analysis of 183 patients, *Am J Cardiol* 52:739, 1983.

40. Kerber RE et al: Ventricular tachycardia rate and morphology determine energy and current requirements for transthoracic conversion, *Circulation* 85:158, 1992.

41. Kerber RE et al: Advance prediction of transthoracic impedance in human defibrillation and cardioversion: importance of impedance in determining the success of low-energy shocks, *Circulation* 70:303, 1984.

42. Kerber RE et al: Self-adhesive preapplied electrode pads for defibrillation and cardioversion, *J Am Coll Cardiol* 3:815, 1984.

43. Ko JK et al: Supraventricular tachycardia mechanisms and their age distribution in pediatric patients, *Am J Cardiol* 69:1028, 1992.

44. Kral MA et al: Automatic implantable cardioverter defibrillator implantation for malignant ventricular arrhythmias associated with congenital heart disease, *Am J Cardiol* 63:118, 1989.

45. Kron J et al: The automatic implantable cardioverter-defibrillator in young patients, *J Am Coll Cardiol* 16:896, 1990.

46. Losek JD et al: Prehospital countershock treatment of pediatric asystole, *Am J Emerg Med* 7:571, 1989.

47. Lown B, Kleiger R, Wolff G: The technique of cardioversion, *Am Heart J* 67:282, 1964.

48. Maron BJ et al: Sudden death in young athletes, *Circulation* 62:218, 1980.

49. Overholt ED et al: Usefulness of adenosine for arrhythmias in infants and children, *Am J Cardiol* 61:336, 1988.

50. Parker JC Jr, Philpot J, Pillow JR: Infantile hematomyelia complicating electrocardioversion, *Arch Pathol Lab Med* 109:370, 1985.

51. Patel AS, Galysh FT: Experimental studies to design safe external pediatric paddles for a DC defibrillator, *IEEE Trans Biomed Eng* 19:228, 1972.

52. Porter CJ, Garson A Jr, Gillette PC: Verapamil: an effective calcium blocking agent for pediatric patients, *Pediatrics* 71:748, 1983.

53. Radford D: Side-effects of verapamil in infants, *Arch Dis Child* 465, 1983.

54. Saalouke MG et al: Electrophysiologic studies after Mustard's operation for d-transposition of the great vessels, *Am J Cardiol* 41:1104, 1978.

55. Sapire DW, O'Riordan AC, Black IFS: Safety and efficacy of short- and long-term verapamil therapy in children with tachycardia, *Am J Cardiol* 48:1091, 1981.

56. Shahar E, Barzilay Z, Frand M: Verapamil in the treatment of paroxysmal supraventricular tachycardia in infants and children, *J Pediatr* 98:323, 1981.

57. Silka MJ et al: Assessment and follow-up of pediatric survivors of sudden cardiac death, *Circulation* 82:341, 1990.

58. Sreeram N, Wren C: Supraventricular

tachycardia in infants: response to initial treatment, *Arch Dis Child* 65:127, 1990.

59. Thompson BM et al: Immediate counter-shock treatment of asystole, *Ann Emerg Med* 13(Part 2):827, 1984.

60. Till J et al: Efficacy and safety of adenosine in the treatment of supraventricular tachycardia in infants and children, *Br Heart J* 62:204, 1989.

61. Till JA, Shinebourne EA: Supraventricular tachycardia: diagnosis and current acute management, *Arch Dis Child* 66:647, 1991.

62. Walsh CK, Krongard E: Terminal cardiac electrical activity in pediatric patients, *Am J Cardiol* 51:559, 1983.

63. Weaver WD et al: Ventricular defibrillation—a comparative trial using 175-J and 320-J shocks, *N Engl J Med* 307:1101, 1982.

64. Winkle RA et al: Long-term outcome with the automatic implantable cardioverter-defibrillator, *J Am Coll Cardiol* 13:1353, 1989.

65. Zipes DP: Electrophysiological mechanisms involved in ventricular fibrillation, *Circulation* 52(suppl 3):120, 1975.

Chapter 9
AEDs: Automatic and Advisory Transchest Defibrillation

Nathan R. Every
W. Douglas Weaver

The automatic external defibrillator (AED) is a device that recognizes and treats ventricular tachyarrhythmias in patients with cardiac arrest without requiring interpretation of the rhythm by medical personnel (Fig. 9-1). The AED has come into widespread use in both the hospital and the prehospital setting in the past decade. Since the first report of the use of the AED in 1979,[12] there has been rapid evolution of this technology with expanded clinical testing in a variety of settings. The widespread acceptance of this technology was illustrated in 1988 when the International Association of Fire Chiefs adopted a proposal to equip every fire truck in the U.S. with an AED.[28] A new chapter on AEDs has been added to the American Heart Association's (AHA) textbook on advanced cardiac life support (ACLS), and the AHA now requires AED instruction as part of ACLS certification.

The rationale for the use and development of the AED comes from observations made during early clinical studies of cardiac arrest. Patient survival to hospital discharge appeared to be most strongly related to the time elapsed between collapse of the patient and the start of basic CPR as well as the time to the first defibrillatory shock.[34] Since these early studies investigators have tried to improve survival after cardiac arrest by training larger segments of the population in the technique of basic CPR as well as shortening the time from collapse to defibrillation through the expanded use of the AED. Because AEDs eliminate the need for training in recognition of rhythm, they make early defibrillation possible by first-responding personnel who are minimally trained.

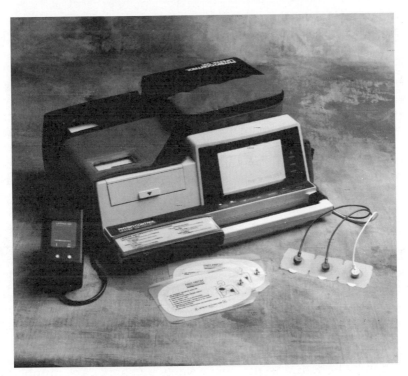

Fig. 9-1. Defibrillator for automatic external use. (From Physio-Control Corporation, with permission.)

RATIONALE

Eighty-five percent of cardiac arrests in high-risk patients are due to tachyarrhythmias.[11] Electric cardioversion or defibrillation is the only effective treatment for these rhythms. In patients with ventricular fibrillation there is a 7% to 10% decline in the probability of survival with each minute that passes between onset of fibrillation and defibrillation. After 10 to 12 minutes without defibrillation, the probability of survival approaches zero.[34] Further evidence for the importance of rapid defibrillation in treating unexpected cardiac arrest came from several observational studies in supervised cardiac exercise programs. The presence of trained personnel and the availability of defibrillators resulted in a combined survival rate of 89% in 101 cardiac arrests.[20,22,24,33]

The traditional approach to improving the availability of prehospital defibrillation was to train paramedics in manual defibrillation. Several studies have indicated improved survival with the addition of paramedic services including manual defibrillation to communities with basic emergency medical technician (EMT) services (basic life support services).[13,15] Unfortunately, paramedic response times are on average 5 to 10 minutes slower than basic EMT response times. In order to decrease the time to defibrillation, a greater number of emergency medical personnel required training.

Training of EMTs in recognition of cardiac rhythm and manual defibrillation techniques had the potential to expand the availability of defibrillation. Studies of the effectiveness of early defibrillation in such programs showed improved survival, with odds ratios ranging from 3.3 to 6.3. As with the paramedics, survival from cardiac arrest appeared to be improved by EMTs trained in defibrillation.[2,14,17,31]

There are several difficulties, however, with this approach. First, the time and cost of initial training for manual defibrillation is high. Second, frequent review of clinical skills is required to maintain proficiency. Third, the frequency of cardiac arrest due to ventricular fibrillation is so low that most EMTs would rarely use their skills. Finally, due to the significant training requirements expansion of the use of defibrillators through training of nonmedical personnel would be unlikely.

The relative ease of training and skill maintenance for AED use solved many of these problems, and the use of AEDs has expanded from EMTs to other large groups of nonmedical personnel including firefighters, police officers, security guards, lifeguards, and public transportation crews. Together this group of individuals are termed "first responders." Although few studies have evaluated the effect of first responders on community survival rates from cardiac arrest, several studies have shown significantly improved survival after community institution of early defibrillation with EMT use of AEDs. In California after passage of legislation that allowed defibrillation by basic EMTs and public safety personnel, the number of individuals eligible to provide basic defibrillation increased to 300,000.[23] Survival rates after this expansion of AED availability were increased (19% of those with witnessed VF and 13% of those that were shocked). Thus through the use of the AED early defibrillation by an expanded group of lay and medical personnel appears possible and may improve survival after cardiac arrest.

APPROPRIATE ENVIRONMENTS

There has been widespread testing of the AED in a variety of clinical settings ranging from paramedic use to lay use by families of survivors of cardiac arrest. Through all of these investigations the goal has been to expand the use of defibrillation and shorten the time from collapse to attempted defibrillation of the victim of cardiac arrest. Institution of community AED use depends on the needs and organization of emergency medical services in that community. Strategies to increase the utilization of AEDs would be different in an urban community with paramedic services in place compared to a rural community that provides only volunteer ambulance services.

In the urban setting the AED has been introduced in conjunction with already established paramedic services that historically utilized manual defibrillation. Due to the length of training for paramedics and the cost to run a paramedic service, the number of paramedics in a given region has been small. Thus response times in some regions have been slow, and this may contribute to lower cardiac arrest survival rates in some cities. The problem of slow response times by paramedics has led to the development of a tiered response system. In this system calls to 911 are answered first by the nearest emergency personnel. These are often EMT-firefighters, who require little extra training to be a first responder. First responders may perform only basic life support, although many emergency systems have trained and equipped first responders with AEDs to provide defibrillation prior to the arrival of paramedics. More sophisticated medical intervention such as intubation and IV medications are still performed by paramedics.

In the tiered response system used in Seattle, firefighters equipped with AEDs arrive an average of 1.7 minutes faster than paramedics. Survival rates from cardiac arrest rose from 19% to 30% when Seattle firefighters were equipped with AEDs.[35] Although different organizational strategies have rarely been compared directly, it appears that the highest survival rates are obtained with a double response system when first responders are equipped with AEDs, and the lowest survival rates are seen with single-response BLS systems.[18]

Despite the high survival rates seen in some urban areas with a tiered response system, many suburban and rural communities have neither the population nor the tax base to support such an emergency system. It has been estimated that an EMT working in a community of 5000 or fewer will be called on to defibrillate a patient only once every 7 years.[31] The AED, due to the ease of training and retention of skills, has a particularly important role in these communities as a more cost-effective solution to reducing the time to defibrillation in victims of cardiac arrest.

AEDs have been shown to be as effective as manual defibrillators in rural communities. Stults et al.[30] found that when AEDs are used, shocks are delivered an average of 1.2 minutes faster than when manual defibrillators are used. Although this time advantage was not correlated with increased survival, the sample size in this study was small. Overall, it appears that AEDs are as effective as and more practical than manual defibrillators and serve the role of increasing the availability of defibrillation in smaller communities that do not have paramedic services.

HOME USE

Due to the success of the AED by emergency medical systems in improving survival rates from cardiac arrest, investigators have attempted to target its use to particularly high-risk individuals such as survivors of cardiac arrest. The 6-month mortality for survivors of cardiac arrest is 20%.[16] Seventy percent of these deaths are due to VF and 70% of the VF deaths occur at home.[26] Placing an AED in the home of these high-risk patients appeared to be a reasonable strategy for improving survival. In simulated conditions laypersons can learn to operate an AED and can provide defibrillatory shocks an average of 8 minutes faster than the typical EMT response time.[27]

The success of this strategy, however, is limited and depends on multiple factors. First, suitable family members must be available to accept instruction in the AED. Moore et al.[27] noted in one study of survivors of cardiac arrest that only 50% of family members were eligible or willing to receive the device and appropriate training. The second factor in layperson resuscitation is that the training must be successful. In general, skill acquisition by family members for the use of the AED has been shown to be excellent; however, retention of skills over the next few months has been poor. A third factor is that the arrest must be witnessed and the witness must recognize the event as an arrest. Finally, the operator and device must perform properly.

Eisenberg et al.[19] found disappointing results with home AED placement in 59 patients having a history of cardiac arrest. In this group there were 10 cardiac arrests and only one of these patients was resuscitated.[19] Other investigators, however, have shown some success in home defibrillator use, albeit in small groups of patients.[5,32]

Success of the implanted cardioverter defibrillator (ICD) for survivors of cardiac arrest makes this patient group less likely to be candidates for targeted AED deployment. Of course, the majority of cardiac arrest victims do not have a history of cardiac arrest and may not be considered at high risk for cardiac arrest. Thus training of nonmedical personnel including security guards, lifeguards, transportation workers, workers at remote settings (oil rigs), and workers in highly populated settings (stadiums) in the use of AEDs may be a more effective use of the AED. Laypersons who are not family members of cardiac arrest victims may be better suited for training in the use of the AED particularly at events where large numbers of people gather. Weaver et al.[36] trained 160 security personnel in a 3-hour course on the operation of the AED for the 1986 World's Exposition in Vancouver. There were six cardiac arrests during the 5.5 months of operation. Two of the arrests were ventricular fibrillation and both patients survived.

TRAINING

One of the chief advantages of the AED is the shorter period of time required for training and maintenance of skills. In contrast to the manual defibrillator, which requires at least a 16-hour course in cardiac rhythm recognition and treatment, as well as quarterly skill review sessions,[1] training for AED use usually consists of a 4-hour course devoted to the operation of the AED according to strict protocol.[4] No attempt is made to teach any aspect of rhythm recognition during AED training. Furthermore, formalized periodic sessions for skills maintenance are not required. Studies of EMT skill retention with the AED have not shown any deterioration over time of performance variables such as time to shock or adherence to protocol.

Frequent review of operation and maintenance of the AED is recommended for users even on an informal basis. Most systems permit a maximum of 90 days between practice drills. These drills should include a performance review of recent episodes of AED use, review of equipment operations and maintenance, review of standing orders, and practice with a rhythm simulator. A quick check of equipment for operation, storage, and maintenance prior to each work shift is also recommended to maximize familiarity with the device.

Most emergency medical systems also require medical director supervision for the training, use, and review of AED operations by emergency and lay personnel. Every event in which the AED is used must be reviewed by the medical director. This includes review of the voice and magnetic recorder that stores information about the device and the operator's performance. Previous studies have shown that most device failures are due to violations of AED protocol or to poor equipment maintenance.[6] These problems can often be identified and remedied on a systemwide basis with careful review of all cardiac arrest cases by the medical director. In circumstances where AEDs are used by laypersons outside the emergency medical system a physician must take responsibility for the training and the use of the AED.

TECHNIQUE OF AED USE

The skills required of the AED user include recognition of cardiac arrest, attachment of the device, and memorization of the treatment sequence.

RECOGNITION OF CARDIAC ARREST

Training in the use of the AED assumes that the trainee has a full knowledge of basic life support (BLS). One recognized reason for failure of the AED has been the inability of the provider to recognize cardiac arrest.[19] This is particularly frequent if the operator is a family member. Patient movement due to seizures or agonal respirations have resulted in failure to recognize cardiac arrest. Thus training must emphasize recognition of cardiac arrest and possible difficulties in making this diagnosis.

OPERATION OF THE AED

Once cardiac arrest has been verified, the operator is required to take the following steps: The AED power is turned on and cables are attached to the monitor/defibrillator pads. Monitor/defibrillator pads are attached to the victim: one pad at the right sternal border, the other over the left lower ribs at the cardiac apex. The rhythm is analyzed by depressing the appropriate button on the AED. The patient should be left untouched during analysis and the operator should count to 15. In most devices the capacitors will charge during the analysis phase. If VF is recognized during the analysis, the device will warn the operator either by synthesized voice or a visible display. In a fully automatic device the first shock will be delivered without operator action. In a semiautomatic device the operator must activate the AED to give a shock after the ventricular fibrillation signal is received. With either device all personnel must be "clear" of the patient during the analysis and shock application.

After the first shock is delivered, CPR is withheld and the analysis control is immediately activated to start another cycle. Verification of cardiac arrest by manual arterial pulse checks should not be done until after the third shock. However, the patient should be quickly assessed for signs of resumed circulation prior to reanalysis with the AED. Depending on the device, the energy for the first shock is 200 J with an automatic increase in the second and third shocks not to exceed 360 J. All subsequent shocks are usually at 360 J. AEDs may be left attached to the patient during transport; however, rhythm analysis and shocks should not be attempted while the vehicle is moving, since motion artifacts in the ECG may produce inaccurate rhythm analysis.

CPR AND AED USE

After a cardiac arrest is verified, CPR is initiated if there is any delay in the arrival or setup of the AED. However, if the device is readily available, it may be advantageous to train operators to immediately attach the device and analyze the rhythm prior to the start of CPR. The basic rule is that the initial three cycles of AED analysis should not be delayed under any circumstances in a patient with verified cardiac arrest.

Standards of CPR allow a maximum of 70 seconds for the diagnosis of VF and the delivery of three shocks. The time between the activation of the rhythm analysis and the delivery of the shock in most AEDs is 10 to 15 seconds. Thus the delivery of three shocks without resumption of CPR is an acceptable standard of care with the AED.

After three successive shocks, the patient is assessed for breathing and pulse. If there is no pulse after the third shock, CPR is resumed or started for 60 seconds. After this period of CPR, the rhythm is again analyzed and shocks 4 through 6 are given without intervening pulse checks. This sequence of 60 seconds of CPR followed by three analysis/shock cycles should be continued until either the patient develops a rhythm which should not be shocked, or until advance support services (paramedics) arrive.

ADVANCED CARDIAC LIFE SUPPORT AND THE AED

Due to the large number of BLS providers now trained in the use of the AED, the interaction between these providers and ACLS-trained personnel has become increasingly important. The ACLS-trained provider has authority at the scene; however, if the ACLS provider has more limited experience with the AED it is essential that these operators work together.

On arrival, the ACLS provider should get a verbal report of the resuscitation effort. In most situations the AED protocols should be continued without interruption until ACLS providers are ready to assume this function. Most AEDs can be manually operated when necessary, and the AED should not be replaced by a manual defibrillator unless the AED does not have a rhythm display.

In the situation where there are two providers available at the scene one should operate the AED and the other should do CPR. If there is a third operator available, the institution of IV access and airway management should proceed simultaneously if possible. Communication between providers is critical since there should be no patient contact during the AED analysis/shock sequences.

VENTRICULAR TACHYCARDIA

Although AEDs are not programmed to deliver synchronized shocks, they will deliver asynchronous shocks to rapid monomorphic or polymorphic ventricular tachycardia with rates greater than the specified cutoff. Assuming that the AED has been appropriately attached to an unconscious, apneic, and pulseless patient, this shock of a patient in nonperfusing ventricular tachycardia is appropriate under current ACLS guidelines.

MECHANICAL RELIABILITY OF AEDS

AEDs have been extensively tested with libraries of recorded rhythms[10] and in numerous field trials.[7,9,25] Although not 100% accurate, AEDs have performed as well as EMTs with manual defibrillators in the treatment of cardiac arrest.[7,9,30]

Sources of error in trials of AEDs included poor equipment maintenance, with broken cable connectors, defective or dirty monitor/defibrillator pads due to improper storage, and improper battery maintenance or charging.[6] These problems should be eliminated by routine maintenance and proper storage procedures. Another source of error is in operator violations of protocol. These include failure to recognize cardiac arrest, failure to use the device properly, and failure to shock the patient when semiautomatic devices are used. These errors should be minimized by periodic review of AED operations and medical director review of all AED uses.

Another source of error with the AED has been with the development of algorithms for the recognition of VF. Presently the analysis of the ECG rhythm is done by a combination of methods. An example of one ECG criteria is as follows:

1. Rate greater than 150 beats per minute.
2. QRS slope.
3 QRS morphology.
4. Amplitude greater than .15mm.
5. Rate variability.
6. Time away from the isoelectric baseline.

The AED assesses the rhythm at 2 to 4 second intervals. If abnormal complexes are detected at more than twice the frequency of any other QRS complex for three consecutive cycles, the AED will be primed to deliver a shock.

Initial assessment of AED recognition of VF showed excellent specificity at or near 100% (only one study showed an episode of inappropriate shock), with sensitivity ranging from 76% to 96%.[8,25,30,35] The major error in the algorithm has been in the recognition of low-amplitude (fine) VF. Weaver et al.[35] noted an increase in sensitivity from 77% to 96% when the algorithm was changed to improve the recognition of fine VF. Specificity remained at 100% with this change. AEDs are not misled by patient movements (seizures or agonal respirations) or artifact.

MAINTENANCE OF THE AED

Routine testing and maintenance of the AED are critical for optimal performance. Engineering personnel should perform a maintenance check on the device every 3 to 6 months; however, routine user maintenance on a daily or shift schedule is necessary for optimal personnel and device performance. Fig. 9-2 is an example of a shift checklist for AEDs.

The Defibrillator Working Group of the Food and Drug Administration identified battery maintenance and replacement as one of the most significant problems affecting AED performance. Emergency medical systems should have a documented plan for battery maintenance and replacement. Nicad batteries are used in approximately 85% of prehospital defibrillators due to their light weight, fast recharge time, and rapid availability of stored energy during defibrillator charging. Lead-acid batteries are used more commonly on crash cart type defibrillators and are preferred in applications of continuously charged and rarely discharged defibrillators (for example, hospital-based). Either type of battery may be affected by extremes of temperature. The box on pp. 192-193 lists the Defibrillator Working Group's recommendations for battery and AED testing.

FULLY AUTOMATIC VERSUS SHOCK-ADVISORY DEFIBRILLATORS

Fully automatic defibrillators require only that the device be properly attached, the power turned on, and the rhythm assessment activated. The operator is not required to activate the device to shock the patient. In shock-advisory or semiautomatic defibrillators there is an extra step in which the operator must first activate the device to analyze the rhythm and then activate the device to shock the patient. Although there are several theoretical and

---

Fig. 9-2. Sample operator's shift checklist for automated external defibrillators (AEDs). (Reproduced with permission from the Defibrillator Working Group of the Center for Devices and Radiological Health, Food, and Drug Administration, rev 1.1d, 2/90.)

AUTOMATED DEFIBRILLATORS: OPERATOR'S SHIFT CHECKLIST

Date: _____   Shift: _____   Location: _____

Mfr/Model No.: _____   Serial No. or Facility ID No.: _____

At the beginning of each shift, inspect the unit. Indicate whether all requirements have been met.
Note any corrective action taken. Sign the form.

	Okay as found	Corrective Action/Remarks
1. Defibrillator Unit		
Clean, no spills, clear of objects on top, casing intact		
2. Cables/Connectors		
a. Inspect for cracks, broken wire, or damage		
*b. Connectors engage securely		
3. Supplies		
a. Two sets of pads in sealed packages, within expiration date *f. Monitoring electrodes		
b. Hand towel *g. Spare charged battery		
c. Scissors *h. Adequate ECG paper		
d. Razor *i. Manual override module, key, or card		
*e. Alcohol wipes *j. Cassette tape, memory module, and/or event card plus spares		
4. Power Supply		
a. Battery-powered units		
(1) Verify fully charged battery in place		
(2) Spare charged battery available		
(3) Follow appropriate battery rotation schedule per manufacturer's recommendation		
b. AC/Battery backup units		
(1) Plugged into live outlet to maintain battery charge		
(2) Test on battery power and reconnect to line power		
5. Indicators/ECG Display		
*a. Remove cassette tape, memory module, and/or event card		
b. Power-on-display		
c. Self-test ok		
d. Monitor display functional		
*e. "Service" message display off		
*f. Battery charging; low battery light off		
g. Correct time displayed set with dispatch center		
6. *ECG Recorder		
a. Adequate ECG paper		
b. Recorder prints		
7. Charge/Display Cycle		
*a. Disconnect AC plug–battery backup units		
b. Attach to simulator		
c. Detects, charges and delivers shock for "VF"		
d. Responds correctly to nonshockable rhythms		
*e. Manual override functional		
f. Detach from simulator		
*g. Replace cassette tape, module, and/or memory card		
8. *Pacemaker		
a. Pacer output cable intact		
b. Pacer pads present (set of two)		
c. Inspect per manufacturer's operational guidelines		
☐ **Major problem(s) identified** (OUT OF SERVICE)		

Applicable only if the unit has this supply or capability

rev 1.0auto,8/891

Signature: _____

Recommendations for Battery and AED Testing*

Nickel-Cadmium Battery Operator Maintenance Checklist

Battery dates—label each battery for date manufactured and date placed in service. Useful life is generally 2 years, though periodic testing and reconditioning can extend this. Maintain traceable record for each battery.

Exercise procedure—perform a reconditioning or exercise procedure (deep discharge/charge three times) of the batteries every 3 months with battery support system available from the manufacturer. Ensure that discharge occurs to the depth specified by the manufacturer.

Battery capacity—check the capacity of the batteries following the exercise procedure every 3 months. They should have greater than 70% of their rated capacity after being run through the exercise procedures. If not, remove battery from service.

Self-discharge test—perform a self-discharge test of the batteries every 6 months. They should self-discharge no more than 25% of measured capacity after 1 week. If they exceed this rate, remove battery from service.

Charge time test—measure the defibrillator charging time on battery power every 3 to 6 months. The defibrillator should charge to maximum rated energy level within 12 seconds with battery at room temperature (20°C to 25°C). If not, remove battery from service.

Energy accuracy test—perform energy accuracy test every 3 to 6 months. Charge to 50 then to 360 J and discharge each time into a 50-ohm load energy meter. To pass, the battery must deliver ± 15% of selected energy; otherwise, remove from service.

Sealed Lead-Acid Battery Operator Maintenance Checklist

Full charging—sealed lead-acid batteries should be kept fully charged. Recharge fully as soon as possible after each use by plugging the defibrillator into a source of AC line power.

---

*These are generic periodic maintenance recommendations that should be performed by the persons responsible for long-term periodic maintenance. While these checks usually will be performed by clinical engineers, they are within the capabilities of most clinical operators, without highly specialized testing equipment. They note the general areas that must be checked on a regular basis. Users should consult clinical engineering or manufacturer's service manuals for specific and complete details. Whenever replacement batteries are not immediately available, mark the defective unit and notify clinical engineering.

Recommendations for Battery and AED Testing–contd.

Constant charging—Keep defibrillator (or battery if separate from the defibrillator) plugged into AC line power during standby periods to provide constant battery charging.

No deep discharge cycling—avoid periodic deep discharge cycling because this may damage lead-acid batteries (unlike nickel-cadmium batteries).

Measure battery voltage—certain defibrillators incorporate circuitry and displays for the measurement of battery voltage and recommended voltage ranges. If such is the case, a monthly check of battery voltage is recommended.

Avoid uncharged batteries—a battery left uncharged for excessive periods (4 to 6 months) may be damaged and require replacement. Certain defibrillators are capable of testing for damage and required battery replacement.

Battery age—check the date code on battery. With proper maintenance, and depending on use, battery life should exceed 2 years and may exceed 5 years.

safety advantages that favor one type of device over another, few studies have compared the two.

TIME TO DEFIBRILLATION

As might be expected, operation of the semiautomatic defibrillator may take longer than the automatic device. In a nonrandomized field trial of 89 episodes of cardiac arrest Bocka et al.[3] found that semiautomatic defibrillation took an average of 26 seconds longer than automatic defibrillation. The effect of this delay on survival, however, could not be identified in this small trial. On the other hand, Papa[29] found no difference in time to shock between the two types of devices for paramedics tested with simulated cardiac arrest. Thus in field conditions operation of the semiautomatic defibrillator may be slower than the automatic defibrillator, although the effect on survival is not known.

SAFETY

The semiautomatic defibrillator has the theoretical advantage of increased safety to both the patient and the operator since the extra step required to administer the shock may prevent an inappropriate shock. However, instances of inappropriate shock have not occurred, probably due to the high specificity of the algorithm to detect VF and the fact that AEDs are only attached to unconscious, pulseless, and apneic patients.

In terms of operator safety the semiautomatic defibrillator allows operators to assure that all personnel are "clear" prior to initiation of the shock. However, most automatic defibrillators have either a voice warning or LCD readout to warn personnel prior to automatic delivery of the shock. Furthermore, training in the use of the AED emphasizes that there should be no patient contact after the analyze-rhythm sequence is initiated. Between 1984 and 1987 there were 13 reports of operator injuries due to AEDs.[21] Most of these injuries were due to violations of operator protocol. Overall there is little evidence of improved safety with the semiautomatic AED although many manufacturers and users prefer this type of device.

CONCLUSION

Through the increased availability of rapid defibrillation the AED has made a modest contribution to improving survival for victims of out-of-hospital cardiac arrest in some communities. It is currently uncertain whether the availability of the AED can be expanded by training more emergency service personnel as well as laypersons in the use of the device and whether such widespread availability would significantly affect outcome. Simpler and less expensive AEDs could make these devices available at any large gathering such as a sporting event as well as at remote locations where emergency response time would be slow. When treated within 1 to 2 minutes, ventricular tachyarrhythmias can be successfully terminated with little or no neurologic sequelae. Along with implantable defibrillators the increased availability of AEDs may be a reasonable approach in lowering morbidity and mortality from sudden cardiac death.

REFERENCES

1. ACT Foundation: Statement on EMT defibrillation, *JEMS* 8:37, 1983.
2. Bachman JW, McDonald GS, O'Brien PC: A study of out-of-hospital cardiac arrest in Northeastern Minnesota, *JAMA* 256:477, 1986.
3. Bocka JJ, Swor R: In-field comparison between fully automatic and semi-automatic defibrillators, *Pre-hospital and Disaster Medicine* 6:415, 1991.
4. Bradley K et al: A comparison of an innovative four hour EMT-D with a "standard" ten hour course, *Ann Emerg Med* 17:613, 1988.
5. Chadda KD, Kammerer R: Early experience with the portable automatic external defibrillator in the home and public places, *Am J Cardiol* 60:732, 1987.
6. Cummins RO et al: Defibrillator failures: causes of problems and recommendations for improvement, *JAMA* 264:1019, 1990.
7. Cummins RO et al: Sensitivity, accuracy and safety of an automatic external defibrillator: report of a field evaluation, *Lancet* 2:318, 1984.
8. Cummins RO et al: Automatic external defibrillators used by emergency medical technicians: a controlled clinical trial, *Circulation* 4:111, 1985.
9. Cummins RO et al: Automated external defibrillators used by emergency medical technicians: a controlled clinical trial, *JAMA* 257:1605, 1987.
10. Cummins RO et al: A new rhythm library for testing automatic external defibrillators: performance of three devices, *J Am Coll Cardiol* 11:597, 1988.
11. de Luna AB, Coumel P, Leclercq JF:

Ambulatory sudden cardiac death: mechanisms of production of fatal arrhythmia on the basis of 157 cases, *Am Heart J* 117:151, 1989.

12. Diack AW et al: An automatic cardiac resuscitator for emergency treatment of cardiac arrest, *Med Instrum* 13:78, 1979.

13. Eisenberg M, Bergner L, Hallstrom AP: Paramedic programs and out-of-hospital cardiac arrest: II. Impact on community mortality, *Am J Public Health* 69:39, 1979.

14. Eisenberg MS, Copass MK, Hallstrom AP: Treatment of out-of-hospital cardiac arrest with rapid defibrillation by emergency medical technicians, *N Engl J Med* 302;1379, 1980.

15. Eisenberg MS et al: Management of out-of-hospital cardiac arrest; failure of basic emergency medical technician services, *JAMA* 243:1049, 1980.

16. Eisenberg MS, Hallstrom AP, Bergner L: Longterm survival following out-of-hospital cardiac arrest, *N Engl J Med* 306:1340, 1982.

17. Eisenberg MS et al: Treatment of ventricular fibrillation: emergency medical technician defibrillation and paramedic services, *JAMA* 251:1723, 1984.

18. Eisenberg MS et al: Cardiac arrest and resuscitation: a tale of 29 cities, *Ann Emerg Med* 19:179, 1990.

19. Eisenberg MS et al: Use of the automatic external defibrillator in homes of survivors of out-of-hospital ventricular fibrillation, *Am J Cardiol* 63:443, 1989.

20. Fletcher GF, Cantwell JD: Ventricular fibrillation in a medically supervised cardiac exercise program: clinical angiographic and surgical correlations, *JAMA* 238:2627, 1977.

21. Gibbs W, Eisenberg MS, Damon S: Dangers of defibrillation: injuries to emergency personnel during patient resuscitation, *Am J Emerg Med* 18:454, 1989.

22. Haskell WL: Cardiovascular complications during exercise training of cardiac patients, *Circulation* 57:920, 1978.

23. Haynes BE et al: A statewide early defibrillation initiative including laypersons and outcome reporting, *JAMA* 266:545, 1991.

24. Hossack KF, Hartwig R: Cardiac arrest associated with supervised cardiac rehabilitation, *J Cardiac Rehab* 2:402, 1982.

25. Jaggarao NS et al: Use of an automated external defibrillator-pacemaker by ambulance staff, *Lancet* 2:73, 1982.

26. Litwin PE et al: The location of collapse and its effect on survival from cardiac arrest, *Ann Emerg Med* 16:787, 1987.

27. Moore JE et al: Layperson use of automatic external defibrillation, *Ann Emerg Med* 16:669, 1987.

28. Murphy DM: Rapid defibrillation: fire service to lead the way, *J Emerg Med Serv* 12:67, 1987.

29. Papa FJ: Time to defibrillation: a controlled laboratory study comparing 3 automatic and semi-automatic defibrillators, *J Emerg Med* 4:318, 1989.

30. Stults KR, Brown DB, Kerber RE: Efficacy of an automated external defibrillator in the management of out-of-hospital cardiac arrest: validation of the diagnostic algorithm and initial clinical experience in a rural environment, *Circulation* 73:701, 1986.

31. Stults KR et al: Prehospital defibrillation performed by emergency medical technicians in rural communities, *N Engl J Med* 310:219, 1984.

32. Swenson RD et al: Automatic external defibrillator use by family members to treat cardiac arrest, *Circulation* 76 (Suppl IV):IV-463 1987 (abstract).

33. VanCamp SP, Peterson RA: Cardiovascular complications of outpatient cardiac rehabilitation programs, *JAMA* 256:1160, 1986.

34. Weaver WD et al: Factors influencing survival after out-of-hospital cardiac arrest, *J Am Coll Cardiol* 7:752, 1986.

35. Weaver WD et al: Use of the automatic external defibrillator in the management of out-of-hospital cardiac arrest, *N Engl J Med* 319:661, 1988.

36. Weaver WD et al: Emergency medical care requirements for large public assemblies and a new strategy for managing cardiac arrest in this setting, *Ann Emerg Med* 18:155, 1989.

Chapter 10
Algorithms for Arrhythmia Analysis in AEDs

Francis M. Charbonnier

Automatic or advisory external defibrillators (AEDs) are the most significant recent advance in external defibrillation. They represent a practical and effective response to the developing concepts of chain of survival and early defibrillation in the 1970s and 1980s.

A number of studies[9,17,20,21] have clearly demonstrated that early defibrillation is the key to achieving large increases in survival rate from cardiac arrest. This has led to the chain-of-survival concept, which is very well described in the American Heart Association's medical/scientific statement "Improving Survival from Sudden Cardiac Arrest: The 'Chain of Survival' Concept."[5] The concept associates optimum survival rate with four linked steps: early access to the emergency medical services system, early cardiopulmonary resuscitation, early defibrillation, and early advanced cardiac care. Early defibrillation is the most critical of these four steps. A position statement by the Emergency Cardiac Care Committee of the American Heart Association, chaired by Dr. R. E. Kerber, states that

> . . . To achieve the goal of early defibrillation, the AHA endorses the position that all emergency personnel should be trained and permitted to operate an appropriately maintained defibrillator; this includes all first responding emergency personnel, both hospital and non-hospital (e.g., EMTs, first responders, fire fighters, volunteer emergency personnel, etc.). To further facilitate early defibrillation, it is essential that a defibrillator be immediately available to emergency personnel responding to a cardiac arrest. Therefore, all emergency ambulances and other vehicles that respond to or transport cardiac patients should be equipped with a defibrillator.[24]

Full implementation of an early defibrillation strategy therefore requires that a very large number of defibrillators be dispersed on vehicles or in the community and be available for use by a very large number of persons with little or no training in resuscitation. Identifying, training, and maintaining the skills of so many people is impractical and costly. Thus effective early defibrillation programs are only feasible with the development of "smart" automatic or advisory defibrillators that are capable of interpreting ECGs, differentiating shockable from nonshockable rhythms, and making shock decisions with a degree of accuracy comparable to that achieved by well-trained paramedics. The success of AEDs and early defibrillation depends on the quality and accuracy of the ECG interpretation algorithms used in AEDs, and considerable efforts have been made over the past 15 years to develop, test, and improve algorithms capable of high sensitivity and nearly 100% specificity for detection of ventricular fibrillation (VF).

ALGORITHMS USED IN THE FIRST AED

The first AED was developed by Dr. A. W. Diack and associates and was described in a 1979 article in *Medical Instrumentation*: "An Automatic Cardiac Resuscitator for Emergency Treatment of Cardiac Arrest."[7] This device represented the first attempt at automatic recognition and treatment of cardiac arrest. The device was designed to identify several conditions requiring intervention, that is, either ventricular fibrillation or rapid ventricular tachycardia or extreme bradycardia or asystole, and to respond by automatically delivering either a defibrillating pulse or a series of pacing pulses. The cardiac resuscitator algorithm will be discussed in some detail because of its pioneering importance and because of innovative attempts at improving sensing and diagnosis, and also to show the use of field testing in evaluating and improving algorithms. Dr. Diack faced problems that have challenged AED algorithm designers ever since and introduced innovative approaches to try to solve these problems.

A prime criterion for identifying a patient condition that requires intervention (defibrillation or emergency pacing) is that the patient be unconscious, pulseless, and not breathing; this cannot be reliably indicated by analysis of the ECG alone. Hence Dr. Diack designed special electrodes to sense several vital signs and improve the accuracy of his diagnosis. His system uses a unique pathway from the base of the tongue to the skin of the epigastrium for both sensing vital signs and delivering the defibrillating or pacing currents. A plastic oropharyngeal airway is fitted with both a transducer to measure air flow and an electrode in contact with the base of the tongue to sense the ECG. The other electrode is incorporated in a pregelled self-adhesive pad placed over the epigastrium near the apex of the heart. The ECG acquired through these electrodes is reasonably similar to a lead II acquired by conventional defibrillators, and the impedance and efficacy of the tongue-epigastrium defibrillation pathway have been shown to be similar to those of the usual external defibrillation pathways.[12] The oropharyngeal airway yielded two important benefits: first, insertion of the airway would normally be prevented by the gag reflex in a conscious patient; hence successful insertion of the airway independently verified the loss of the midbrain functions that maintain consciousness, breathing, and the gag reflex. Second, the airway contained a transducer that measured air flow and breathing.

The algorithm and the logic decision for the automatic cardiac resuscitator (ACR) are shown in Fig. 10-1.

The decision to treat requires satisfaction of two sequential criteria. The first criterion ("feature classifier") is based on air flow measurements: if air flow is greater than 120 cm^3 per breath, at a rate greater than five breaths per minute, the algorithm presumes that unconsciousness is due to a cause other than cardiac arrest, for example, a stroke or insulin reaction, and the device will not treat. The second criterion is based on a rather elementary analysis of ECG rate and amplitude. If the ECG rate is greater than 200 bpm (later changed to 150 bpm) and the amplitude is greater than 0.15 mV, VF or shockable VT (ventricular tachycardia) is declared and a defibrillating shock is delivered. If the ECG rate is below 25 bpm or if the amplitude is less than 0.15 mV, extreme bradycardia or asystole is declared and the device automatically paces at a fixed rate of 72 bpm. If the ECG rate is between 25 and 200 bpm, the device does not intervene.

A constant concern is that poor electrode contact may distort the ECG signal, reduce its amplitude, or inject noise, causing the algorithm to fail. Hence it is essential to verify good electrode contact before analyzing the ECG. In the ACR, as in most subsequent AEDs, good electrode contact is verified by measuring the impedance between the electrodes and preventing ECG analysis and device intervention when the impedance exceeds a preselected value (for example, 200 ohms).

A common dilemma in algorithm design is that the ECG analysis period should be short so that shock decisions are not delayed, but ECG analysis over a short period is vulnerable to error because large statistical fluctuations in rate and amplitude may occur and because noise and artifact may be mistaken as beats, producing fictitious high heart rates. This dilemma is usually resolved by breaking up the ECG into short analysis segments of typically 2 to 4 seconds individual duration, analyzing successive segments, comparing the individual segment results, and requiring majority decisions to declare a shockable rhythm. For instance, the ACR analyzes consecutive 2.4 second segments of ECG. VF is declared if three VF detections are made within 15 seconds.

The ACR was extensively tested in the early and mid 1980s. The first paper by Jaggarao[11] reported the correct use of the ACR on 11 patients (5 defibrillated and 6 paced) with 5 survivors. However, one patient received an inappropriate defibrillation shock, and fine VF (amplitude less than approximately .35 mV) was not recognized or treated, reducing the sensitivity of the device.

Dr. R. O. Cummins reported the use of the ACR by paramedics.[3] The ACR defibrillated 13 of 16 patients in VF (81% sensitivity) and did not shock any of

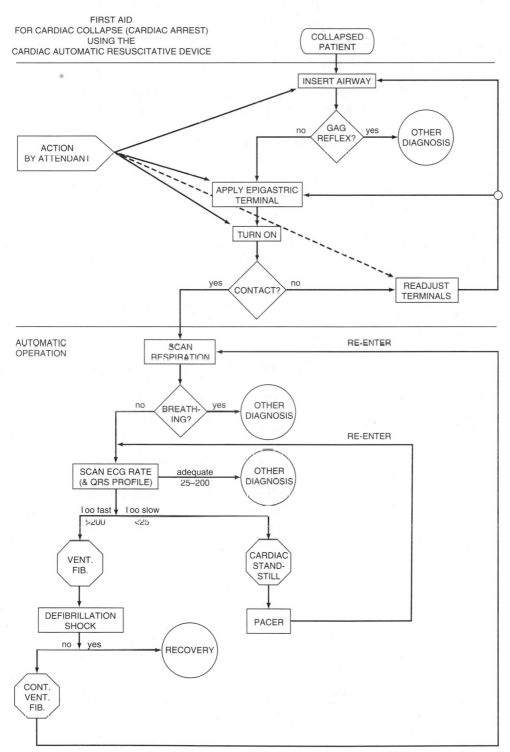

Fig. 10-1. Logic decision tree for automatic cardiac resuscitator.

21 patients in non-VF rhythms, including 13 cases of asystole (100% specificity). Of course, the small size of that patient database reduces the accuracy of these sensitivity and specificity figures.

Another study by Roskovec,[15] of patients in the electrophysiology laboratory, showed that the algorithm performed well for coarse ventricular fibrillation but made fairly frequent inappropriate decisions, both false negatives by failing to recognize fine VF and false positives by defibrillating high rate supraventricular and ventricular tachycardias.

These problems clearly showed that the ECG algorithm was not sophisticated enough. It was also found that patients in VF may experience agonal contractions that produced apparent airflow and breathing so that the breathing detection algorithm sometimes prevented the device from defibrillating actual VF.

These field studies led to a thorough redesign of the ACR, implemented in the Heart Aid Model 95 automatic external defibrillator-pacer (AEDP) from Cardiac Resuscitator Company. This device is well described in Dr. A. L. Aronson's paper: "The Automatic External Defibrillator Pacemaker: Clinical Rationale and Engineering Design."[2] Two alternative electrode systems are offered: the standard defibrillator system with self-adhesive electrode pads in either AA or AP position, intended for users competent to recognize unconscious, pulseless, and apneic patients, and the previous tongue-chest system (with air flow detector), intended for completely untrained users. The ECG analysis algorithm was considerably improved and is shown in Fig. 10-2. The ECG detection and analysis is now performed by two separate detectors: a "QRS" slope detector, which is highly sensitive to very high slope signals such as R waves but tends to reject lower slope signals, and a general wave detector called V-Fib detector, which detects all waves regardless of slope. The outputs of these two detectors are analyzed and compared for successive 2.4 second segments. A "positive" interval occurs when the output count of the VF detector is six or more and is more than twice the QRS detector count. Capacitor charging begins if a second positive interval occurs within the next 7.2 seconds (three segments). VF is declared and a defibrillation shock is delivered if a third positive interval is identified within the 7.2 seconds following the start of charging. Shockable VT is declared if no breath is detected for 12 seconds and positive intervals occur in the same sequence as for VF, a positive interval (for VT) occurring when the QRS detector count exceeds 7 (within 2.4 seconds, that is, rate > 200 bpm). Finally, pacing is initiated when no breath is detected for 12 seconds and both VF and QRS detectors show 0 or 1 count over a 4.8 second interval (that is, rate < 25 bpm).

Stults[16] compared the accuracy and efficacy of the new AEDP with that of standard defibrillators when used by trained EMTs. In a preliminary test Stults analyzed the response of the AEDP to 205 cardiac arrest and other rhythms previously recorded from actual patients in the field and annotated by a trained ECG professional. The AEDP demonstrated 92% sensitivity and

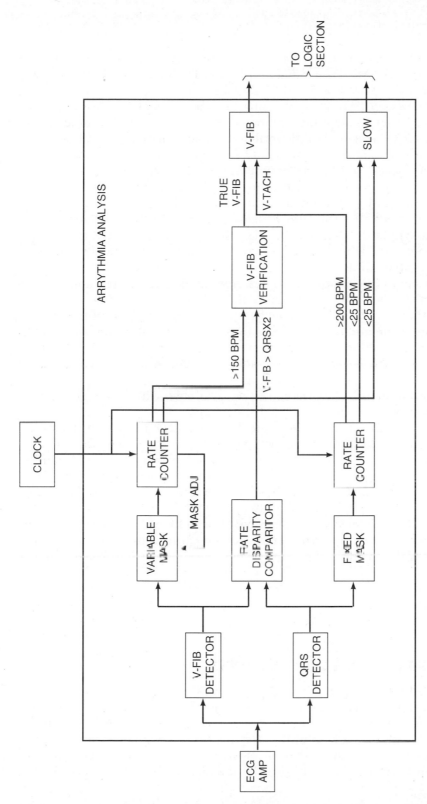

Fig. 10-2. Block diagram of ECG analysis section for automatic external defibrillator-pacemaker. (From Aronson AL, Haggar B: The automatic external defibrillator pacemaker: clinical rationa e and engineering design, *Med Instrum* 20:27, 1986.

100% specificity for VF. Comparison of the AEDP with ambulance technicians showed lower AEDP sensitivity for VF (AEDP 83% vs. technicians 98%), but higher specificity (100% vs. 94%). AEDPs were more successful at terminating VF (97% vs. 70%). Hospital admission and survival rates were similar.

Cummins,[4] in a similar study, compared the performance of trained EMTs using either AEDP or standard defibrillators. The sensitivity for VF was 78% AEDP vs. 76% standard, the specificity for non-VF rhythms was 100% vs. 95%, and the successful VF termination rate was 62% vs. 57%.

Hence these various studies led to the conclusion that the improved algorithms used in the AEDP resulted in values of sensitivity, specificity, defibrillation efficacy, and survival rates at least comparable to those achieved by EMTs using standard defibrillators. These studies also suggested that further improvements in AED performance may be achieved by further refining the ECG analysis algorithms.

Our purpose in this chapter is to describe the general design and features of VF detection algorithms, to describe their development using appropriate databases, then their bench and field testing, to indicate the importance of signal conditioning and quality checks to improve algorithm performance in an often difficult and noisy environment, to indicate the lessons learned from field testing and the resulting improvements in algorithm performance, and to speculate briefly on possible directions for future algorithm improvements.

AEDs from four manufacturers are now available, with more likely to follow in the future: Heart Start 1000 and Heart Start 3000 from Laerdal, which use algorithms derived from CRC and First Medical Devices, respectively; LifePak 300 from Physio-Control; First Medic 610 from SpaceLabs (formerly First Medical Devices Co.); and Responder 1200 from Marquette (formerly Tem Tech). Though the various algorithms differ in significant details, they share the same goals, general design structure, and essential features. Hence the description given here is generally applicable to the various algorithms currently used. These algorithms continue to be field tested and assessed with the purpose of correcting errors and designing future improvements. Most devices currently on the market are intended for use primarily by qualified first responders who are required to verify that the patient is unconscious, pulseless, and in cardiac arrest before attaching the electrodes. Most devices are also advisory rather than fully automatic, that is, they display a shock or not shock recommendation but require the operator to actually deliver the shock.

ALGORITHM PERFORMANCE MEASURES

Computerized interpretation of ECGs is a familiar problem. There have been a number of successful implementations in interpretive cardiographs and ambulatory monitoring systems. However, these algorithms use ECG traces from several leads and are optimized for their specific application. Therefore the well-known general pattern recognition methods used for ECG interpretation are also used in AEDs but must be tailored to optimize results in that specific application. In a standard diagnostic ECG interpretation problem, one must be able to identify and differentiate a very large number of morphologies and rhythm classifications, and limited sensitivity and specificity must be accepted for certain diagnoses. For AEDs one seeks only to determine whether an ECG sample represents a shockable or nonshockable rhythm; that is, there are only two classes. The performance of the algorithm is measured by using an annotated database, a collection of a large number of diverse ECG samples that have been reviewed and annotated by a cardiologist to provide the correct classification, and comparing the algorithm's classification to that of the gold standard (cardiologist) in a "truth table" (Table 10-1).

The sensitivity of the algorithm is the number of correct shock decisions as a percentage of the total number of truly shockable rhythms, that is,

$$Se = \frac{A}{A + C}$$

The positive predictive accuracy is the number of true positive classifications divided by the total number of shock decisions, that is,

$$PPA = \frac{A}{A + B}$$

The specificity is the number of true negatives (nonshockable rhythms correctly classified) divided by the total number of nonshockable rhythms, that is,

$$Sp = \frac{D}{B + D}$$

Table 10-1
Truth Table

Algorithm classification \ Gold standard classification	Shockable rhythm	Nonshockable rhythm
Shockable	A	B
Nonshockable	C	D

A, the number of true positives, i.e., truly shockable rhythms that the algorithm correctly classified as shockable. B, the number of false positives, i.e., nonshockable rhythms that the algorithm wrongly classified as shockable. C, the number of false negatives, i.e., shockable rhythms that the algorithm wrongly classified as nonshockable. D, the number of true negatives,

Finally, the prevalence is the number of truly shockable rhythms as a percentage of the total population, that is,

$$P = \frac{A + C}{A + B + C + D}$$

Ideally, AEDs should have both 100% sensitivity and 100% specificity. This is not possible in the real world and a trade-off exists between sensitivity and specificity. This trade-off is controlled by choosing classifier values and by choosing between "and," "or," or more complex decision logic algorithms when multiple features are used.

Whereas specificity basically describes the quality of the algorithm in avoiding false positive decisions, in practice we usually are more concerned with the PPA, which indicates the percentage of shock decisions that were correct. PPA depends on both specificity and prevalence. If prevalence is low, a much higher specificity is needed to maintain an acceptable PPA. For example, assume that sensitivity and specificity are both 90%: if $P = 50\%$, PPA is also 90%; if $P = 90\%$, PPA is 99%; but if $P = 10\%$, PPA is only 50%, and if $P = 1\%$, PPA is only 10%. Hence, at a prevalence of 50%, a PPA of 90% requires a specificity of 90% but, at a low prevalence of 5%, a PPA of 90% requires a much higher specificity of 99.5%.

Fortunately, in the case of AEDs the prevalence (that is, the percentage of all patients to whom the AED is applied who are truly shockable) is fairly high, ranging 30% to 70%. For instance, Weaver[23] reports that in a study including 620 patients in out-of-hospital cardiac arrest, the first rhythm recorded by first responders was VF 40%, VT 1%, asystole 36%, EMD 17%, and other rhythms 6%. With a prevalence of the order of 50%, a Sp of 95% yields an equally high PPA of 95%.

ALGORITHMS FOR AEDS AND ICDS

Automatic implantable defibrillators were first developed by Mirowski in the early 1970s. These devices gradually evolved to add synchronized cardioversion for high-rate VT and pacing modalities (for example, burst pacing) for treatment of early VT. The latter devices are often called pacer-cardioverter-defibrillators (PCDs). In this chapter the term *ICD* will be used for all members of this family of implantable devices.

The first algorithms for both AEDs and ICDs were developed in the late 1970s, and at first glance one may think that algorithms for the two devices would be very similar since they deal primarily with VF detection. In fact, the algorithms are quite different.

ICDs continuously sense the heart rhythm using bipolar signals (electrograms) from epicardial electrodes or endocardial (transvenous) electrodes, depending on the form of surgery used to implant the ICD. The position of the sensing electrodes is adjusted at implantation to provide strong signals (of the order of 10 to 15 mV) with high-frequency content, and individual beats are easily detected, at least for rhythms other than VF. Whereas the initial goal of ICDs was to detect and shock VF, it was soon realized that VF was often the end stage of a progression of arrhythmias, preceded by moderate rate then rapid ventricular tachycardia. Whereas sustained VT is normally treated by synchronized cardioversion with an external defibrillator, it was found that alternative techniques such as antitachycardia pacing or, failing that, very-low-energy synchronized cardioversion were quite effective in treating VT at an early stage and preventing it from degenerating into VF. Consequently the present third-generation ICDs emphasize detection of early VT and provide a tiered response depending on the characteristics of the arrhythmia detected. Even in third-generation ICDs a single bipolar signal is obtained in the ventricles, and the determination of VT or VF is based simply on rate or cycle length. The highly variable amplitude of the electrogram in VF makes reliable beat count and rate measurements difficult, and without the use of morphology analysis it is often difficult to differentiate ventricular from supraventricular tachycardias. Hence a fairly high false positive rate, resulting in inappropriate shocks, is reported for ICDs. Further improvements in ICD algorithms, possibly using dual chamber sensing to get atrial/ventricular timing information, or comparing the time of arrival and the direction of activation fronts at separate sensors, are under study and will certainly advance the state of the art.

The situation is very different with AEDs. By the time an AED is brought to the side of a patient in cardiac arrest the arrhythmia has usually progressed to VF or even asystole, the surface ECG signals are relatively weak and often contaminated by noise and artifact, and the device responds with a shock decision for all shockable rhythms (that is, synchronized cardioversion is not attempted for VT).

GENERAL DESIGN AND VALIDATION OF AED ALGORITHMS

The general procedure for designing and testing AED algorithms includes a number of sequential steps:

1. Define the shockable and nonshockable rhythm classes.
2. Select the general structure of the algorithm.
3. Develop a comprehensive annotated database (gold standard or truth). Use that database to evaluate and select the features and classifiers to be used in the algorithm and define all the measurements required to extract and quantify the features used in the algorithm.
4. Define the amount of signal conditioning and the quality checks that are necessary for ensuring good algorithm performance on noisy signals.
5. Bench test the algorithm: Using databases independent from the database used for algorithm development, measure the sensitivity of the algorithm for all shockable rhythms and the specificity for all nonshock-

able rhythms. Revise the algorithm design if the results do not meet pre-selected goals.

6. Subject the AED algorithm to extensive field testing to ensure that the performance in a complex and varied environment meets the goals.

7. When a number of AEDs are routinely used in the field, ensure that they are capable of detailed event recording so that these records can be used for medical review and for ongoing testing and improvement of the algorithms.

These steps will now be described in detail. We will be limited in some of the specifics by a developing and regrettable trend in medical electronics. Whereas 20 years ago inventions were often shared and patent protection seldom sought, by the 1980s intellectual property had become extremely important. Patents are aggressively sought to get a competitive advantage. Many features of current products and algorithms are either patented or held as trade secrets, and hence cannot be given in this book.

CHOICE OF SHOCKABLE RHYTHMS

The general medical consensus is that VF should be shocked, VT that causes the patient to be pulseless and unconscious should also be shocked, and all other rhythms including asystole should not be shocked. The case of asystole is controversial. It could be argued that if the patient is truly in asystole the prognosis is extremely poor and no great harm would result from delivering a shock (though a shock will almost certainly produce no benefit). The concern however is that the patient may only appear to be in asystole, for example, because of faulty ECG detection, so that a shock should not be given. Hence AED algorithms are designed for high specificity and do not shock apparent asystole.

There is a continuum from coarse VF to fine VF to asystole with noise superimposed. The boundary between coarse and fine VF is usually set at 0.2 mV average amplitude. Detection of VF becomes progressively more difficult as the amplitude decreases, and interpretation of noisy asystole as fine VF becomes more likely. Various algorithms have set different limits on the amplitude boundary between fine VF and asystole. More aggressive algorithms choose a lower boundary (for example, 0.08 mV) whereas conservative algorithms choose a higher boundary (0.15 or 0.2 mV). Of course, the lower boundary results in greater sensitivity but lower specificity, though this reduced specificity is more acceptable since it occurs only for asystole.

The definition of shockable VT is more difficult because the best criterion, an unconscious and pulseless patient, cannot be measured on the ECG. All algorithms use a rate criterion for identifying shockable VT. The general cardiology definition of VT specifies a rate greater than 120 bpm. Patients in VT at a relatively low rate, for example, 140 bpm, usually have a pulse and are conscious; hence should not be shocked. Most patients in VT at a rate of 180 or 200 bpm suffer severe hemodynamic compromise, are pulseless and unconscious. Thus the higher the VT rate, the more likely that the patient should be shocked. The problem is that the VT rate at which the patient becomes unconscious varies greatly from one patient to another and even from time to time for a given patient. Thus a criterion for shockable VT that is based on rate alone will necessarily result in limited sensitivity for shockable VT or low specificity for nonshockable VT. This problem cannot be avoided in fully automatic defibrillators intended for bystander or home use because the unskilled operator is not expected to be able to determine whether the patient has a pulse. In this case the rate threshold for shockable VT is usually set quite high, for example, 160 to 180 bpm, to increase specificity. The problem is not severe for advisory defibrillators used by better trained first responders or EMTs. In this case the responder is qualified to identify cardiac arrest and is instructed to apply the electrodes and to activate the defibrillator only after verifying that the patient is in cardiac arrest. Under such conditions any VT detection by the algorithm is clearly a shockable rhythm. Hence several algorithms set a low-rate threshold for shockable VT, for example, 150 or even 120 bpm, and usually add a morphology criterion, for example, QRS duration greater than 160 mS, to reject supraventricular tachycardia.

SELECTION OF ALGORITHM DESIGN

We need to distinguish between only two classes of ECG rhythms, shockable or not. The problem is therefore a two-class pattern recognition problem. The different methods of pattern recognition can be divided into two general approaches, statistical (decision-theoretic) methods and syntactic methods. The basic ideas behind the two approaches are similar. In order to classify the signal the distinguishing characteristics of each class of signals are first learned from a set of signals with known classification. These characteristics are then used in the pattern recognition process to classify unknown signals. In the case of statistical pattern recognition the distinguishing characteristics are a measured set of features, classifiers, and decision rules. In the case of syntactic pattern recognition the distinguishing characteristics are a set of "language" primitives and an associated grammar. Only statistical pattern recognition methods will be discussed since they have a sound theoretical basis, have been widely used in all types of pattern recognition and particularly ECG analysis, and are used in all the present AED algorithms.

In the statistical approach the classification is based on a set of selected measurements, called "features," that are extracted from the input signal. These features are chosen to provide clustering among individual samples of a class and the best possible separation between classes so that the classifier can unambiguously assign a given incoming signal to the correct class. The statistical approach can therefore be broken down into two subproblems, measuring features of the signal and classifying the signal based on these features. The design problem is selecting the best set of features to measure and then choosing the classifier value to optimally classify the feature set.

Fig. 10-3 depicts the statistical pattern recognition process. The lower half of the figure depicts the process of training the pattern recognition system while the upper half of the figure shows how the system is then used to classify an unknown signal.

During the development of the algorithm, signals with known classification are used to identify a number of features that are chosen by using some measure of class separability and selecting the set of features that maximize this measure. Once the feature set is chosen, the classifier is designed, which divides the feature space into least overlapping regions, one for each pattern class.

In classifying an unknown input signal the signal is first checked for quality and is processed to identify and remove noise. This processing step, common to any pattern recognition method, is extremely important and may improve the performance of the algorithm very significantly.

The specific choice of features and classifiers, and the decision algorithms selected when multiple features are used, have a determining effect on algorithm performance. The general considerations and trade-offs will be illustrated before discussing specific AED algorithms.

Consider first the simplest case of a single feature F (for instance, rate, wave duration, amplitude, etc.), which is continuously variable and can be measured, and two classes only, A and B. Using the annotated development database, hence knowing the correct classification, we measure the feature on every ECG segment and plot the distribution for each class as illustrated in Fig. 10-4, A. In this case the feature value falls between F_1 and F_2 for all members of class A and between F_3 and F_4 for class B. The single feature F perfectly separates the two classes, and a classifier value such as F_0 (anywhere between F_2 and F_3) will yield 100% sensitivity and specificity.

Unfortunately, this seldom happens. The situation of Fig. 10-4, B is much more likely. The two distributions overlap and there is no classifier that pro-

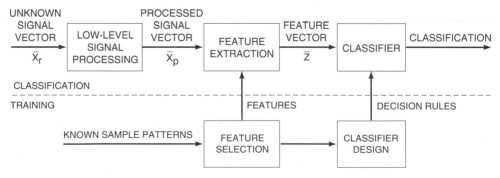

Fig. 10-3. Statistical pattern recognition classification method.

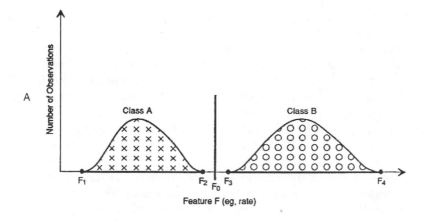

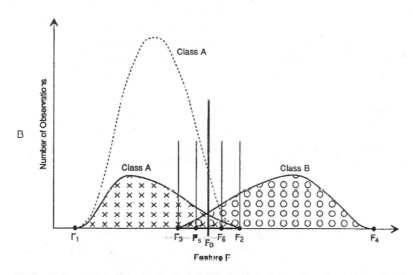

Fig. 10-4. Schematic illustration of feature clustering for the case of one feature F and two classes, A and B. **A**, Separate clusters. **B**, Overlapping clusters.

vides complete separation. Assuming that classes A and B represent nonshockable and shockable rhythms respectively, we can achieve 100% sensitivity but reduced specificity (approximately 70%) by choosing classifier F_3, or 75% sensitivity and 100% specificity by choosing classifier F_2, or any other preferred combination of sensitivity and specificity by choosing an intermediate classifier value such as F_5 (high sensitivity) or F_6 (high specificity), or F_0. Classes A and B have similar populations in Figs. 10-4, *A*, and 10-4, *B*; hence prevalence is roughly 50%. We see readily that if prevalence were lower (for example, classes A' and B), the specificity would remain the same for any given classifier but the positive predictive accuracy would be much lower.

Because a single feature rarely separates the two classes, most algorithms measure and use several features for better classification. Consider for instance two features F and G and the two-dimensional plot of Fig. 10-5. The two classes provide two two-dimensional clusters. Feature F provides a relatively poor separation (low sensitivity at F_2, low specificity at F_1) and feature G provides an even poorer separation so that either feature alone would yield a very poor classification. However, since we now have two features we can combine their results to reach a decision, and we can chose the classifier values F_0 and G_0 and the combination logic to increase either sensitivity or specificity: for instance, if we require that both features be positive for class B, we will have low sensitivity (diagonally shaded area) but almost 100% specificity (crosshatched area). If we only require that either feature be positive, we achieve nearly 100% sensitivity but low specificity. We can use a more sophisticated combination by recognizing that in the favorable case of Fig. 10-5 there is a correlation between the values of the two features F and G so that the two clusters have almost no overlap in two-dimensional feature space and that a one-dimensional classifier line such as MN provides high values of both sensitivity and specificity (vertically and horizontally

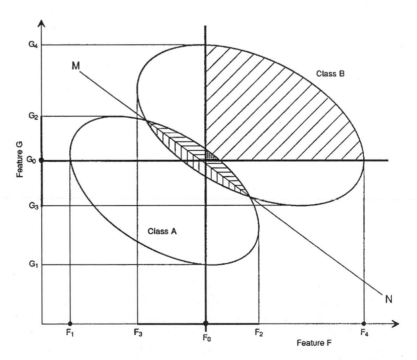

Fig. 10-5. Schematic two-dimensional feature clustering for the case of two features, F and G, and two classes, A and B.

shaded areas). Of course, there could be different shapes and orientations of the clusters where the two-dimensional classification with a line classifier is not substantially better than the product of two one-dimensional classifications.

These general concepts are clearly applicable to the case of n features, leading to class clusters in n-dimensional space and the possibility of an effective $(n-1)$-dimensional classifier surface to provide very high sensitivity and specificity.

DEVELOPMENT OF AED ALGORITHMS

A comprehensive high-quality ECG database is needed to develop an ECG algorithm. Developers of ECG analysis programs for ambulatory ECG monitoring have benefited from the availability of three standard annotated databases (from the American Heart Association [AHA], the Massachusetts Institute of Technology [MIT], and the European Society of Cardiology [ESC]). These databases are internationally accepted and in some cases are even divided into a published teaching database and an undisclosed testing database for independent third-party testing of algorithm performance. Unfortunately these standard databases were not acquired under conditions (choice of lead, filtering, sample rate, etc.) that apply to AEDs. Also the standard databases contain numerous examples of all nonshockable rhythms but only a few or no examples of VF or shockable VT. Hence these standard databases are not sufficient for AED algorithm development or testing, and every AED manufacturer has had to develop and annotate their own databases for development and testing.

Craig Edwards[8] gives a good example of the database and algorithm development process at First Medical Devices Co., which is representative of the process generally followed. Three independent ECG databases were developed to support the design activities and laboratory testing of the algorithm; one of these databases was for algorithm development and the other two were for algorithm testing.

The largest database was created to support the algorithm design process and included many types of rhythms from a variety of sources that were collected and stored on FM magnetic tape. Then these sequences of ECGs were digitally sampled 100 times per second, and each value was stored in a computer as an eightbit word. Next the data were edited into 8200 ECG segments of 3 second duration. Each segment was annotated with the assistance of medical personnel as "shock," "no shock," or "noise." There were 1800 shock segments and 6400 no-shock segments. Those segments with significant artifact from CPR or tape splices were not included. The segments identified as VF or VT (more than 180 beats per minute) were labeled as shockable and requiring defibrillation. All other rhythms, including asystole and VT with less than 180 beats per minute, were defined as no-shock segments. Noise was defined as a segment with no recognizable ECG rhythm present and was not shocked.

Once an annotated database is available for algorithm development, a number of possible features are measured and classifier values adjusted to determine the effectiveness of these features. For instance, features in some form in all present AED algorithms include: isoelectric content, average rate, number of beats and narrow complexes detected, and variability of time interval between adjacent complexes (beats).

ISOELECTRIC CURRENT

Isoelectric content measures what proportion of the ECG signal lies within a band close to the zero baseline, as shown in Fig. 10-6, which is based on technical documentation from an AED manufacturer. It is clear that a normal sinus rhythm (NSR) has a high proportion of the signal within a narrow iso-electric band (that is, has a high isoelectric content), whereas a VF or VT sig-nal has a much lower isoelectric content. Hence isoelectric content is a good feature candidate. While selection of isoelectric content as a feature is straightforward, it is important to filter the ECG signal in order to eliminate noise, artifact and reduce baseline wander, then to make a good determina-tion of the isoelectric line, that may contain some residual baseline wander. Then one chooses the optimum width of the isoelectric band, and finally one

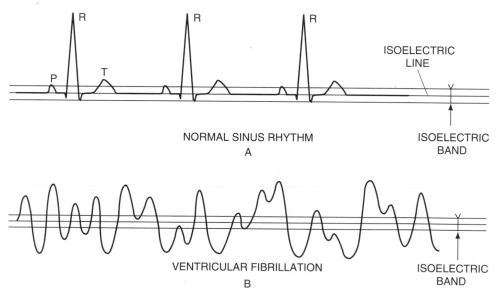

Fig. 10-6. Illustration of isoelectric content as a VF detection feature. Determine iso-electric line and select width of isoelectric band. Measure the percentage of time when the signal is within the isoelectric band. The percentage is high for normal sinus rhythm (e.g., 90%). The percentage is much lower for VT or VF (e.g., 30%).

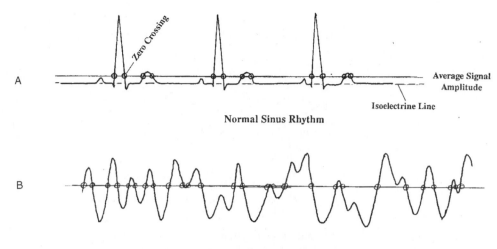

Fig. 10-7. Illustration of zero crossings measure as a VF detection feature. Determine the average signal amplitude line (zero line) and count the number of zero crossing points where the ECG signal crosses the zero line. Few zero crossings for NSR, many for VF.

adjusts the value of the isoelectric content classifier that yields the best trade-off between sensitivity and specificity.

AVERAGE RATE

Average rate is obtained by counting the number of zero-point crossings, as shown in Fig. 10-7. Clearly the number of zero-point crossings increases from NSR to VT to coarse VF to fine VF so that average rate is a clear feature candidate. Here again the effectiveness of the feature will depend on good signal conditioning to minimize noise, good filtering to reduce baseline wander, and good positioning of the isoelectric line used to determine zero point crossings.

BEAT DETECTION

Accurate QRS or beat detection is the first objective of all ECG analysis programs, and the techniques for accurate QRS detection are well tested. One utilizes the fact that at least one wave (generally the R wave) in the QRS complex has a large amplitude and a very short duration, hence is characterized by a uniquely high slope, as shown in Fig. 10-8. Therefore the ECG is searched for very narrow waves (for example, < 160 nsec) with very high slopes (for example, > 20mV/sec). If no or very few such waves are found, it can be assumed that there are no QRS complexes and therefore the patient is

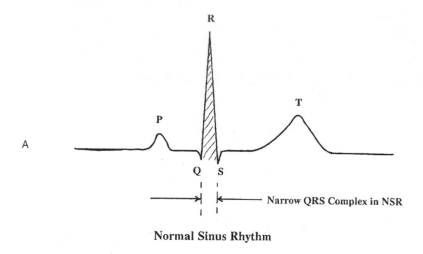

Fig. 10-8. Illustration of the search for narrow-width, high-slope waves for QRS detection. QRS complex is characterized by narrow base, large amplitude (hence very high slope) and shape more triangular than sinusoidal. Search for complexes (waves) with these characteristics.

in VF or at least wide-complex VT. If many such waves are found, they may include QRS complexes and also sharp VF or VT waves, and further analysis is required to rule VF in or out. Of course, good signal conditioning and filtering is essential since large noise or artifact may be mistaken for narrow complexes, that is, R waves.

VARIABILITY

If the number of narrow complexes detected exceeds a preset value, the variability of the time interval between successive narrow complexes is analyzed, as shown in Fig. 10-9, to determine whether the narrow complexes are R waves (low variability) or VF waves (high variability). Here again good signal conditioning to remove artifact is essential, since an NSR with artifact may yield a high number of narrow complex detections and high variability (because of random artifact timing), which would cause false positive VF detection.

After the features have been selected and the classifier values optimized, the features are organized in a logic decision sequence, as illustrated in Fig. 10-10 based on a particular manufacturer. In Fig. 10-10 four features were retained, and the logic combination requires that three or four of these features meet preset criteria before a shock decision is made. Hence the decision chart aims at achieving high specificity (at some expense in sensitivity). The choice of features and their logic organization will vary from one manufacturer to another, as illustrated in Fig. 10-11, which is based on a patent from another manufacturer.[13] The sequential features and classifiers used in this

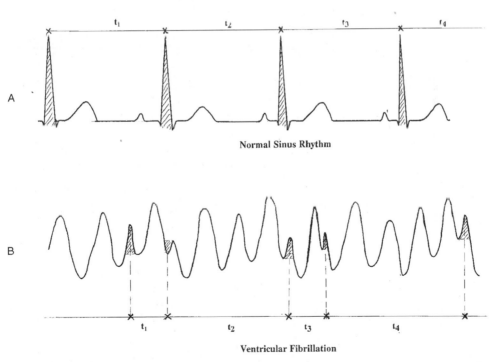

Fig. 10-9. Illustration of variability of time interval between consecutive narrow peaks as a VF detection feature. Analyze series of time intervals t_j between complexes tentatively identified as QRS complexes—t_j series has low variance for NSR, high variance for VF.

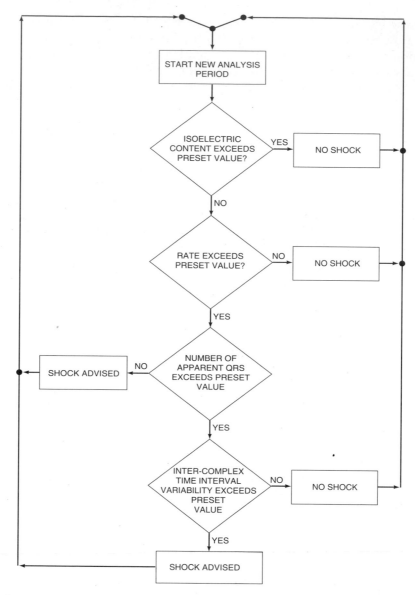

Fig. 10-10. Simplified shock decision flow chart for an AED. The logic combination of feature classification aims at high specificity.

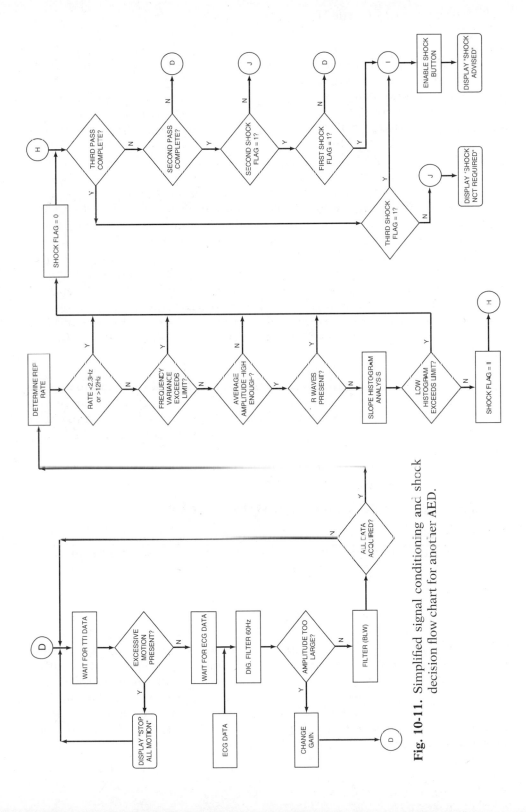

Fig. 10-11. Simplified signal conditioning and shock decision flow chart for another AED.

decision logic tree are: *average rate*, which must be between 2.3 and 12 Hz; *frequency variance*, which must be less than a preset level; *average amplitude*, which must exceed a preset value for the analysis to continue; *beat detection*, with an algorithm specifically searching for QRS complexes; *slope histogram*, where the slope of the ECG is measured at every sampled point of the ECG, all slopes are sorted in a histogram, and the relative frequency of low slope values is tested. The slope histogram measurement is similar to the isoelectric content measurement of the previous algorithm.

Based on a patent description[19] another algorithm uses a more complex analysis and measures a much larger number of features of both the ECG signal and its derivative (including ECG amplitude, order, and rate; frequency content and regularity; rate of change index; maximum to median amplitude ratio; noise content; number of peaks detected; slice index; minimum-maximum amplitude, peaks and order in the derivative signal; noise sum and noise ratio).

Instead of the single sequential decision tree shown in Figs. 10-10 and 10-11, the algorithm computes a value from a proprietary mathematical formula that incorporates all of the feature values and classifies the ECG signal into one of four classes: noise, asystole, and either no treat or treat (that is, shockable rhythm).

In all algorithms the analysis is made very rapidly, usually in a second or less, on very short ECG segments (2.4 to 4 seconds duration). Recognizing the possible errors on such short segments the analysis is repeated on successive segments and the shock decisions on successive segments are compared. A final shock decision requires majority agreement between individual segment decisions. Usually two out of three shock decisions are sufficient, but some algorithms require that the last segment decision or the last two segment decisions be positive before a shock is advised.

SIGNAL CONDITIONING AND QUALITY CHECKS

A cardinal rule in AEDs is that bad data cause bad decisions. Hence the ECG signals are subjected to quality checks and the analysis does not begin unless the quality checks are passed. Even then careful signal conditioning is applied to reduce baseline wander (hence better define the isoelectric line) and to reduce noise and artifact; the ECG gain is also optimized.

All algorithms measure impedance between the electrodes, by the usual method of injecting a low-amplitude rf current in the electrode circuit. The average impedance is measured and compared to a preselected high value, for example, 150 or 200 ohms. Since the maximum range of patient transthoracic impedance is approximately 25 to 120 ohms, a reading above 150 or 200 ohms clearly indicates very poor electric contact between the electrodes and the patient, hence an unreliable ECG signal. In such a case the ECG analysis algorithm does not proceed and no decision is made, the operator being informed by a message on the display.

In at least some algorithms the impedance is measured dynamically so that both its average value (to verify good electrode contact) and its time fluctuations may be analyzed. It is known that patient motion due to spontaneous movement, CPR, patient transport, or any other cause may introduce artifacts in the ECG that can cause faulty analysis of the ECG and inappropriate shock decisions. Patient motion also causes dynamic changes in a patient's transthoracic impedance (TTI). In at least one algorithm the dynamic impedance is continuously measured and analyzed for evidence of patient motion. If motion is detected, ECG analysis is interrupted as long as motion continues so that any possibly motion-distorted ECG data is excluded from the analysis.

In principle a precise dynamic impedance measurement could have considerable value since respiration and cardiac contractions will modulate the impedance at their respective rates, providing evidence and a rough measure of breathing rate and volume and cardiac rate and output. A patient's transthoracic impedance (TTI) ranges from 25 to 125 ohms with an average value of approximately 70 ohms. Cyclical variations of TTI due to breathing are of the order of 5 to 10 ohms for forced breathing, 1 to 2 ohms for normal tidal volume breathing, and about 0.5 ohm for rapid shallow breathing. Cyclical variations of TTI associated with normal cardiac contractions are of the order of 0.1 to 0.5 ohms and can be readily seen on a clean signal, particularly when a concurrent ECG signal is available for time correlation. However, cyclical TTI variations associated with shallow breathing or cardiac contractions are difficult to identify on noisy tracings. Hence it does not appear that dynamic impedance measurements by AEDs are sufficiently precise and noise free to provide an independent criterion for detecting or ruling out VF through the presence or absence and the amplitude of periodic TTI variations due to respiration or cardiac contractions.

Following impedance-based quality checks for electrode contact and motion, careful signal conditioning is used to improve signal quality and facilitate ECG analysis. This includes at least:

1. High-pass filtering to minimize baseline wander. A relatively high-frequency cutoff, usually 2 Hz, is used since it effectively suppresses BASE-LINE WANDER but does not attenuate VF or VT signals where frequencies of 2 to 8 Hz predominate.
2. Low-pass filtering with a relatively low cutoff frequency, usually 20 Hz. The purpose is to remove high-frequency noise or muscle artifact, which may be confused for QRS complexes, without attenuating VF or VT signals.
3. Notch filter at 50 or 60 Hz to eliminate line frequency noise.

BENCH AND FIELD TESTING OF AED ALGORITHMS

Bench testing using independent databases follows the development of algorithms and signal conditioning techniques. The results have been quite satisfactory for all algorithms currently in use. However, it was soon recognized that bench testing could only provide partial answers and that extensive field testing was necessary for full validation of the algorithms.

For instance, Weaver et al.[22,23] tested AEDs used by first responding firefighters and found that the sensitivity for VF and shockable VT was substantially less than had been predicted from bench testing. The bench testing database had been acquired with defibrillators from the same manufacturer as those subsequently used in clinical testing, and used similar bandwidth and filtering but different electrodes. The field testing results showed a much lower sensitivity for all three shockable rhythms: coarse VF, fine VF, and VT. Possible reasons for this difference were estimated. The detection failures were analyzed and the algorithms were modified, yielding a large increase in sensitivity for all three rhythms, without loss of specificity, as shown in Table 10-2. The three tests included approximately 1000 ECG segments each, with a comparable distribution between VF, VT, and nonshockable rhythms.

These results clearly show the need for extensive field testing before an algorithm can be finalized and insure good performance.

The only published comparative evaluation of the three AEDs then on the market was performed by Cummins et al.[6] in 1988. The three devices were tested on a database collected in prehospital defibrillator programs in Iowa and in King County, Washington and included 102 segments of VF and 144 segments of other rhythms (IVR, VT, SVT, and asystole) for patients presumed to be in cardiac arrest. The results are summarized in Table 10-3.

The three devices were also compared for different classes of VF (extracoarse, medium, and fine) and for specific non-VF rhythms. The general con-

Table 10-2
Bench and Field Testing of AED Algorithms (Sensitivity for shockable rhythms and Specificity for other rhythms)

	Fine VF (<0.2 mV)	Coarse VF (>0.2 mV)VT	VT	Other Rhythms
Bench test	76%	95%	86%	96%
1st field test	15%	62%	22%	99%
2nd field test	65%	92%	60%	98%

Table 10-3
Device Performance

Device	A	B	C	Significance
Average Se for VF (coarse or fine)	88%	92%	93%	NS
Average Sp for all other rhythms	91%	95%	90%	NS
Overall accuracy	90%	94%	91%	NS

Se, sensitivity; sp, specificity.

clusion was that VF sensitivity was approximately 90%, non-VF specificity was 90% to 95%, that there were no statistically significant differences between the three devices, and that the overall performance was good, that is, at least equal to that of EMTs or paramedics using conventional defibrillator monitors.

FUTURE ALGORITHM DEVELOPMENT

The foregoing discussion indicates that following improvements based on field testing, the present algorithms show good performance and demonstrate the usefulness of AEDs for early defibrillation by minimally trained first responders. Some further refinements are of course possible, but it seems unlikely that further major improvements in overall accuracy will be achieved under present conditions, that is, with algorithms based entirely on short segments of a single ECG lead, using only features that are easily measured and rapidly analyzed.

However, there are various possibilities currently under study that may become practical in the future and may allow major improvements.

1. There is a continuing interest in the independent detection of cardiac arrest with a non-ECG sensor. This was the purpose of the oropharyngeal airway and airflow detector used in 1979 in the first AED. This independent sensor was later abandoned because it was prone to false negative errors, hence reduced the VF sensitivity of the device below that achieved with ECG detection alone. However, the sensor technology may improve; alternatively, effective measurement of blood pressure, blood flow, or cardiac output may be feasible, or dynamic impedance measurement accuracy may be improved sufficiently to allow reliable detection and assessment of breathing and cardiac contractions by impedance methods.

2. Acquisition and analysis of several leads of ECG would clearly increase the reliability of ECG measurements and feature classifiers, though this would require additional electrodes.

3. The ECG features used to identify VF are relatively simple, even if accurate measurements are difficult on low-quality, noisy signals. More sophisticated methods have been suggested to differentiate VF from VT and from other rhythms. For instance, frequency-domain analysis has shown that power spectra for VF are clearly differentiated from those for other rhythms, leading to effective classification.[14] Auto-correlation techniques may also be used with good results.[10] Finally, Thakor has suggested a very interesting technique in which the ECG signal is analyzed for a certain period with three possible conclusions: definitely class A (for example, VF), definitely class B, or uncertain—more data/analysis needed, in which case the ECG acquisition and analysis continues until a definite conclusion is reached.[18]

Whereas these techniques have the potential for higher sensitivity and specificity, there are two practical obstacles to their implementation in AEDs: (1) Most of these techniques are computer-intensive, taxing the capability of present microprocessors for real-time applications. With the steady increase in microprocessor speed and computing power this will not be a problem in the future. (2) Most of these techniques require analysis of a long segment of ECG, hence are in conflict with the desire for very rapid analysis and shock decision.

REFERENCES

1. American Heart Association: Automated external defibrillation. In *Textbook of advanced cardiac life support,* ed 2, Dallas, 1992, The Association.
2. Aronson AL, Haggar B: The automatic external defibrillator pacemaker: clinical rationale and engineering design, *Med Instrum* 20:27, 1986.
3. Cummins RO et al: Sensitivity, accuracy and safety of an AED, *Lancet* 2:318, 1984.
4. Cummins RO et al: Automatic external defibrillators used by EMTs: a controlled clinical trial, *JAMA* 257:1605, 1987.
5. Cummins RO et al: Improving survival from sudden cardiac arrest: the "chain of survival" concept, *Circulation* 83:1832, 1991.
6. Cummins RO et al: A new rhythm library for testing AEDs: performance of 3 devices, *J Am Coll Cardiol* 1:597, 1988.
7. Diack AW et al: An automatic cardiac resuscitator for emergency treatment of cardiac arrest, *Med Instr* 13:78, 1979.
8. Edwards DC: Development of a decision algorithm for a semi-automatic defibrillator, *Ann Emerg Med* 18:39, 1989.
9. Eisenberg MS et al: Treatment of out of hospital cardiac arrest with rapid defibrillation by EMTs, *N Engl J Med* 302:1379, 1980.
10. Guillen SG et al: VF detection by auto correlation peak analysis, *J Electrocardiol* 22:253, 1989.
11. Jaggarao NSV et al: Use of AEDP by ambulance staff, *Lancet* 2:73, 1982.
12. Kerber RE et al: Evaluation of a new defibrillation pathway: the tongue-epigastric route, *J Am Coll Cardiol* 2:966, 1983; *J Am Coll Cardiol* 4:253, 1984.
13. Morgan CB et al: Interactive portable defibrillator. U.S. Patent 4610254, September 1986.
14. Nolle FM et al: Evaluation of a frequency-domain algorithm to detect VF, *Comp Cardiol* 337, 1989.
15. Roskovec A et al: Safety and percentage of a portable AEDP, *Clin Cardiol* 6:527, 1983.
16. Stults KR, Brown DD, Kerber RE: Efficacy of an automatic external defibrillator in the management of out of hospital cardiac arrest: validation of the diagnostic algorithm and initial clinical experience in a rural environment, *Circulation* 73:701, 1986.
17. Stults KR et al: Pre-hospital defibrillation performed by EMTs in rural communities, *N Engl J Med* 310:219, 1984.
18. Thakor NV et al: VT and VF detection by a sequential hypothesis testing algorithm, *IEEE Transactions on BME* 37:837, 1990.
19. Vandehey ME: Defibrillator ECG interpreter, U.S. Patent 4919144, April 1990.
20. Weaver WD et al: Factors influencing survival after out of hospital cardiac arrest, *J Am Coll Cardiol* 7:752, 1986.
21. Weaver WD et al: Improved neurologic recovery and survival after early defibrillation, *Circulation* 69:943, 1984.
22. Weaver WD et al: Use of the AED in the management of out of hospital cardiac arrest, *N Engl J Med* 319:661, 1988.
23. Weaver WD et al: AEDs: importance of field testing to evaluate performance, *J Am Coll Cardiol* 10: 1259, 1987.
24. Kerber RE: AHA Position Statement on Early Defibrillation, *Circulation* 83: 2233, 1991.

Chapter 11
Effects of Drugs on Defibrillation Threshold

Charles F. Babbs

Timely electrical defibrillation by application of a strong electric shock to the heart either through internal transventricular or external transthoracic electrodes is ordinarily safe and effective therapy for an otherwise lethal disturbance of cardiac rhythm. Occasionally, however, drug interventions can influence defibrillation success. Since patients at high risk for ventricular fibrillation are likely to be receiving drug therapy for cardiovascular disease—including antiarrhythmic drugs—it is important to understand the interactions of these agents with the process of electrical defibrillation. This chapter reviews the manner in which selected cardiac drugs influence the electric shock intensity required for ventricular defibrillation and in turn the probability of the return of spontaneous circulation.

According to the most widely accepted theory of electrical defibrillation[8,65,70] (Chapters 1, 2, 3) the passage of an electric shock on the order of 100 mA/cm^2 through the ventricles for 2 to 20 msec will simultaneously stimulate most ventricular muscle cells, causing potentially excitable cells in the path of propagating fibrillation wavelets to become refractory for a brief interval thereafter. This sudden electrical intervention stops the self-propagation of the multiple random waves of excitation that constitute fibrillation. The minimum measured shock intensity in a set of repeated trials that is able to abolish fibrillation is defined as the *defibrillation threshold*.* Owing to anatomic variations in heart size, ventricular filling, lung volumes, and respiratory motion, as well as biochemical and physiologic variations in tissue pO_2, tissue pH, and extracellular potassium concentration, measured threshold

---

*The operational definition of defibrillation threshold and the methods for measuring it are presented in detail in Chapter 1 of this volume.

values will vary in the neighborhood of ± 10% in a given individual[3] and up to 50% in a population of individuals of roughly the same body mass.[15,60] Drugs too can cause further changes in defibrillation threshold. The most clinically worrisome agents are those that raise threshold and so reduce the probability of resuscitation from an otherwise lethal state.

When it is technically possible to deliver a clearly suprathreshold shock through either external transthoracic electrodes or internal transcardiac electrodes at surgery, drug-induced increases in defibrillation threshold are usually of little clinical significance,[9] since the margin of safety for defibrillation energy is so large: twentyfold, when the indicator of untoward effects is microscopically detectable damage, and 320-fold when the indicator of untoward effects is death.[7] The advent of the implantable cardioverter defibrillation (ICD), however, has created a clinical setting in which defibrillation energy will always be fundamentally limited by (1) the desire to keep implanted devices as small as is reasonably possible, (2) the desire to make battery life as long as possible, and (3) the desire to make the sensation or discomfort experienced by the patient receiving a shock as little as possible. In this setting delivery of defibrillation shocks that are consistently just above threshold, but not excessively above threshold, becomes a design criterion for ICDs, and systematic changes in threshold produced by drug therapy become much more meaningful and clinically important. Such drug interactions with the electrical energy used for defibrillation are especially likely since many patients treated with ICDs either require chronic antiarrhythmic drug therapy or receive acute antiarrhythmic drug therapy with the onset of symptoms.[25] To the extent that an unwise choice of antiarrhythmic drugs causes threshold elevation in a patient with small defibrillation threshold margins, drug interactions with ICD function could prove to be undesirable or even fatal.

As subsequently reviewed in detail, drugs that act at the cellular level to narrow the gap between the transmembrane resting potential and the threshold firing potential of fibrillating cardiomyocytes are expected to decrease the electrical defibrillation threshold by making it easier to electrically stimulate the requisite critical mass of myocardium. Conversely drugs that widen this gap are expected to increase defibrillation threshold by making it more difficult to electrically stimulate a critical mass of myocardium. A review of relevant membrane physiology suggests that drugs that alter the sodium or potassium conductances of cell membranes, or the ratio of intracellular to extracellular sodium or potassium concentration, should influence the gap between the transmembrane resting potential and the threshold potential of individual cardiac muscle cells and in turn alter the defibrillation threshold. This working hypothesis[8] is now supported by much experimental data. Accordingly the present chapter includes, first, a review of electrical events during defibrillation at the cellular level where drugs must ultimately act; second, a discussion of a transmembrane ionic current model to predict drug

effects on defibrillation threshold; and third, a comparison of theoretical predictions with experimental and clinical data.

MECHANISM OF ELECTRICAL DEFIBRILLATION

SIMPLIFYING ASSUMPTIONS

Although extremely high currents and voltages appear across the heart and
thorax during ventricular defibrillation, the electrical stimulus at the cellular
level is physiologic and inherently nontoxic if properly applied. When considered at this level, the actions of drugs upon transmembrane ionic conductances and equilibrium potentials can influence the effectiveness of electrical
ventricular defibrillation in an understandable and predictable manner. Such
understanding is aided by three fundamental assumptions. The first is that
the essential requirement for defibrillation is excitation of a critical mass of
the nonrefractory cells in the fibrillating myocardium, for which Zipes[70] originally and Witkowski and coworkers[65] more recently have provided good evidence. Owing to the essentially chaotic nature of established ventricular
fibrillation, described in Chapter 1, it is also quite reasonable to assume that
at any instant during fibrillation, individual myocardial cells may be found in
any phase of polarization (Fig. 11-1), as has been demonstrated experimentally by Sano and coworkers.[56] If in turn fibrillation is conceived as the presence of numerous randomly oriented wavefronts of depolarization, in three-
dimensional space, spreading throughout the myocardium, as represented in
Fig. 11-2, electrical defibrillation requires simultaneous excitation of the cells
just ahead of each propagating wavefront. These cells would be found either
in phase 4 of the action potential or in the latter part of phase 3, as defined in
the tracing for cell D in Fig. 11-1. Using this conceptual framework, one's
understanding of the chaotic, three-dimensional myocardium may be simplified somewhat by the realization that in order to defibrillate it is not necessary to excite those cells in the fibrillating muscle mass that are already
refractory to excitation in phases 0, 1, 2, or the midportion of phase 3. In this
sense the problem reduces to one of field stimulation of nonrefractory cardiomyocytes. A third simplifying assumption that is useful in understanding
drug effects in defibrillation is that it is necessary only to depolarize one side
of the cell membrane of each cardiac muscle cell to the extent of the difference between the resting (phase 4) transmembrane potential and the cellular
firing threshold. This stimulus would be sufficient to excite fully recovered
cells in phase 4 as well as to prolong the refractory periods of cells just emerging from relative refractoriness in late phase 3.[59]

THE ACTION OF DEFIBRILLATING CURRENT AT THE CELLULAR LEVEL

Although electrical defibrillation requires the passage of high total current
and the development of high total voltage between the defibrillating elec-

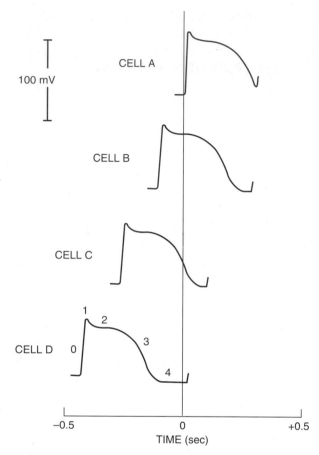

Fig. 11-1. Conceptual description of the temporal dispersion of individual myocardial action potentials within a fibrillating ventricular muscle mass. Action potentials of four hypothetical cells, *A, B, C,* and *D,* are indicated as functions of time. Phases 1 through 4 of the action potential are indicated on the tracing for cell *D.* During fibrillation cells may be found in any stage of polarization at any instant in time. Phase 4 is usually abbreviated (Cells *A* and *C*), and often excitation can occur in the latter part of phase 3 (cell *A*). The amplitude of the action potentials in fibrillation is about 75 mV. (From Sano, T, Tsuchihihashi H, Shinamoto T: Ventricular fibrillation studied by the microelectrode method, *Circ Res* 6:41, 1958.)

trodes, at the cellular level the magnitudes of the shock-induced electrical events are much less dramatic and much more physiologic. Consider an idealized, uniform current field passing transversely through a bundle of myocardial fibers, as sketched in Fig. 11-3, *A.* Here each member of the bundle represents a cell or a syncytial grouping of cells. Now imagine a thin rectangular slab of tissue, one cell layer thick, that is perpendicular to the cur-

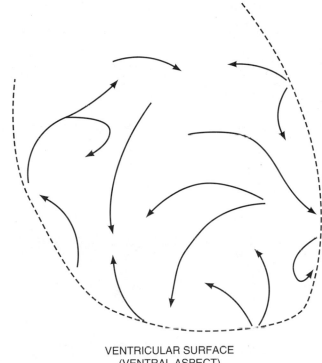

VENTRICULAR SURFACE
(VENTRAL ASPECT)

Fig. 11-2. Conceptual description of the spatial dispersion of multiple, random wavelets of depolarization traversing the ventricles during fibrillation. Heads of arrows indicate the wavefront of each wavelet and its direction of propagation. Tails of arrows indicate the length of refractory tissue trailing each wavefront. When a wavefront encounters a refractory strip, it will split into daughter wavefronts or become extinguished. In sustained fibrillation successive generations of wavelets are always able to spread into areas of excitable myocardium. In theory an effective defibrillator shock simultaneously excites and renders refractory the tissue just ahead of a sufficient number of wavefronts to abolish or encapsulate their further propagation.

rent field, containing muscle cells, extracellular fluid, blood vessels, and connective tissue (Fig. 11-3, *B*). Within the slab the long axes of the muscle cells are perpendicular to the flow of electric current. Let the dimensions of this slab of ventricular tissue be 20 μm thick, the approximate diameter of a typical ventricular muscle fiber, and 1 cm² in surface area.

The action of defibrillating current at the cellular level can be appreciated by considering the DC equivalent circuit elements of the 1 cell thick slab, as shown in Fig. 11-3, *C* and *D*. The resistive component of the slab consists of the electrolyte-filled extracellular space, which comprises about 30% of the volume of mammalian ventricular muscle.[34] The capacitive component con-

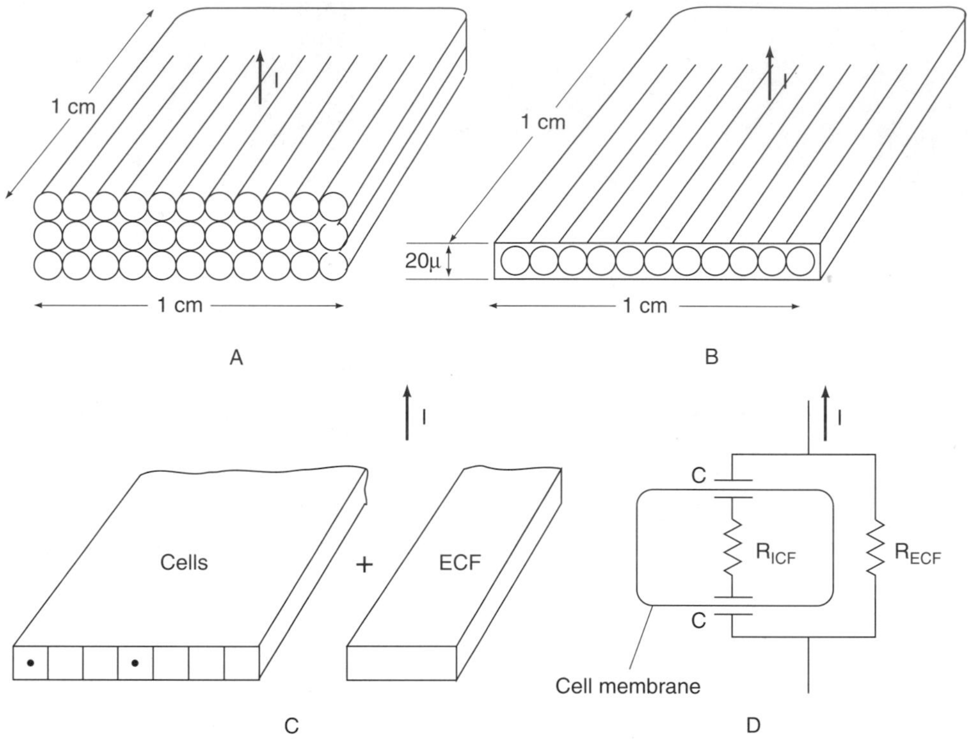

Fig. 11-3. Scheme for analysis of the action of defibrillating current within the myocardium. **A**, Bundle of myocardial fibers oriented perpendicular to electric current field, *I*. **B** and **C**, Hypothetical tissue element 1 cm² in cross-sectional area and one cell diameter in thickness, containing cells and extracellular fluid. **D**, Equivalent circuit for hypothetical tissue element.

sists of muscle and connective tissue cells, comprising about 70% of ventricular volume, which are surrounded by relatively high-resistivity, insulating cell membranes. By definition two conductors separated by an insulator constitute a capacitance. In the present case the extracellular and intracellular fluid layers are the conductors, and the lipid-rich cell membranes are the insulators. Classically the cell membranes of cardiac muscle have been modeled as parallel resistive-capacitive networks,[66] but in the present application membrane resistance is so large with respect to the extracellular fluid resistance (2000 ohms for 1 cm² versus 0.4 ohms for 1 cm²) that membrane resistance can be ignored for DC shocks and the membranes considered as purely capacitive, as shown in Fig. 11-4. This sketch represents the equivalent electrical circuit elements of the stimulated cardiac tissue slab.

If a direct current pulse is now applied to the network depicted in Fig. 11-4, current will flow initially onto the series capacitors, causing them to charge. This charging of membrane capacitance will tend to depolarize the cathodal sides and hyperpolarize the anodal sides of the cells. The time for membrane capacitors to charge maximally is about three to five "RC" time constants, after which nearly all of the current flows through the extracellular fluid resistance and the final voltage across both series capacitors is equal to the voltage drop across the extracellular resistance. Taking values of R and C from the literature,[2] the time constant for charging of membrane capacitance in this model may be computed on the order of 5×10^{-6} sec. This very short charge time is negligible with respect to the duration of defibrillation shocks—several thousand microseconds—and so is not a limiting factor compared to the biological time constant for voltage-dependent activation of sodium conductance, which is on the order of 0.5 msec.[27,44] The biological time constant requires that normally the cathodal side of the cell must remain above the firing potential for more than a millisecond before sodium activation will become sufficient to cause rapid sodium inrush, depolarization, and refractoriness.

Thus during the first 5 µseconds of a defibrillatory shock the membrane capacitances become fully charged, and thereafter current flows preferentially around the cells rather than through them.[37] Electrophysiologically the essential result of the passage of current through cardiac tissue via macroelectrodes is the redistribution of charge across the membranes of cardiomyocytes in the field. This charge redistribution results in hyperpolarization of the anodal sides and depolarization of the cathodal sides of the cells, as shown in Fig. 11-4, *B*. For example, if a 60 mV potential difference appearing across the cell is divided equally across the series membrane capacitors, then 30 mV will appear across the anodal side of a symmetrical cell and 30 mV will appear across the cathodal side of the cell, owing to charge redistribution in

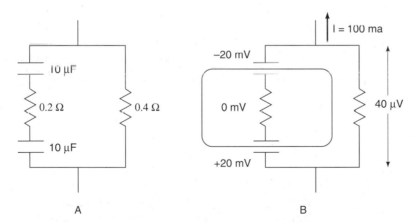

Fig. 11-4. Equivalent circuit for DC electrical stimulation of cardiomyocytes in a hypothetical slice of myocardium 1 cm² in cross-sectional area and one cell diameter in thickness. **A,** Approximate values of the circuit elements. **B,** Voltage changes produced during passage of an electric current of near threshold intensity perpendicular to the plane of the slice.

the electric field. In turn, the anodal side of the cell will be hyperpolarized by 30 mV and the cathodal side will be depolarized 30 mV. If such a change is large enough to bring the transmembrane potential on the cathodal side of the cell from a resting potential of approximately −90 mV to the firing threshold of approximately −60 mV for the duration of the shock, then voltage-dependent sodium channels on that side will open and an action potential—with subsequent refractoriness—will be generated.

FIBER ORIENTATION

In the foregoing equivalent circuit model the major factor in field stimulation of the cell is the magnitude of the transcellular voltage difference. This difference is critically dependent on the size, geometry, and orientation of the cell. It is greater for larger-diameter cells and also greater for long cylindrical cells that are oriented parallel rather than perpendicular to the imposed electric field. Given equal voltage division across the anodal and cathodal membrane capacitances the change in transmembrane potential created by the shock is one half the voltage gradient in the tissue multiplied by the span, h, of the cell in the direction of the field (Fig. 11-5). For a cylindrically shaped cell the span can be related geometrically to the angle, Θ, of tilt, as shown in Fig. 11-5, B, according to the expression

$$h = d \cos \Theta + L \sin \Theta$$

where d is the diameter of the cell and L is the length of the cell. For a typical cardiomyocyte the length-to-diameter ratio L/d is about 5/1. If the myocardial fibers are tilted rather than perpendicular to the direction of current flow, their span in the direction of the field would be greater, and in turn a greater voltage difference would develop across the membrane capacitances, causing correspondingly greater changes in the transmembrane potential.

Using the simple mathematical model in Fig. 11-5 it is interesting to compute the fiber orientation, Θ, corresponding to defibrillation threshold voltage gradients determined from animal experiments. Witkowski, Penkoske, and Plonze[65] measured the voltage gradients generated by defibrillatory shocks in dog hearts instrumented with 40 epicardial electrodes connected to special-purpose direct-coupled amplifiers able to withstand the strong signals generated by defibrillation trials. They found that the highest epicardial voltage gradient minimum for an unsuccessful defibrillation attempt was 8.5 V/cm. That is, defibrillation threshold was 8.6 V/cm. This value is virtually identical to that measured by Niebauer et al.[52] for similar trapezoidal waves, who found threshold voltage gradients of 8.2 to 8.5 V/cm for monophasic trapezoidal current pulses delivered to isolated dog hearts suspended in an isoresistive saline tank in which the resistivity of the bath was matched to that of the blood perfused heart, creating an approximately uniform current density field. In both experimental studies a shock of 8.6 V/cm or greater always

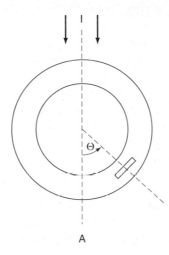

A

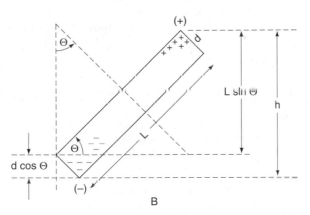

B

Fig. 11-5. A cylindrical model of the left ventricle to estimate geometric effects of fiber orientation upon the relationship between the threshold transmembrane potential of individual cardiomyocytes and the defibrillation threshold voltage gradient in intact hearts. Most myocytes are tilted at some angle, Θ, with respect to the current field. Because they are longer than they are wide, up-field and down-field sides of the cell span a distance, h, greater than the cell diameter and are charged to a greater degree than if Θ were 0. The effective voltage difference across the cell is equal to the voltage gradient in V/cm multiplied by the span h. Theoretically this voltage difference is divided equally across the membrane capacitances at the positive and negative ends of the cell. In a uniform current field a voltage gradient of > 8.5 V/cm will defibrillate normal dog hearts *in vivo* and *in situ*. Cardiomyocytes angled at 25° or more will be depolarized by > 25 mV in an 8.5 V/cm field, whereas muscle fibers at shallower angles will be depolarized less. By geometry, cells angled at > 25° constitute about 72% of the ventricular muscle mass for transventricular shocks delivered perpendicular to the long axis of the left ventricule, assuming a cylindrical model. This fraction of cells, which would be excited by a threshold shock, corresponds to the critical mass of myocardium that must be depolarized to abolish fibrillation experimentally.

defibrillated the ventricles. Interestingly, the value of 8.5 V/cm, corresponding to 17 mV/20μ, would not be sufficient to depolarize a fully recovered normal cardiomyocyte in phase 4, assuming that the cell is 20 μm in diameter and oriented perpendicular to the current field ($\Theta = 0, h = d$). However, if the cell is tilted to an angle of 25 degrees, h becomes 60 μm for a 20 μm diameter, 100 μm long cell. The corresponding transcellular voltage difference is 51 mV, inducing a 25 mV depolarization on the cathodal side of a symmetrical cell, approximately that necessary to stimulate. Cells tilted at an angle greater than 25 degrees also would be stimulated.

In a cylindrical model of the left ventricle (Fig. 11-5, *B*) cells angled at greater than 25° would constitute about 72% of the muscle mass. Such cells may represent the critical mass of the ventricles defibrillated by threshold shocks in a uniform field in Niebauer's experimental studies. This value agrees with the critical mass value from Zipes's[70] work, in which 72% of the ventricular muscle mass had to be depolarized by injection of KCl solution into multiple coronary artery branches in order to achieve defibrillation. This estimate also agrees with the original observations of Garrey,[35] who reported in 1914 that experimental fibrillation ceased when "three fourths" of the mass of an isolated, fibrillating heart was pared away surgically. When fiber orientation is taken into account in this way, the concept of a critical mass and the concept of excitation of nonrefractory myocytes can be unified to produce a simple theoretical explanation of the mechanism of electrical ventricular defibrillation.

Thus theoretical analysis and experimental results are consistent with the hypotheses that (1) a critical mass of fibrillating myocardium must be rendered simultaneously refractory by field stimulation provided by the defibrillatory shock and (2) the process of field stimulation induces depolarization of membrane capacitances of individual cardiomyocytes, tilted at a critical angle Θ or greater, in a manner expected from classical membrane physiology. Given this model of the mechanism of defibrillation, it is now possible to develop concepts to predict and understand drug interactions with defibrillating current.

THE IONIC CURRENT MODEL

Assuming that cardiac defibrillation is essentially large-scale electrical stimulation of nonrefractory areas in the fibrillating muscle mass, the action of cardiac drugs can be understood in terms of their influence on the transmembrane sodium and potassium currents, I_{Na} and I_K, according to electrophysiologic mechanisms first proposed by the present author over a decade ago,[8] and subsequently confirmed by a variety of experimental studies. In brief, drugs can change defibrillation threshold by altering the degree of membrane depolarization that is required to initiate an action potential in individual, nonrefractory cardiac muscle cells. The required degree of depolarization can be expressed as the "gap" between resting membrane potential and cellular threshold potential for self-sustaining sodium channel activation, $E_{th} - E_r$. These values are determined by the balance of ionic sodium and potassium currents as functions of the transmembrane potential, E_m, as shown in Fig. 11-6, A. Here gNa and gK denote sodium and potassium conductances of the membrane, E_{Na} and E_K denote Nernst equilibrium potentials,[12,19] I_{Na} denotes inward sodium current, and I_K denotes outward potassium current. The solid curve denoting sodium current is concave upward because of the voltage dependence of fast sodium channels. That is, gNa is not a constant but rather a voltage-dependent variable representing a fundamental intrinsic property of excitable membranes. Depolarization itself induces a sudden increase in gNa, while at this precontraction stage gK is essentially unchanged. The sodium and potassium current curves therefore cross at two points, at which inward sodium current and outward potassium current are equal. One point represents a stable equilibrium—the resting membrane potential, E_r. The other point is an unstable equilibrium—the cellular firing threshold, E_{th}. These two points divide the transmembrane potential domain into three zones, labeled *1, 2,* and *3* in Fig. 11-6.

The intensity of the electrical stimulus required to excite the ventricular muscle cell is related to the width of zone 2. As illustrated in Fig. 11-6, B, if E_m is transiently driven away from the stable equilibrium value, E_r, by a depolarizing stimulus into zone 2, it will return to E_r, driven by the net ionic current, since outward potassium current exceeds inward sodium current in zone 2. However, if E_m is driven past the cellular firing threshold by a depolarizing stimulus into zone 3, an action potential will be initiated because inward sodium current will grow progressively greater than outward potassium current, and the cell will become completely depolarized and refractory. The intensity of the stimulus required to excite the cell in this way depends upon the extent of zone 2, as measured by the difference $(E_{th} - E_r)$.

This ionic current model sets the stage for the prediction of drug effects upon defibrillation threshold. As can be readily imagined with reference to Fig. 11-6, A, drugs that increase gK or decrease gNa will widen zone 2, and so increase the strength of the stimulus required for excitation. In turn these drugs will increase the defibrillation threshold. Drugs that decrease gK or increase gNa will narrow zone 2 and reduce the defibrillation threshold. A recent example of this effect has been provided experimentally by Echt and coworkers,[26] who tested defibrillation energy requirements (measured in terms of the energy, E_{50}, required for 50% successful defibrillation during multiple trials in anesthetized dogs) before and after infusions of cesium chloride, a known potassium channel blocker. From Fig. 11-6 one would predict that an agent that decreases gK, reducing the slope of the dashed line representing outward potassium current, would reduce defibrillation threshold. This effect was observed by Echt et al. following cesium infusion.

In other fundamental studies[6] the present author and his coworkers have demonstrated the ionic mechanism illustrated in Fig. 11-6 by manipulating

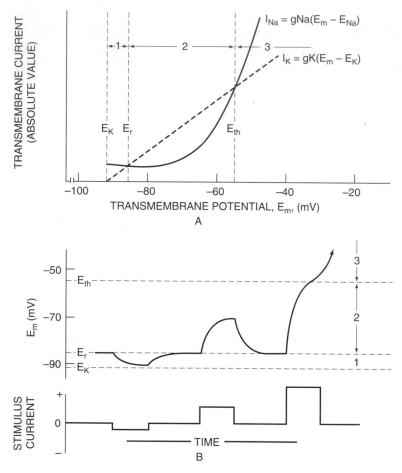

Fig. 11-6. Semiquantitative ionic current model for understanding drug effects in defibrillation in terms of the balance of inward sodium and outward potassium currents. **A**, Absolute values of sodium and potassium currents as a function of transmembrane potential, E_m. Zones 1, 2, and 3 of the E_m domain are identified. The crossing points of the sodium and potassium curves define two equilibrium states: one at the resting membrane potential, E_r, the other at the cellular threshold potential, E_{th}. Approximate normal values for E_r and E_{th} are shown. **B**, effects of alterations in membrane potential caused by brief DC shocks. If E_m is transiently driven into zone 1 or zone 2, it will return to the stable equilibrium value, E_r. If E_m is driven into zone 3, an action potential will be generated.

transmembrane potassium currents in a different way. In these experiments we used infusions of KCl in anesthetized dogs to induce a shift of the potassium equilibrium potential, E_K. The value of E_K depends most importantly upon the log ($[K_o]/[K_i]$), where $[K_o]$ and $[K_i]$ represent extracellular and intracellular potassium concentrations. Normally $[K_o] \cong 4\ mEq/L$, $[K_i] \cong 150\ mEq/L$, and $E_K = -60$ log ($[K_o]/[K_i]$) $= -94$ mV. Moderate elevation of extracellular potassium concentration, $[K_o]$, makes E_K less negative, shifting the dashed line for potassium current in Fig. 11-6, A to the right without changing its slope. This effect decreases the extent of zone 2 and increases excitability. Experimentally infusion of potassium chloride in dogs was shown to lower defibrillation threshold[6] (Fig. 11-7). Indeed at a critical level of $[K_o]$ spontaneous defibrillation occurs, as would be predicted qualitatively by the ionic current model in Fig. 11-6. Extremely high levels of $[K_o]$, which cause a shift of the potassium current line completely to the right of the sodium current curve, make the cell inexcitable because a normal resting potential cannot be restored. This latter state is induced by cardioplegic solutions used to immobilize the heart at surgery and is the physiologic basis of chemical defibrillation achieved by injection of KCl solutions into the coronary circulation.

The experiments of Tacker et al.[62] using the short-acting cardiac glycoside ouabain may also be interpreted along similar lines. Cardiac glycosides are now known to work by inhibiting membrane-bound Na^+/K^+ ATPase in the heart.[45] Inhibition of inward potassium pumping would be expected to alter the log($[K_o]/[K_i]$), by increasing K_o locally near the outer membrane surfaces of affected cardiomyocytes. As a result the potassium equilibrium potential, E_K, would be made less negative, shifting the potassium current curve in Fig. 11-6 slightly to the right and decreasing the extent of zone 2. This electrophysiologic change would be expected to decrease defibrillation threshold even though one ordinarily thinks of the digitalis glycosides as proarrhythmic agents. In fact Tacker et al.[62] found that ouabain transiently and dose-dependently reduced transchest defibrillation threshold in dogs. Thus in all of the foregoing studies various manipulations of potassium conductance and the potassium equilibrium potential confirm the ionic current model of direct current defibrillation.

Several diligent groups of investigators over the past two decades have studied a variety of antiarrhythmic drugs to determine their effects on ventricular defibrillation threshold in healthy anesthetized dogs. With relatively minor exceptions, consistent with the axiom of pharmacology that no drug has only one effect, the actions of cardiac drugs on the defibrillation threshold can be understood in terms of basic electrophysiology and their effects upon ionic channel currents. With reference to the ionic current model in Fig. 11-6 and to the width of the excitatory gap between E_r and E_{th} one can make the following predictions about the effects of antiarrhythmic drugs based upon their ionic mechanisms of action: (1) a pure sodium current blocking drug or a pure potassium current enhancing drug would raise defibrillation

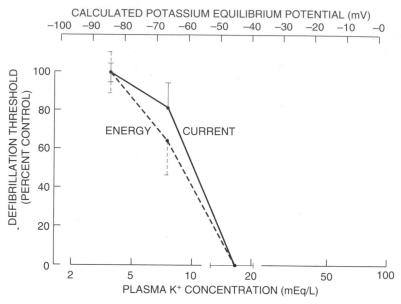

Fig. 11-7. Effects of potassium infusion upon transventricular defibrillation threshold in pentobarbital anesthetized dogs. Defibrillation threshold fell during potassium intoxication. The percent decrease in defibrillation threshold was linearly related to the logarithm of the extracellular potassium concentration $[K_o]$ and to the potassium equilibrium potential E_K, calculated from measured extracellular and intracellular potassium concentrations of ventricular muscle. In dogs supported by left ventricular bypass in order to maintain the circulation during potassium intoxication, the values of $[K_o]$ and E_K required for spontaneous, potassium-induced defibrillation (electrical defibrillation threshold = 0) were 16.6 mEq/L and −46 mV, compared to normal values in this animal model of 3.9 mEq/L and −84 mV. Error bars represent standard deviations. The abscissa is broken to indicate standard deviation of potassium concentration for spontaneous defibrillation (horizontal error bars). Results are similar whether threshold shock strength was measured in terms of current or energy. (Redrawn with permission from Babbs CF et al: Dependence of defibrillation threshold upon extracellular/intracellular K' concentrations, *Electro-cardiology* 13:7, 1980.)

threshold by increasing the excitatory gap of recovered, nondepolarized cells that are spatially positioned just ahead of the various fibrillation wavelets; (2) a pure sodium current enhancing drug or a pure potassium current blocking drug would reduce threshold by decreasing the excitatory gap.

MEASURES OF DEFIBRILLATION EFFICACY

THRESHOLD DISTRIBUTIONS VS. PERCENT SUCCESS CURVES

Before addressing the results of experimental studies of the interaction of drugs with defibrillating shocks it is necessary to review methodological and

conceptual controversies regarding the best measure of the electrical requirement for defibrillation, which were presented in detail in Chapter 1. The minimum shock strength required to accomplish defibrillation is described in the
classical literature as the defibrillation threshold[13,63] and is related conceptu-
ally to threshold phenomena at the cellular level, according to the theoretical
framework just presented. Well-defined experimental protocols for determination of defibrillation threshold have been developed[13] and the temporal stability and reproducibility of threshold data in animals have been established.[3]
However some investigators, most notably Schuder and coworkers[38] in the
1970s and Winkle and coworkers[20,30] in the 1980s, have argued that defibrillation data are best expressed not in terms of a threshold but rather in terms of
a percent success vs. shock strength curve. Such a curve may be obtained in
more time-consuming experimental protocols in which percent success is
determined directly during multiple repeated trials and logistic regression or
similar techniques are used to reconstruct the underlying percent success vs.
energy dose curve. Those favoring the latter approach have argued that there
is no true threshold because the resulting percent success data do not jump
abruptly from 0% to 100% as a function of energy. These authors have tended
to use the term *defibrillation threshold* in quotes,[29,30] as if inviting the reader to
join them in the select group of those who know better.[58] On the other hand
those favoring the original concept of defibrillation threshold (the present
author among them) consider it unremarkable that modest changes in measured threshold values (typically about ±5 percent in current and ±20 percent
in energy)[3] occur on repeated determinations in the same animal, owing to
changes in chest dimensions and impedance, changes in instantaneous ventricular filling with persistent atrial contractions, and even changes in the
random pattern of fibrillatory wavelets themselves.[37] Such physiologic and
biologic variability is described by the standard deviation of threshold measurements reported in experimental studies.

The literature on drug interventions in defibrillation can thus be sorted
into two camps, those reporting defibrillation threshold (DFT) and those
reporting the electrical dose for 50% successful defibrillation (E_{50}). Fortunately, for the purpose of interpreting the literature these two terms are actually equivalent in all essential respects because a shock of median threshold
intensity will defibrillate on 50% of experimental trials. The equivalence of E_{50}
and DFT data is shown mathematically later in this chapter and has been
confirmed experimentally by Bourland and coworkers[14] (Fig. 11-8). In general
the scaled integral of the histogram representing the distribution of measured
threshold values as a function of shock strength is the same as the percent
success curve. In turn the mean threshold shock strength under given experimental conditions is a good estimate of the E_{50}. Conversely the scaled derivative of the percent success curve is the same as the distribution of threshold
values. The mathematics of this type of equivalency are well established in
pharmacology and are isomorphic with the equivalency of the distribution of
sensitivities of individual animals to a given drug and the cumulative dose-
response curve.[39] Accordingly in the following discussion of specific agents

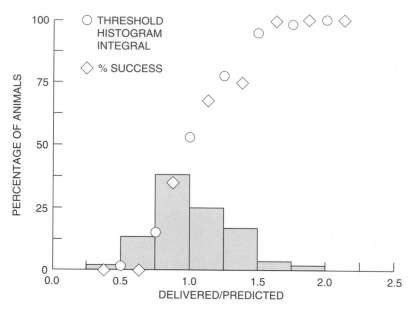

Fig. 11-8. Experimental demonstration of the relationship between defibrillation threshold and percent success data. Bourland and coworkers (Bourland JD et al: Ventricular defibrillation threshold: its relationship to the chance of defibrillating a subject, *Proceedings AAMI 17th Annual Meeting,* May 9-12, 1982), analyzed first-shock percent success and threshold data from 60 experiments in 8 to 60 kg dogs in which defibrillation shocks were delivered by intracardiac catheter electrodes (right ventricle to superior vena cava). To compare data from animals of different size, shock intensity was expressed as a fraction of threshold current predicted from body weight using the expression $I = aW^b$, where I is defibrillation threshold current, W is body weight, and a and b are constants determined from a least-mean-squares fit. The solid histogram represents the distribution of measured threshold values; the circles represent the integral of the threshold distribution; and the diamond symbols represent the percentage of animals successfully defibrillated on the first shock. The first shock success curve and the cumulative threshold curves are very similar. Median threshold shock is equivalent to the E_{50}.

drug-induced changes in DFT and drug-induced changes in the median effective dose or E_{50} are interpreted as representing the same underlying biologic events.

SINGLE FIBRILLATION VS. MULTIPLE FIBRILLATION PROTOCOLS

Another methodological issue of current concern is related to the interpretation of clinical studies of defibrillation threshold performed during cardiac surgery. Traditionally defibrillation threshold values have been computed using only first-shock data.[13] After induction of fibrillation, a test shock is

Table 11-1
Comparison of Single Fibrillation—Multiple Shock Technique with Multiple Fibrillation—First Shock Technique in 7 Dogs

Body weight (kg)	Threshold current ratio (SF/MF)	Threshold energy ratio (SF/MF)
6.0	0.99	0.85
6.0	0.89	0.83
7.7	1.00	0.98
12.0	1.04	1.01
16.1	1.06	1.10
23.7	0.98	1.01
22.5	1.11	1.28
mean	1.01	1.01
S.D.	0.07	0.15

SF, single fibrillation technique; MF, multiple fibrillation technique.

given, followed if necessary by a rescue shock of known effectiveness. Only results of the first shock are counted, and so multiple, repeated episodes of fibrillation are required to establish threshold. This precaution was deemed necessary in early work because the extent to which prior unsuccessful shocks or prolonged fibrillation duration would influence the success of subsequent shocks was not known. Multiple fibrillation first-shock protocols became established and were widely used in animal studies. In clinical studies, however, especially those involving defibrillation at cardiac surgery, there is a great incentive to minimize the total time involved in taking defibrillation threshold data, especially for protocols that do not directly benefit the individual patient and that prolong the "pump time" and the duration of anesthesia. The most efficient and ethically reasonable protocol for experimental defibrillation would involve only a single fibrillation episode and multiple shocks, beginning with an anticipated subthreshold shock and proceeding with stepwise increases in shock intensity until defibrillation is achieved. The question then arises as to whether one can validly compare data from single fibrillation, multiple shock studies with data from traditional multiple fibrillation, and first shock studies.

Table 11-1 summarizes the results of a direct comparison of the two approaches* performed in the author's laboratory in 1976 for transchest defibrillation in pentobarbital-anesthetized dogs. Five alternate trials of each technique were tested in seven animals weighing 6 to 24 kg. The mean ratio of single fibrillation to multiple fibrillation threshold current was 1.01, and the mean ratio of single fibrillation to multiple fibrillation threshold energy was also 1.01. The correlation coefficient, r, for mean threshold current determined by the two techniques in the seven dogs was 0.990. The corresponding

*Previously unpublished.

correlation coefficient for threshold energy was 0.975. Thus the two methods give essentially equivalent results, a finding recently confirmed by Hahn and coworkers[40] using a percent success–based experimental paradigm. Thus in reviewing and interpreting literature including both earlier animal studies and more recent human data, one need not be concerned about artifactual differences between single fibrillation versus multiple fibrillation protocols.

EFFECTS OF SPECIFIC CARDIAC DRUGS ON DEFIBRILLATION

QUINIDINE

The original reports of Woolfolk[67] in 1966 demonstrating a dose-related increase in energy requirements for ventricular defibrillation in dogs administered quinidine (14 to 42 mg/kg, IV) and of Babbs[5] in 1979 demonstrating the time-action curve for DFT elevation by high-dose (50 mg/kg) intravenous quinidine were the first to describe the effects upon defibrillation of DFT elevation by this prototypic class IA sodium channel blocker (Fig. 11-9). At more moderate doses of 10 mg/kg threshold elevation in experimental studies has ranged from zero[24] to 20%[21] in energy. As in the case of most drugs studied in the field of defibrillation, complete dose-response relationships are not available from any single laboratory. This state of affairs is not surprising, since defibrillation studies must necessarily be done in larger animals, such as dogs, with hearts large enough to sustain fibrillation.[36] The use of larger animals rather than rats or mice makes the cost of dose-response studies with adequate numbers of animals in each group quite discouraging. Nonetheless, an appreciation for dose-response relationships can be gained from a meta-analysis of various published studies in which the effective dose is reduced to a single bolus or loading dose equivalent in mg/kg and the response is reduced to the percentage change in threshold energy, or the equivalent change in E_{50}.

Fig. 11-10 shows the results of such a metaanalysis for quinidine. Each data symbol represents a different published study. Results for non-drug-treated controls in the various quinidine studies are plotted at zero dose. This combined summary of published animal studies shows rather clearly a dose-related threshold elevation by quinidine, as would be expected for a sodium channel blocking agent from the ionic current model. The effects are minimal, however, until the dose exceeds 10 mg/kg. Clinically, administration of a single large oral dose of 600 mg in a 70 kg patient may be useful to determine whether the drug will be effective in controlling ventricular arrhythmias, and therapeutic plasma levels range from 2 to 5 µg/ml or 5 mg/kg of plasma water. In children 6 mg/kg body weight every 6 hours is recommended.[11] Accordingly only modest elevations in defibrillation energy requirements would be expected at clinically realistic doses of quinidine. Similarly Deeb and coworkers[22] found that procainamide, often considered an alternative to quinidine,[31] had no effect on internal defibrillation threshold at therapeutic concentrations. Nonetheless, in the case of quinidine, the combined theoretical consid-

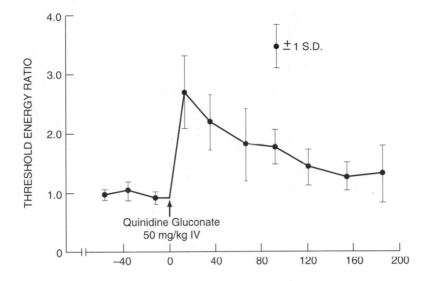

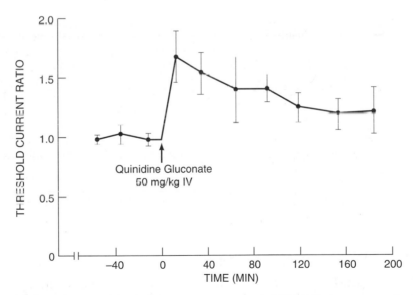

Fig. 11-9. Time course of high-dose intravenous quinidine effect on transchest ventricular defibrillation threshold in normal, pentobarbital anesthetized dogs. Data from reference 5. Each data point represents the mean value for five dogs. The absolute threshold values corresponding to 1.00 on the vertical axes were 0.94 J/kg delivered energy and 1.21 amp/kg peak current. (Redrawn with permission from Babbs CF, Whistler SJ, Geddes LA: Elevation of ventricular defibrillation threshold in dogs by antiarrhythmic drugs, *Am Heart J* 98:435, 1979.)

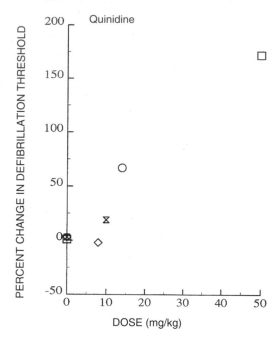

Fig. 11-10. Metaanalysis of dose-response relationships for quinidine. Each data symbol represents a different published study: circles (Woolfolk DI et al: The effect of quinidine on electrical energy required for ventricular defibrillation, *Am Heart J* 72:659, 1966), squares (Babbs CF, Whistler SJ, Geddes LA: Elevation of ventricular defibrillation threshold in dogs by antiarrhythmic drugs, *Am Heart J* 98:H435, 1979), diamonds (Dorian P et al: Effect of quinidine and bretylium on defibrillation energy requirements, *Am Heart J* 112:19, 1986), hour glass (Dawson AK, Steinberg MI, Shapland JE: Effect of class I and class III drugs on current and energy required for internal defibrillation, *Circulation* 27:384, 1985 [abstract]).

erations and higher dose experimental data are probably sufficient to discourage its use in patients with ICDs.

ENCAINIDE AND O-DEMETHYL-ENCAINIDE

Encainide is a newer class IC antiarrhythmic agent whose ionic mechanism of action is also predominantly sodium channel blockade.[72] From the limited experimental data available the effects of this agent upon defibrillation are much more dramatic and disturbing than those of quinidine. Encainide and its active metabolite O-demethyl-encainide greatly increase E_{50} values in experimental canine studies, doubling defibrillation energy requirements in what are clinically realistic doses, given the interspecies differences in tissue sensitivity between dogs and humans.[29] Even more disturbing from a practical standpoint is that 4 of 13 dogs given encainide or O-demethyl-encainide in

Winkle's study could not be defibrillated, even with shocks 20 times predrug baseline intensities. Interestingly a related metabolite, 3-methoxy-O-demethyl-encainide (MODE), was found to produce a much smaller and statistically insignificant elevation of E_{50}. Evidently very small alterations of the structure of the compound can have large effects upon activity, an observation that is consistent with a receptor-specific molecular action such as sodium channel blockade.

FLECAINIDE

Hernandez and coworkers[42] studied the effects of the encainide-like antiarrhythmic drug flecainide on defibrillation thresholds in anesthetized dogs using nontruncated exponential pulses delivered through two epicardial patch electrodes in an electromechanical configuration that mimicked an ICD. Flecainide infusion increased E_{50} from 6.5 to 11.4 J, and the flecainide-treated animals experienced additional side effects of the drug, including severe hypotension and ventricular fibrillation resistant to defibrillation. Accordingly both theory and experimental data tend to discourage use of encainide and flecainide in patients who remain at risk of ventricular fibrillation and whose ventricles are likely to be defibrillated by energy-limited devices such as ICDs.

LIDOCAINE

Although lidocaine is a well-known local anesthetic that can act upon nerves in higher concentrations by blocking sodium channels, its cardiac action at the lower concentrations achieved systemically when it is administered as an antiarrhythmic agent are due predominantly to an increase in outward potassium conductance.[12] Accordingly lidocaine is considered a class IB (formerly class II) antiarrhythmic agent. Lidocaine shortens action potential duration either by increasing gK or to a lesser degree by decreasing gNa.[12] According to the ionic current hypothesis illustrated in Fig. 11-6, a clear prediction can be made that these effects upon ionic currents, both separately and together, should raise the shock intensity required for excitation of nonrefractory muscle and in turn for defibrillation.

Experimentally a reasonably linear dose-response relationship can be inferred from a metaanalysis of five published studies of the interaction of lidocaine with defibrillation shocks in pentobarbital anesthetized dogs (Fig. 11-11). The correlation coefficient, $r = 0.779$, for the combined dose-response scattergram is less than that for quinidine ($r = 0.971$); however measurable elevations do occur at therapeutic doses. In the experiments of Echt and coworkers[26] in which plasma lidocaine concentrations were determined, lidocaine clearly increased defibrillation energy requirements at therapeutic plasma concentrations. This effect upon threshold occurred despite a regularization of the waveform morphology in the right ventricular electrogram toward a less chaotic pattern.

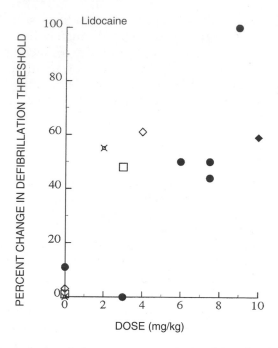

Fig. 11-11. Metaanalysis of dose-response relationships for lidocaine. Each data symbol represents a different published study: filled circles (Echt DS, Cato EL, Coxe DR: pH-dependent effects of lidocaine on defibrillation energy requirements in dogs, *Circulation* 80:1003, 1989), squares (Babbs CF, Whistler SJ, Geddes LA: Elevation of ventricular defibrillation threshold in dogs by antiarrhythmic drugs, *Am Heart J* 98:H435, 1979), filled diamond (Kerber RE: Effect of lidocaine and bretylium on energy requirements for transthoracic defibrillation: experimental studies, *J Am Coll Cardiol* 7:397, 1986), open diamond (Dorian P et al: Lidocaine causes a reversible, concentration-dependent increase in defibrillation energy requirements, *J Am Coll Cardiol* 8:327, 1986), crossed circle (Chow MSS et al: The effect of lidocaine and bretylium on the defibrillation threshold during cardiac arrest and cardiopulmonary resuscitation, *Proceedings of the Society for Experimental Biology and Medicine* 182:63, 1986).

In other experiments[26] the increase in defibrillation threshold by lidocaine was enhanced in the presence of acidosis and reversed in the presence of alkalosis, a finding consistent with the hypothesis that only the ionized form of the drug (pK_a 7.9) interacts with ion channels. Interestingly if one computes the proportion of lidocaine in the ionized, positively charged form using blood pH data, the pK_a of the drug, and the relationship

$$\frac{[L]}{[LH^+]} = 10^{pH - pK_a}$$

one finds that when the proportion of positively charged lidocaine increased from 76% to 83% during experimental acidosis, the E_{50} current and voltage (proportional to the square root of the energy) increased by 20%. Conversely when the proportion of positively charged lidocaine decreased from 94% to 65%, the threshold current and voltage decreased by 32%. These findings indicate a roughly proportional relationship between the amount of ionized lidocaine in the system and the effects of the drug on defibrillation field strength. Such findings provide strong experimental evidence that lidocaine alters defibrillation threshold by understandable ionic mechanisms.

Despite multiple and well-repeated animal studies, however,[5,17,23,26,48] clinical trials in humans[47] have not shown a clear or statistically significant effect of lidocaine upon defibrillation threshold (Table 11-2). This discrepancy could well be explained simply by the dose effect seen in Fig. 11-11, since the loading doses of 2 to 8 mg/kg IV in the canine studies that showed threshold elevation exceed the usual clinical doses. Further, in the settings in which lidocaine is usually used, such as in the control of ventricular arrhythmias in patients hospitalized for acute myocardial infarction, external defibrillation with more than adequate reserve energy is always available. Hence the adverse consequences of modest threshold elevation by lidocaine can be circumvented by the use of slightly higher energy. Thus compared to many controversial issues in cardiology the interaction of lidocaine with defibrillation shocks is a relatively well-studied and well-understood phenomenon, which need not be of concern in the acute care of the cardiac patient.

BRETYLIUM

The interpretation of bretylium effects in defibrillation is rendered difficult by the drug's multiple modes of action, including initial stimulation of catecholamine release with marked hypertension (during perfusing rhythms), followed by delayed antifibrillatory effects after uptake of the drug by the myocardium.[24] In addition to the original study of Tacker et al.,[64] Chow and coworkers[17] also found a slight decrease in ventricular defibrillation threshold after bretylium administration, which in the latter study did not reach statistical significance. A similar effect was observed by Kerber and coworkers,[48] who found that a 7 mg/kg intravenous dose of bretylium caused a 25% fall in defibrillation threshold in pentobarbital anesthetized dogs. However, Koo and coworkers[50] tested two doses of intravenous bretylium (10 and 30 mg/kg), which produced large changes in heart rate and arterial blood pressure and found no effects upon defibrillation threshold during a subsequent 4-hour monitoring period. Since all reports indicate either no change or a small decrease in threshold after bretylium, an overview of the literature clearly suggests little influence of this drug (Fig. 11-12), with little evidence of a dose-related effect. Unlike class I antiarrhythmics, bretylium, a class III agent, has never been shown to significantly increase threshold. The experimental class III agent, clofilium, has been shown to have a similar effect upon defib-

Table 11-2
Transventricular Defibrillation Thresholds in Patients Undergoing Open Heart Surgery

	Threshold current (amps)	Threshold energy (watt-seconds)
Controls	11.4	6.9
(no drug)	7.5	3.1
	4.1	1.2
	8.8	4.2
	7.7	2.9
	9.1	4.2
	6.8	3.1
	8.8	3.3
	10.9	5.8
	5.5	1.6
	10.7	6.1
	12.3	6.8
	12.9	7.9
	11.1	6.6
	0.8	0.1
	12.2	7.8
	4.0	1.7
	5.6	1.7
mean (n = 18)	8.3	4.2
S.D.	3.4	2.5
Lidocaine	5.5	1.9
(2 mg/kg IV)	5.8	1.7
	5.2	1.3
	16.2	14.6
	8.3	2.8
	9.4	4.6
	8.4	3.9
	13.7	8.0
	7.3	2.7
	8.2	3.4
	18.4	21.3
	12.2	8.2
mean (n = 12)	9.9	6.2
S.D.	4.3	6.1

Patients were studied at the Houston Veterans Administration Hospital from 6/6/78 to 7/16/79 to determine if lidocaine at clinical doses alters direct transventricular defibrillation threshold during open heart surgery. Prior to discontinuation of cardiopulmonary bypass, during which spontaneous or electrically induced ventricular fibrillation was sustained, damped sinusoidal waveform shocks of 1.5, 5, 10, 20, or 40 watt-seconds were delivered in rapid succession through paddle electrodes matched to heart size until ventricular defibrillation was achieved (single fibrillation–multiple shock technique). Defibrillation threshold was estimated as the mean of the shock intensity that defibrillated and the greatest shock intensity that did not: that is, (hit + miss)/2. Delivered energy was calculated from peak voltage, peak current, and the internal resis-

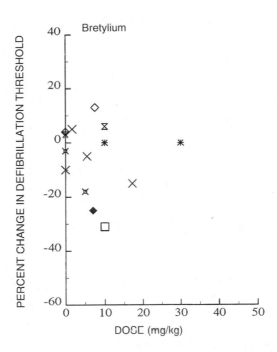

Fig. 11-12. Metaanalysis of dose-response relationships for bretylium. Each data symbol represents a different published study: square (Tacker WA et al: The effect of newer antiarrhythmic drugs on defibrillation threshold, *Crit Care Med* 8:177, 1980), star (Koo CC, Allen D, Frank-Pantridge J: Lack of effect of bretylium tosylate on electrical ventricular defibrillation in a controlled study, *Cardiovasc Res* 18:762, 1984), open diamond (Dorian, P et al: Effect of quinidine and bretylium on defibrillation energy requirements, *Am Heart J* 112:19, 1986), solid diamond (Kerber RE: Effect of lidocaine and bretylium on energy requirements for transthoracic defibrillation: experimental studies, *J Am Coll Cardiol* 7:397, 1986), crosses (Tacker WA et al: The effect of newer antiarrhythmic drugs on defibrillation threshold, *Crit Care Med* 8:177, 1980), crossed circle (Chow MSS et al: The effect of lidocaine and bretylium on the defibrillation threshold during cardiac arrest and cardiopulmonary resuscitation, *Proceedings of the Society for Experimental Biology and Medicine* 182:63, 1986).

---

tance, inductance, and capacitance of the defibrillator, as described by Babbs and Whistler.[4] Other details were as reported previously.[9] For the combined study groups visually estimated heart weight was 538 g, bypass time was 56 minutes, perfusion pressure was 76 mmHg, blood pH was 7.4, and serum potassium was 4.1 mEq/L (mean values). These parameters were not different for lidocaine treated vs. non–drug-treated patients. Although mean threshold energy was approximately 50% greater in lidocaine-treated patients, the study was discontinued because of the clinically satisfactory low-energy requirements in both groups and because of the high variability among patients, which would have dictated an exceedingly large study population to demonstrate a statistically significant drug effect.

rillation threshold,[64] with less depression of arterial blood pressure after defibrillation.

AMIODARONE

Fogoros, Fiedler, and Elson[33] have proposed a strategy for the selective use of amiodarone and the implantable defibrillator for the prevention of sudden death, and in the year 1987 half (304/618) of patients implanted with Intec Systems' ICD were being treated with amiodarone, either alone or in conjunction with other antiarrhythmic drugs.[30] This class III agent has the theoretical advantage of not being a pure sodium channel blocking agent, and the drug was originally considered to have a low incidence of side effects and toxicity. Electrophysiologic actions, including prolongation of action potential duration and effective refractory period without prolongation of QRS duration of the cardiac electrogram, suggest an ionic mechanism related to decreased potassium conductance.[71] Long-term toxicity, however, has tended to dampen enthusiasm for its use.[28,30] In experimental studies high-dose (10 mg/kg) intravenous amiodarone decreases defibrillation energy by about 20% in dogs, whereas chronic, oral amiodarone has no effect.[30] Although not ideal from the standpoint of toxicity, amiodarone is the only drug in clinical use that has been shown both to increase fibrillation threshold and to decrease defibrillation threshold.

VERAPAMIL AND OTHER CALCIUM ENTRY BLOCKERS

In contrast to the unimpressive effects of lidocaine upon defibrillation threshold in human patients, Jones and coworkers[47] found a clear elevation in threshold by about 50% in energy following 10 mg IV doses of verapamil in a small series of 12 patients, suggesting a need for caution in the use of verapamil in patients with ICDs having small defibrillation threshold margins at the time of implantation. In contrast Kerber and co-workers,[48] studying a different calcium entry blocker, found no effect upon defibrillation success of infusions of nisoldipine sufficient to reduce blood pressure either 10 or 20%. Since the various calcium entry blockers have widely differing chemical structures and therefore a wide spectrum of ancillary effects, it is reasonable to suggest that the verapamil effect upon defibrillation may not be related to calcium currents per se, but rather to sodium or potassium currents at higher doses, as suggested by the abrupt upturn in the composite dose-response curve in Fig. 11-13. This interpretation is consistent with the more comprehensive study of Hite, Kerber, and their coworkers,[43] who found that verapamil and diltiazem reduced percent successful defibrillation as a function of energy (that is, increased E_{50}), while nifedipine did not. All three drugs, however, were effective in blunting the apparent adrenergic response to the cardiac fibrillation-arrest-defibrillation sequence, an observation possibly related to their α receptor blocking activity.[43] However, Capparelli[16] noted that resus-

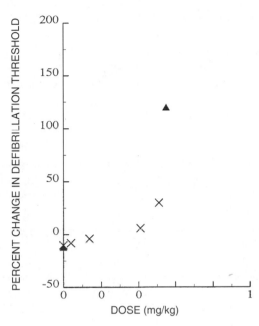

Fig. 11-13. Metaanalysis of dose-response relationships for verapamil. Each data symbol represents a different published study: crosses (Tacker WA et al: The effect of newer antiarrhythmic drugs on defibrillation threshold, *Crit Care Med* 8:177, 1980), filled triangles (Hite PR et al: Effect of calcium channel blockers on hemodynamic responses to defibrillation, *Am Heart J* 117:569, 1989).

citation success was improved in animals with electrically induced ventricular fibrillation by prior administration of the calcium entry blocker diltiazem. Because of the various structural types of calcium entry blockers, their various secondary effects, and their possible nonlinear dose-response curves, as suggested by Fig. 11-13, a simple description of the interaction of calcium blockers with defibrillation may not be possible. Clearly large numbers of patients with cardiac disease are taking oral calcium entry blockers, and no obvious and dramatic correlation—either positive or negative—with resuscitation success has been noted. At present the interactions of calcium blockers with electrical defibrillation, if any, remain unclear.

ADRENERGIC AGENTS

Defibrillation is often required in profoundly altered adrenergic states. On the one hand ventricular fibrillation and low-output tachycardias treated by ICDs occur during shocklike states of inherently increased adrenergic activity, or in the case of CPR exogenously administered catecholamines. Adrenergic responses are quite likely to be important if not absolutely necessary for hemodynamic recovery following defibrillation, especially if fibrillation persists for more than 30 seconds.[1,68,69] On the other hand adrenergic blocking drugs such as propranolol and selective α_1 or α_2 blocking agents are increasingly used in treating angina and hypertension in patients who may be at high risk for ventricular fibrillation. These considerations have led many investigators to contemplate and study the influence of adrenergic agents upon defibrillation threshold.

The problem is confounded experimentally however by the dramatic effects of such agents upon the cardiovascular system, which could in themselves also alter defibrillation success. For example, profound peripheral vascular constriction by alpha adrenergic agents given to an experimental animal just before the induction of fibrillation for the purpose of threshold testing would greatly increase peripheral vascular resistance. The resultant afterload on the ventricles would produce a state of increased myocardial oxygen demand prior to fibrillation. At the same time coronary arteriolar constriction may well reduce myocardial oxygen supply or at least counteract the effects of raised perfusion pressure. This functional state rather than the direct effects of adrenergic receptor stimulation may well alter the measured threshold—an idea that is supported by experimental observations that local ischemia produced by coronary artery ligation or plastic bead embolization raises defibrillation threshold.[10,61]

Similarly alpha adrenergic stimulation of veins during fibrillation may squeeze blood from the periphery into the heart, increasing ventricular filling and heart size, so as to have geometric effects upon wall stress, electrical current distributions, electrical impedance of the heart, and other factors influencing defibrillation success through mechanisms unrelated to adrenergic receptor stimulation per se. Conversely alpha blockers given to an intact animal may permit electrical defibrillation but inhibit recovery of the circulation thereafter, especially if fibrillation time exceeds 10 to 30 seconds.[1,68]

Despite such experimental difficulties there have been several partial investigations into the role of exogenous and endogenous adrenergic agents in defibrillation. Fig. 11-14 shows results of an early and previously unpublished study from the author's laboratory, in which transchest defibrillation threshold in pentobarbital anesthetized dogs was measured following intravenous infusions of the classical mixed $\beta_1 + \beta_2$ agonist isoproterenol over a wide range of logarithmically spaced doses. Fibrillation was induced electrically and the infusion stopped at the time of maximal blood-pressure response to the drug, indicating adequate tissue distribution. Then threshold was determined rapidly by repeated trials of incremented shock strength, beginning with a subthreshold shock. Because isoproterenol even in high doses causes only modest decreases in mean blood pressure with increased pulse pressure, and because isoproterenol augments rather than reduces myocardial perfusion, the confounding issues of secondary ischemia are avoided. In this way the effects of intense adrenergic stimulation were studied in partial isolation from other variables. No effect upon threshold was found. Similarly others in general have failed to note profound effects of adrenergic status or drug ther-

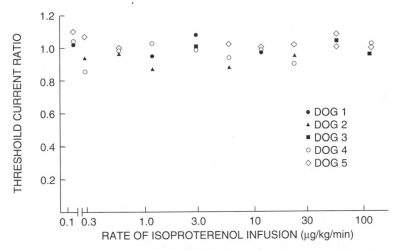

Fig. 11-14. Effect of isoproterenol infusion on transchest defibrillation threshold in pentobarbital-anesthetized dogs. Each data point represents a measured threshold value in a single animal. Threshold is unaltered by intense adrenergic stimulation caused by isoproterenol infusion at rates 30 times in excess of that producing a maximal blood pressure response (3 µg/kg/min). Saturation of cardiac beta adrenergic receptors does not alter defibrillation threshold.

apy.[54,55] The finding of Ruffy and coworkers[55] of increased threshold with the beta blocker propranolol may be readily attributed to this agent's quinidine-like antiarrhythmic effect, which is unrelated to its interaction with adrenergic receptors.[12]

Although adrenergic drugs do not appear to have profound effects on the electrical dose required to abolish fibrillation, the effects of adrenergic agonists and blockers on hemodynamic recovery following a brief period of cardiac arrest are important and have been well documented experimentally.[42,43,49,53,68] Agents with alpha blocking or other antiadrenergic activity may be especially dangerous in patients likely to suffer cardiac arrest and resuscitation—even by an ICD—because they impair perfusion of the brain and heart during cardiopulmonary resuscitation and slow recovery of blood pressure and coronary perfusion after defibrillation.

SUMMARY AND CONCLUSIONS

Drug effects upon defibrillation can be best understood at the cellular level where drugs act. Recognizing that no drug has a completely pure and singular ionic mechanism of action and that other effects such as induction of adrenergic blockade or postdefibrillation hypotension may substantially alter success, the results of many published reports are nonetheless essentially consistent with the ionic current model and with the hypothesis that the actions of drugs upon the transmembrane ionic currents in nonrefractory

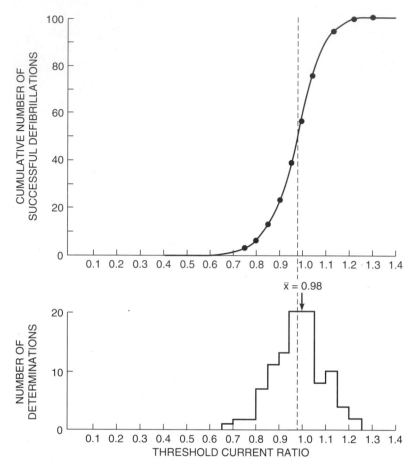

Fig. 11-15. Derivation of the relationship between defibrillation threshold data and percent success data. Actual data are shown for 100 transchest defibrillation attempts in five pentobarbital-anesthetized dogs as described in reference 3. To combine data from different animals each animal's threshold current was normalized by the mean threshold current for that animal to obtain the threshold current ratio (abscissa). For individual animals threshold data, measured to 10% tolerance in current, vary about the mean value measured in a given animal as shown in the bottom histogram. The mean threshold current ratio for the population is 0.98, corresponding to the median effective dose, or E_{50} (*dashed lines*). Half of the animals would be defibrillated by this current dose, since half have thresholds at or below this value. The remainder of the percent success curve is obtained by integration of the threshold histogram. The mean threshold value is a good estimate of the E_{50}; the mean threshold value plus 1.3 standard deviations is a good estimate of the E_{90}.

myocytes determine their effects upon electrical defibrillation threshold. The conclusions drawn from experimental studies are not dependent upon the methodological differences related to the use of external versus internal electrodes for defibrillation, the use of DFT versus E_{50} as a measure of defibrillation energy requirements, or the use of single fibrillation, multishock protocols versus multiple fibrillation, first-shock protocols.

An important limitation of most laboratory studies of the interactions of drugs with electrical ventricular defibrillation however is that with a few exceptions only normal animals with healthy hearts have been studied. Typically ventricular fibrillation is neither produced nor accompanied by myocardial ischemia, although myocardial ischemia itself has been shown to elevate defibrillation threshold in the canine model.[10,61] Possible interactions between drug effects and pathophysiology have simply not been studied. Additionally most drug studies are acute in nature, utilizing the intravenous route for clarity and simplicity. Effects of oral medications, as might be given to patients with ICDs, have been little studied. Chronic oral therapy may raise the tissue concentrations of certain metabolites, which theoretically might have more potent effects upon threshold than the parent compounds. However this consideration is entirely speculative. No such potent metabolites are presently known.

Despite these limitations there is a reasonably large and easy-to-interpret data base describing the interactions of drugs with defibrillating current in a number of animal models and clinical settings. The results obtained from many independent laboratories are consistent with the conceptual framework outlined in Figs. 11-3 and 11-6. According to this conceptual framework the defibrillating shock induces a current and voltage field in the muscle, which at the cellular level and remote from the edge effects of electrodes induces physiologic depolarization and hyperpolarization of membrane capacitances, depending on the orientation of the cell with respect to the field. Resting membranes that are depolarized sufficiently to reach the cellular threshold for sodium activation become excited and are subsequently rendered refractory for roughly the duration of the induced action potential. The simultaneous excitation of nonrefractory islands of tissue in the paths of multiple fibrillation wavelets extinguishes their self-propagation.

Drug interventions that widen the gap between resting membrane potential and threshold potential of individual nonrefractory myocytes tend to increase the field strength required to defibrillate. Conversely drug interventions that narrow the gap reduce the required field strength. Antiarrhythmic drugs that have a "local anesthetic" activity related to sodium channel blockade do not reduce the defibrillation threshold and should not be given for this purpose. At higher doses such agents clearly elevate defibrillation energy requirements, however measured. Lidocaine, which both decreases sodium conductance and increases potassium conductance in cardiac fibers, has been shown consistently to elevate defibrillation threshold, as would be predicted from Fig. 11-6. However some newer agents such as bretylium and amiodarone, which act by decreasing potassium conductance and increasing action potential duration, may have the dual advantage of reducing defibrillation threshold while preventing recurrent episodes of fibrillation. Hemodynamic recovery after defibrillation is also important for return of spontaneous circulation, and the ancillary effects of cardiac drugs upon adrenergic tone in particular can influence overall resuscitation success. In general the interactions of most cardiac drugs at ordinary clinical doses with defibrillation shocks produce modest effects upon energy requirements and the speed of recovery of the circulation. However in special situations in which energy is limited drug interactions such as those between class I antiarrhythmics and defibrillating current can be clinically important and potentially fatal.

In particular, use of the implantable cardioverter defibrillators (ICDs) in patients with recurrent, life-threatening arrhythmias[25,51] has rekindled clinical interest in drug interactions with defibrillation, because energy delivery by such implanted devices is fundamentally limited and because the majority of patients with ICDs also receive concomitant antiarrhythmic drug therapy. A drug that increases defibrillation threshold, therefore, might well have an unwanted, paradoxical effect: although the incidence of lethal arrhythmia may be reduced, the drug might also render the device ineffective, removing the patient's safety net in the event that a serious ventricular rhythm were to occur. Therapy with the wrong drug could defeat the purpose of the device, making worthless the cost, risk, and discomfort of its implantation. On the other hand therapy with a drug that decreases defibrillation threshold would on the average improve the effectiveness of the device, although such an effect could not be relied upon consistently, owing to variable patient compliance with the therapeutic regimen and variable drug concentration in the myocardium as a function of time.

Presently this issue poses a clinical dilemma in the management of patients with ICDs, since no ideal, main-line agents that both reduce the risk of fibrillation and also reduce defibrillation threshold are available and widely accepted for this application. It is certainly reasonable to exclude encainide and flecainide because of their profound effects on threshold. These newer class IC agents may increase defibrillation threshold to a greater degree than other antiarrhythmic agents. Lidocaine can increase defibrillation threshold dose-dependently and reversibly in animals.[5,23] However similar effects have not been observed at clinically usual doses in man.[41,47] Evidently the lidocaine effect at clinical doses in humans is minimal compared to the variability in defibrillation energy requirements among patients (Table 11-2). Further, when lidocaine is given acutely in the hospital setting, where back-up external defibrillation is available, concerns about its effects upon defibrillation threshold should be minimal. Class III antiarrhythmics including bretylium, clofilium, and amiodarone all slightly lower defibrillation threshold. However their chronic toxicity makes them less than ideal for combined use with ICDs for the prevention of sudden cardiac death. Adrenergic agonists and blockers of various types appear to have little direct effect upon defibrillation threshold, although such agents can profoundly alter recovery of the circulation after defibrillation,[53,57,69] owing to their actions on vasomotor tone and blood flow distribution during the arrest-resuscitation sequence. Although there is no ideal drug for arrhythmia prophylaxis in patients with ICDs, low- or normal-dose quinidine or procainamide, or newer agents such as amiodarone, are likely to have few untoward effects upon the success of ventricular defibrillation.

In general the dual hypotheses that defibrillation happens because of simultaneous stimulation of a critical mass of nonrefractory myocardium and that drugs may influence the process of electrical defibrillation by their effects upon transmembrane ionic currents within this critical mass have held up well following a decade of laboratory and clinical studies. These concepts are likely to be useful in predicting and understanding the interactions of future drugs with cardiac defibrillation.

APPENDIX: THRESHOLD VS. PERCENT SUCCESS CURVES

Consider an experiment in which a defibrillation threshold value is determined in an animal model of electrically induced fibrillation by testing shocks of decreasing intensity until failure to defibrillate is observed. In such protocols most investigators have defined defibrillation threshold as the lowest first-shock intensity that actually defibrillated but was no more than 10% greater than a shock that did not defibrillate.[13] If one repeats this experiment many times in the same stable, anesthetized animal, defibrillation threshold data will vary somewhat, owing to factors such as the random placement of shocks within the 10% tolerance window, changes in chest geometry and impedance with respiration, and the random pattern of fibrillation wavelets progressing through the ventricular muscle mass at the instant the shock is applied. As a result the measured threshold values from a single animal will be distributed as shown in the histogram of Fig. 11-15 (*bottom*). To express the data in terms of percent success, it is only necessary to integrate the histogram and scale the result to 100%. This integration is based upon the following thought experiment, given the histogram data. If a test shock were applied that is greater than or equal to 10% of the measured threshold values, it would defibrillate 10% of the time. If a test shock were applied that is greater than or equal to 50% of the measured threshold values, it would defibrillate 50% of the time, etc. In turn the median threshold value is the shock strength that would defibrillate 50% of the time, which is a good estimate of the median effective dose or E_{50} value. For symmetrical distributions, such as those in Fig. 11-15, the mean is an excellent and unbiased estimator of the median,[18] and so we can say that the mean threshold value for a given individual is equivalent to the E_{50}. This mathematically reasonable concept has been confirmed experimentally (Fig. 11-8) in a study in which both methods of determining the minimum shock strength for defibrillation were directly compared.[14] Thus the histogram of defibrillation threshold data and the cumulative percent success curve are equivalent descriptors of the same biologic phenomenon; one curve can be obtained from the other by either differentiation or integration.

When the large number of threshold values required to form a complete histogram is not available, the percent success curve can still be estimated from the mean and standard deviation of a smaller number of threshold measurements (for example, 3 to 5), assuming a Gaussian distribution of the underlying threshold histogram. Then the mean threshold value plus one half standard deviation is the shock strength corresponding to 69% success; the mean threshold value plus one standard deviation is the shock strength corresponding to 84% success; the mean threshold value plus 1.3 standard deviations is the shock strength corresponding to 90% success; and the mean threshold value plus two standard deviations is the shock strength corresponding to 98% success. By drawing a smooth curve through these points (and symmetrically for the 2%, 10%, 16%, and 31% points) it is possible to reconstruct a good estimate of the entire percent success curve in a given subject under stable conditions. Conversely if experimental data are reported only in terms of percent success, the mean threshold and standard deviation can be determined from 50%, 16%, and 84% success points of an interpolated percent success curve.

REFERENCES

1. Abboud FM, Pansegrau DG, Mark AL: Autonomic responses to ventricular defibrillation. In *Proceedings, cardiac defibrillation conference*, 11-15, West Lafayette, Ind., 1975, Purdue University.
2. Babbs CF: Drug induced changes in ventricular defibrillation threshold, Ph.D. Thesis, Purdue University, December 1977.
3. Babbs CF, Whistler SJ, Yim GKW: Temporal stability and precision of ventricular defibrillation threshold data, *Am J Physiol* 95:331, 1978.
4. Babbs CF, Whistler SJ: Evaluation of the operating internal resistance, inductance, and capacitance of intact damped sine wave defibrillators, *Med Instrum* 12:34, 1978.
5. Babbs CF, Whistler SJ, Geddes LA: Elevation of ventricular defibrillation threshold in dogs by antiarrhythmic drugs, *Am Heart J* 98:H345, 1979.
6. Babbs CF et al: Dependence of defibrillation threshold upon extracellular/intracellular K$^+$ concentrations, *J Electrocardiology* 13:7, 1980.
7. Babbs CF et al: Therapeutic indices for damped sinusoidal defibrillator shocks: effective, damaging, and lethal electrical doses, *Am Heart J* 99:734, 1980.
8. Babbs CF: Alteration of defibrillation

threshold by antiarrhythmic drugs: a theoretical framework, *Crit Care Med* 9:362, 1981.
9. Babbs CF et al: Human transventricular defibrillation threshold, *Proceedings, 16th Annual AAMI Meeting*, May 1981.
10. Babbs CF et al: Effects of myocardial infarction on catheter defibrillation threshold, *Med Instrum* 17:18, 1983.
11. Ballin JC: *AMA Drug Evaluations*, American Medical Association, Chicago, 1980.
12. Bigger JT, Hoffman BH: Antiarrhythmic drugs. In Gilman AG, editor: *Goodman and Gilman's the pharmacological basis of therapeutics*, ed 6, Macmillan, New York, 1980, pp 761-792.
13. Bourland JD, Tacker WA, Geddes LA: Strength-duration curves for trapezoidal waveforms of various tilts for transchest defibrillation in animals, *Med Instrum* 12:38, 1978.
14. Bourland JD et al: Ventricular defibrillation threshold: its relationship to the chance of defibrillating a subject, *Proceedings AAMI 17th Annual Meeting*, May 9-12, 1982.
15. Campbell NPS et al: Transthoracic ventricular defibrillation in adults, *Br Med J* 2:1379, 1977.
16. Capparelli EV et al: Diltiazem improves

resuscitation from ventricular fibrillation in dogs, *Clin Res* 35:226A, 1987 (abstract).

17. Chow MSS et al: The effect of lidocaine and bretylium on the defibrillation threshold during cardiac arrest and cardiopulmonary resuscitation, *Proceedings of the Society for Experimental Biology and Medicine* 182:63, 1986.

18. Cooper BE: *Statistics for experimentalists*, Oxford UK, 1969, Permagon Press.

19. Coraboeuf E: Ionic basis of electrical activity in cardiac tissues, *Am J Physiol* 234:H101, 1978.

20. Davy JM: Is there a defibrillation threshold? *Circulation* 70 (Suppl II): II-406, 1984 (abstract).

21. Dawson AK, Steinberg MI, Shapland JE: Effect of class I and class III drugs on current and energy required for internal defibrillation, *Circulation* 72:384, 1985 (abstract).

22. Deeb GM et al: The effects of cardiovascular drugs on the defibrillation threshold and the pathological effects on the heart using an automatic implantable defibrillator, *Ann Thorac Surg* 35:361, 1983.

23. Dorian P et al: Lidocaine causes a reversible, concentration-dependent increase in defibrillation energy requirements, *J Am Coll Cardiol* 8:327, 1986.

24. Dorian P et al: Effect of quinidine and bretylium on defibrillation energy requirements, *Am Heart J* 112:19, 1986.

25. Echt DS et al: Clinical experience, complications and survival in 70 patients with the automatic implantable cardioverter/defibrillator, *Circulation* 71:291, 1985.

26. Echt DS, Cato EL, Coxe DR: pH-dependent effects of lidocaine on defibrillation energy requirements in dogs, *Circulation* 80:1003, 1989.

27. Ehrenstein G: Ion channels in nerve membranes, *Physics Today*, 33, October 1976.

28. Ewy GA: Management of the complications of acute myocardial infarction. In Ewy GA, Bressler R, editors: *Cardiovascular drugs and the management of heart disease*, New York, 1982, Raven Press, pp 521-568.

29. Fain ES et al: Effects of encainide and its metabolites on energy requirements for defibrillation, *Circulation* 73:1334, 1986.

30. Fain ES, Lee JT, Winkle RA: Effects of acute intravenous and chronic oral amiodarone on defibrillation energy requirements, *Am Heart J* 114:8, 1987.

31. Fenster PE: Clinical use of antidysrhythmic agents; procainamide, quinidine, and disopyramide. In Ewy GA, Bressler R, editors: *Cardiovascular drugs and the management of heart disease*, New York, 1982, Raven Press, pp 115-129.

32. Fishler M, Thakor N: Cellsim: a cellular model of defibrillation, *Am Heart J* 124:833, 1992 (abstract).

33. Fogoros RN, Fiedler SB, Elson JJ: Prevention of sudden death: a strategy for the selective use of amiodarone and the automatic implantable defibrillator, *Circulation* 72:385, 1985 (abstract).

34. Frank JS, Langer GA: The myocardial interstitium: its structure and its role in ionic exchange, *J Cell Biol* 60:586, 1974.

35. Garrey WE: The nature of fibrillary contraction of the heart, *Am J Physiol* 33:397, 1914.

36. Geddes LA et al: The electrical dose for ventricular defibrillation with electrodes applied directly to the heart, *J Thorac Cardiovasc Surg* 68:593, 1974.

37. Geddes LA, Baker LE: *Principles of applied biomedical instrumentation*, New York, 1975, Wiley-Interscience.

38. Gold JH et al: Transthoracic ventricular defibrillation in the 100 kg calf with unidirectional rectangular pulses, *Circulation* 56:745, 1977.

39. Goldstein A, Aronow L, Kalman SM: *Principles of drug action: the basis of pharmacology*, ed 2, New York, 1974, John Wiley.

40. Hahn SJ: Multiple epicardial shocks during a fibrillation episode do not alter characteristics of defibrillation probability curves, *Am Heart J* 124:832, 1992 (abstract).

41. Haynes RE et al: Comparison of bretylium tosylate and lidocaine in management of out of hospital ventricular fibrillation: a randomized clinical trial, *Am J Cardiol* 48:353, 1981.

42. Hernandez R et al: Effects of flecainide on defibrillation thresholds in the anesthetized dog, *J Am Coll Cardiol* 14:777, 1989.

43. Hite PR et al: Effect of calcium channel blockers on hemodynamic responses to defibrillation, *Am Heart J* 117:569, 1989.

44. Hodgkin AL, Huxley AF: A quantitative description of membrane current and its

application to conduction and excitation in nerve, *J Physiol* 117:500, 1952.

45. Hoffman BF, Bigger JT: Digitalis and allied cardiac glycosides. In Gilman AG, editor: *Goodman and Gilman's the pharmacological basis of therapeutics*, ed 6, New York, 1980, Macmillan.

46. Jones DL et al: Bretylium decreases and verapamil increases defibrillation threshold in pigs, *Circulation* (submitted).

47. Jones JL et al: Effects of lidocaine and verapamil on defibrillation in humans, *J Electrocardiol* 24:299, 1991.

48. Kerber RE: Effect of lidocaine and bretylium on energy requirements for transthoracic defibrillation: experimental studies, *J Am Coll Cardiol* 7:397, 1986.

49. Kieso RA, Fox-Eastham K, Kerber RE: Effect of nisoldipine on hemodynamic responses to defibrillation, *Am Heart J* 121:834, 1991.

50. Koo CC, Allen D, Frank-Pantridge J: Lack of effect of bretylium tosylate on electrical ventricular defibrillation in a controlled study, *Cardiovasc Res* 18:762, 1984.

51. Mirowski M, Reid PR, Winkle RA: Mortality in patients with implanted automatic defibrillators, *Ann Intern Med* 98:585, 1983.

52. Niebauer MJ et al: The efficacy and safety of defibrillation with 10-millisecond trapezoidal waves of different tilts, *Med Instrum* 18:119, 1984.

53. Pearson JW, Redding JS: Influence of peripheral vascular tone on cardiac resuscitation, *Anesth Analg* 44:746, 1965.

54. Rattes MF et al: Adrenergic effects on internal cardiac defibrillation threshold, *Am J Physiol* 22:H500, 1987.

55. Ruffy R, Schechtman K, Monje E: Beta-adrenergic modulation of direct defibrillation energy in anaesthetized dog heart, *Am J Physiol* 17:H674, 1985.

56. Sano T, Tsuchihashi H, Shimamoto T: Ventricular fibrillation studied by the microelectrode method, *Circ Res* 6:41, 1958.

57. Stephenson HE: Pharmacology of resuscitation—vasopressors, Chapter 46, in *Cardiac arrest and resuscitation*, St Louis, 1974, CV Mosby.

58. Strunk W, White EB: *The Elements of Style*, New York, 1979, Macmillan.

59. Sweeney RJ, Gill RM, Reid PR: Effect of shock duration on refractory period extension by defibrillation shocks, *Am Heart J* 124:835, 1992 (abstract).

60. Tacker WA et al: Energy dosage for human trans-chest electrical ventricular defibrillation, *N Engl J Med* 290:214, 1974.

61. Tacker WA et al: Electrical threshold for defibrillation of canine ventricles following myocardial infarction, *Am Heart J* 88:476, 1974.

62. Tacker WA et al: Alteration of electrical defibrillation threshold by the cardiac glycoside, ouabain, in *Proceedings, Cardiac Defibrillation Conference*, 129-133, West Lafayette, Indiana, 1975, Purdue University.

63. Tacker WA, Geddes LA: Electrical criteria for defibrillation: current, energy and charge and the requirements for damped sinusoidal current. In *Electrical defibrillation*, Boca Raton, Florida, 1980, CRC Press.

64. Tacker WA et al: The effect of newer antiarrhythmic drugs on defibrillation threshold, *Crit Care Med* 8:177, 1980.

65. Witkowski FX, Penkoske PA, Plonsey R: Mechanism of cardiac defibrillation in open-chest dogs with unipolar DC-coupled simultaneous activation and shock potential recordings, *Circulation* 82:244, 1990.

66. Woodbury WJ: Cellular electrophysiology of the heart. In Hamilton WF, editor: *Handbook of Physiology, vol I, sect 2, "Circulation,"* Washington DC, 1962, American Physiological Society.

67. Woolfolk DI et al: The effect of quinidine on electrical energy required for ventricular defibrillation, *Am Heart J* 72:659, 1966.

68. Yakaitis RW, Otto CW, Blitt CD: Relative importance of alpha and beta adrenergic receptors during resuscitation, *Crit Care Med* 7:293, 1979.

69. Yakaitis RW et al: Influence of time and therapy on ventricular defibrillation in dogs, *Crit Care Med* 8:157, 1980.

70. Zipes DP et al: Termination of ventricular fibrillation in dogs by depolarizing a critical amount of myocardium, *Am J Cardiol* 36:37, 1975.

71. Zipes DP, Troup PJ: New antiarrhythmic agents, *Am J Cardiol* 41:1005, 1978.

72. Zipes DP, Prystowsky EN, Heger JJ: Electrophysiology and pharmacology of aprindine, encainide, and propafenone, *Ann New York Acad Sci* 432:201, 1984.

Chapter 12
Cardiac Damage from Transchest and ICD Defibrillator Shocks

John F. Van Vleet
W.A. Tacker, Jr.

Most of the adverse responses to defibrillator shocks described in this chapter can be characterized as irreversible. Such responses are exemplified by mortality or myocardial necrosis. Other changes such as S-T segment shifts are not by themselves indicators of irreversible damage. The propensity of alternating current (AC) defibrillating shocks to cause more damage than direct current (DC) defibrillating shocks contributed in part to the abandonment of AC defibrillation, but several of the early descriptions of AC-induced necrosis led to our present understanding of the damage process.[22,27,32,45,47] In this chapter attention is directed mostly toward the response to DC shocks.

MORTALITY

Electric shocks for defibrillation can produce death in three ways. The first is by precipitating ventricular fibrillation when a relatively weak shock is applied during the ventricular vulnerable period. If the ventricular fibrillation is not converted back to a functional rhythm, death will occur. A different phenomenon can also cause fibrillation. When an extremely powerful shock is applied, the phenomenon of intractable fibrillation may follow, in which case the ventricles are apparently in a state of fibrillation that will not respond to a defibrillating shock. The third mechanism leading to death is cardiogenic shock. Several etiologic factors may cause failure, such as electromechanical dissociation, conduction block, damage to contractile fibers, or functional destruction of a large mass of ventricular tissue.

259

MYOCARDIAL NECROSIS

Delivery of large suprathreshold defibrillation shocks may produce morphologic alterations in cardiac tissue.* The lesions are well documented at the gross, microscopic, and ultrastructural levels.

GROSS MORPHOLOGIC ALTERATIONS

The appearance and distribution of these alterations vary somewhat with the various shock delivery systems. Thus the lesions may be different for (1) transchest shocks, (2) open-chest shocks applied by electrodes on the cardiac surface, and (3) shocks delivered internally be devices such as an automatic implantable cardioverter-defibrillator (ICD) by either epicardial patch electrodes and/or intracavitary electrode catheters. The findings for these three types of defibrillator systems will be presented separately.

Damage from Transchest Shocks

Van Vleet et al.[61] described the progression of morphologic changes in dogs from 2 hours to 8 weeks after excessively strong transchest shocks. Shocks of threshold intensity produced no morphologic changes. With stronger shocks, white zones of damage were grossly visible on the right and left ventricular free walls, more or less in a direct path between the electrodes. These lesions appear 2 hours to 1 day after shocking. The most striking change in progression of the gross lesions at 2 days, 4 days, and 2 weeks after shocking is a change to yellowish white, dry areas of necrosis and calcification.

The lesions are usually located in the anterior wall of the left and/or right ventricle (Figs. 12-1 to 12-6; Plate 2, **A** to **H**). Lesions also appear above the cardiac apex on either side of the left anterior descending coronary artery. The damage is most often subepicardial; but it may extend deep into or throughout the free wall of the ventricles (Figs. 12-4 and 12-5, *B*; Plates 2, **E** and **G**). Similar areas of damage may be on the posterior wall of the right ventricle near the posterolateral margin of the heart. The atria are not usually affected. The transmural lesions usually occur in the thinnest part of the affected free wall, where trabecular structure provides easy access for current to reach the low-resistivity blood in the affected chamber.

Epicardial lesions appear as pale areas that sometimes contain red, hemorrhagic patches (Figs. 12-3, *A* and *B*; Plates 2, **C** and **D**). In many instances the myocardial damage is localized around coronary vessels suggesting that current is shunted through vessels, causing a high current density around them.

Not all lesions are transmural as can be shown by sectioning the myocardium (Figs. 12-4 and 12-5, *B*; Plates 2, **E** and **G**). Less extensive lesions appear near the epicardium and may be deeper with stronger shocks, affect-

Text continues on p. 265.

*References 24, 25, 38, 40, 41, 44, 51, 53, 62, 64.

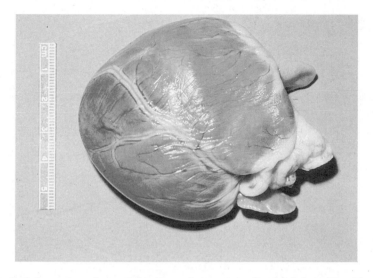

Fig. 12-1. Left lateral surface of the heart from an unshocked dog. (See Plate 2, **A**.)

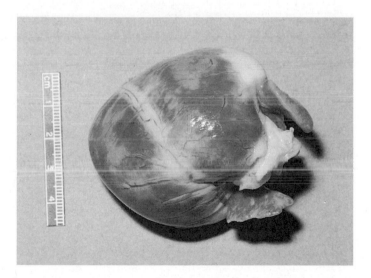

Fig. 12-2. Myocardial necrosis in a dog given a large single transthoracic shock (20 A/Kg body weight) 1 day previously. Large pale areas of necrosis are present in the right and left ventricular walls. (See Plate 2, **B**.)

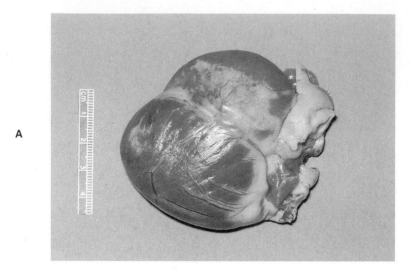

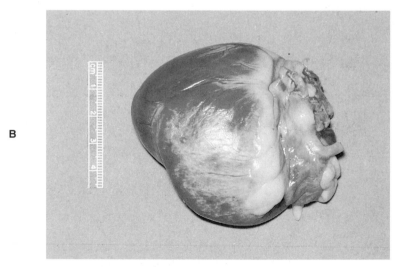

Fig. 12-3. A, Left lateral surface of the heart of a dog that received a large single transthoracic shock (16.7 A/Kg body weight) 2 days previously. **B**, Right lateral surface of the same heart. Prominent yellowish-white areas of right and left ventricular necrosis are seen with several reddish areas of hemorrhage. (See Plates 2, **C** and **D**.)

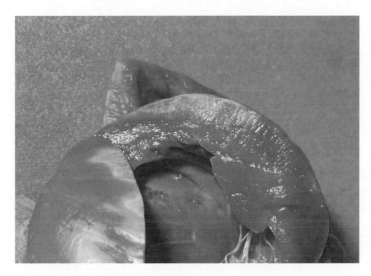

Fig. 12-4. Incised left ventricular wall shows pale areas of myocardial necrosis extending up to one third of the wall thickness. Dog received a large single transthoracic shock (15.2 A/Kg body weight) 2 days previously. (See Plate 2, **E**.)

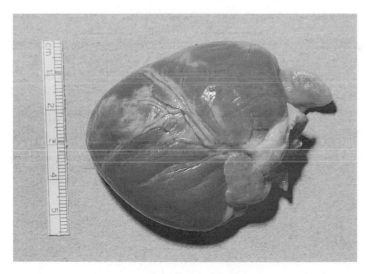

Fig. 12-5. A, Left lateral surface of the heart of a dog given a large single transthoracic shock (15 A/Kg body weight) 4 days previously has irregular pale areas of myocardial necrosis in the left and right ventricular walls. (See Plate 2, **F**.)

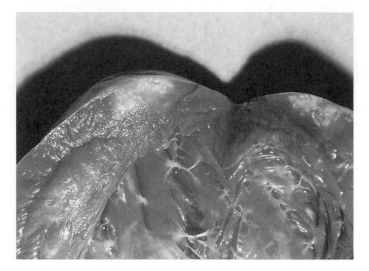

Fig. 12-5. B, Incised left ventricular wall has pale subendocardial areas of necrosis. (See Plate 2, **G.**)

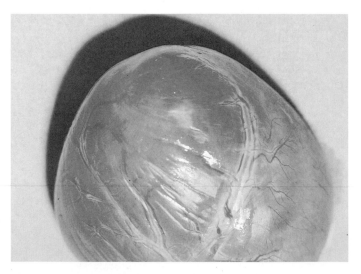

Fig. 12-6. Irregularly shaped pale area of postnecrotic scarring is seen in the left ventricular apex in the heart of a dog given a large single transthoracic shock (15 A/Kg body weight) 8 weeks previously. (See Plate 2, **H.**)

ing the endocardium last. Only with very strong shocks and transmural damage is the septum involved.

After 2 weeks lesions appear as white areas on the epicardial surface. Eight weeks after shocking, the damaged areas are small, pale, shrunken, and firm areas of scarring (Fig. 12-6; Plate 2, **H**).

Damage from Open-chest Shocks Delivered by Electrodes on the Cardiac Surface

The lesions produced when the shocks are applied directly to the surface of the heart share most of the characteristics of the transchest shock lesions.[10,58] No necrosis is seen when a threshold shock is delivered. When higher-intensity shocks are applied, there are a few differences from the lesions seen with transchest shocks, including inflammatory changes produced by the thoracotomy, pericardiotomy, and mechanical trauma of the epicardium.

Immediately after application of excessively strong shocks, tissue under the electrode may become somewhat pale, swollen, and turgid, presumably as a result of tissue edema. The lesions are similar for either electrode polarity (positive or negative). After 48 hours, the damage is grossly evident, characterized by a white ring of myocardial necrosis and calcification that corresponds to the perimeters of the electrodes on the outer surface of the heart (Fig. 12-7, *A*). The necrotic tissue is white, chalklike, dry, and firm. The rings of necrosis may include the atria if they are included in the current path because large electrodes are used. Epicardial lesions induced by the pericardiotomy procedure in dogs cause parietal pericardial and epicardial surfaces to become lightly adhered to each other by a thin film of fibrin, and occasional fibrin tags and small blood clots may be present. Concentrated in the same area may be epicardial, ecchymotic hemorrhages and underlying areas of pallor and swelling that blend gradually into adjacent, normal-appearing areas. Lesions may be predominantly subepicardial or transmural. Fig. 12-7, *B* shows a transmural lesion. Some lesions are mineralized by 48 hours and appear yellowish white, dry, and firm.

Damage from Internal Shocks Delivered by Implanted Defibrillator Patches and Catheters

Reports in the literature describing the gross lesions produced by these devices are sparse. The lack of reports may be a reflection of limited experience with these units in animals and human patients but may also be the result of lack of production of gross lesions. These devices are able to effectively defibrillate with relatively low shock strengths and thus may avoid the high current densities responsible for myocardial necrosis.

The several reports in dogs[8,12,15] and human patients[2,48] do not describe gross lesions from shocks delivered by epicardial patches. In our studies (Van Vleet et al., unpublished observations) we have observed gross lesions in dogs given large suprathreshold shocks by epicardial patches. Pale streaks of subepicardial necrosis may be present beneath the wire coils and around the

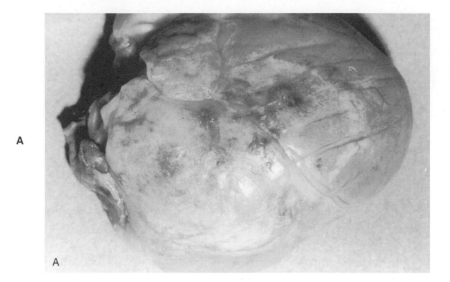

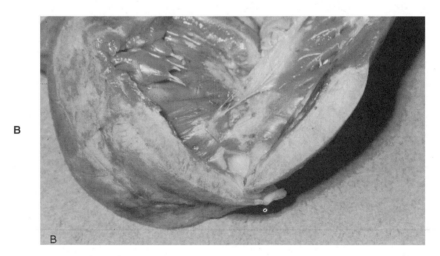

Fig. 12-7. A, Left lateral surface of the heart of a dog that received a large single shock (60 A/Kg body weight) 2 days previously on the surface of the heart. A pale rim of necrosis is seen at the area of contact with the periphery of the paddle. Multiple red areas of hemorrhage are present. **B,** Incised right ventricular wall reveals pale areas of full-thickness myocardial necrosis.

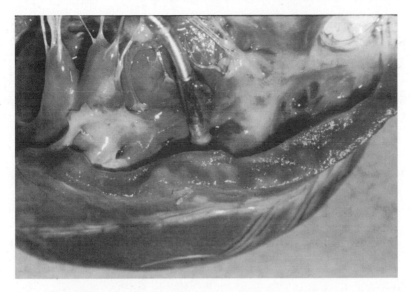

Fig. 12-8. Disseminated pale areas of myocardial necrosis are present in the right ventricular wall near the lodgement site of a defibrillator electrode catheter. The dog had received multiple near-threshold shocks at 0, 5, 12, and 26 weeks after implantation.

periphery of the attached patches when examined several days following delivery of multiple large shocks in safety studies. Dogs given near-threshold shocks generally do not have any gross evidence of myocardial damage.

In our dog studies (Van Vleet et al., unpublished observations) and in those by others[4,23,36,57] of catheter-mounted defibrillator electrodes implanted in the ventricular cavities, gross lesions have been described. Damage was detected in animals given multiple and generally large suprathreshold shocks. The lesions varied from small, pale subendocardial areas in the right ventricular free wall and ventricular septum adjacent to the catheter electrode to occasional full-wall areas of necrosis of the right ventricular wall (Fig. 12-8). Lerman et al.[36] observed areas of subendocardial hemorrhage adjacent to the catheter electrode.

MICROSCOPIC ALTERATIONS

The predominant alteration in areas of myocardial damage after very strong shocks is necrosis of cardiac muscle cells. The lethal injury to myocytes is manifested by alterations termed either hyaline necrosis, contraction-band necrosis (termed myofibrillar degeneration by some), or granular necrosis. Fibers with hyaline necrosis are swollen, hypereosinophilic-staining, and lack cross striations (Fig. 12-9). Contraction-band necrosis is distinctive as affected fibers have a "shredded" appearance with scattered transverse bands

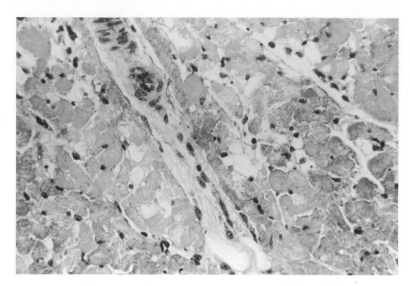

Fig. 12-9. Acute myocardial necrosis in a section of left ventricle from a dog given a large single transthoracic shock (15 A/Kg body weight) 2 days previously. The necrotic myocytes are disrupted, but a myocardial arteriole remains intact. (Hematoxylin and eosin stain; magnification × 400.)

or disks of hypercontracted, eosinophilic, contractile material (Fig. 12-10). Myocytes with granular necrosis have disrupted sarcoplasm with abundant scattered basophilic granules (Fig. 12-11) that represent mineralized mitochondria as confirmed by electron microscopy. All types of necrotic fibers have a persistent "tube" of external lamina that will remain in the condensed stromal tissue following loss of myocytes. Necrotic myocytes have nuclear alterations typical of lethal cellular injury with either shrunken dense pyknotic nuclei or disrupted nuclei termed karyorrhexis. The interstitial tissues are distended by edema, and focal hemorrhage may be present in areas with severe damage.

The distribution of necrosis in the myocardium is directly related to the type of defibrillator utilized. With transchest and epicardial surface defibrillation (either by open-chest electrode placement or by internal defibrillation by implanted patches), the lesions tend to be concentrated in the subepicardial region. With catheter-mounted electrodes the lesions are concentrated in the subendocardial area. Necrosis is most severe in areas of high current density such as occur adjacent to epicardial or endocardial leads or in the general path for current to pass through the heart between leads on the chest wall. Necrosis is frequently seen microscopically surrounding small myocardial blood vessels because current seems to flow preferentially along the low-resistivity column of blood.

The extent of necrosis in the myocardium may vary from diffuse involvement to focal damage or loss of individual cardiac muscle cells. In tissue sections collected from areas of grossly observed pallor the damage is often dif-

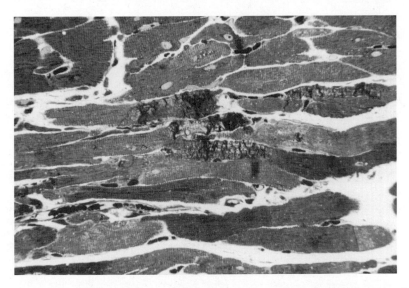

Fig. 12-10. Section of right ventricular myocardium has scattered necrotic fibers with contraction band necrosis. Dog received a single large transthoracic shock (15 A/Kg body weight) 2 days previously. (Toluidine blue stained plastic-embedded section; magnification × 400.)

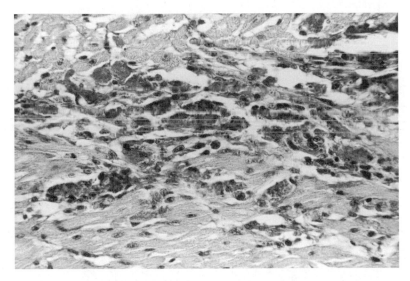

Fig. 12-11. Disseminated myocardial necrosis with mineralization in the left ventricle of a dog given a large single transthoracic shock (15 A/Kg body weight) 4 days previously. The necrotic myocytes are basophilic and disrupted. (Hematoxylin and eosin stain; magnification × 400.)

Table 12-1
Defibrillation-induced Sequential Cardiac Morphologic Alterations

Lesions	Time After Shock							
	Immediate	2 Hours	1 Day	2 Days	4 Days	2 Weeks	8 Weeks	
• Macroscopic (lesions concentrated in free walls of ventricles in a path between the electrodes; depth and width of lesions directly related to shock strength)	Pale, turgid, biventricular areas (±)	White biventricular areas	Same as at 2 hours	Yellowish white biventricular areas	Same as at 2 days	Pale, depressed, (±) biventricular areas	Same as at 2 weeks	
• Microscopic (major findings in areas of macroscopic alterations)	Myocardial edema	Myofibrillar degeneration with contraction bands, sarcoplasmic hyalinization and vacuolization, edema	Same as at 2 hours	Same as at 2 hours plus calcification of necrotic muscle fibers	Same as at 2 days, plus macrophage infiltration, fibroblast proliferation	Loss and atrophy of muscle fibers, fibrosis, stromal collapse	Same as at 2 weeks	
• Ultrastructural	Intracellular edema, mitochondrial degeneration, sarcoplasmic vacuolization	Contraction-band necrosis, mitochondrial densities, interstitial edema	Same as at 2 hours with neutrophilic infiltration	Same as at 1 day with mineralization of mitochondria	Same as at 2 days except macrophage infiltration replaces neutrophilic invasion; persisting tubes of external lamina of necrotic myocytes	Occasional macrophages, activated fibroblasts, collagen accumulation	Same as at 2 weeks with scattered atrophic myocytes with myocytolysis	

±, May be present or absent.

fuse in areas of high current density such as near electrodes and may even extend full-wall in the affected chamber. Shock-induced damage of lesser severity may produce only single or scattered small foci of necrosis in areas of high current density. With even smaller shocks only scattered individual necrotic fibers may be present. Similarly, in hearts with severe damage from large shocks, scattered necrotic fibers may be found in areas of the myocardium that are distant from the site(s) of high current density.

Van Vleet et al.[61] have characterized the sequential myocardial alterations in dogs exposed to very intense transthoracic shocks (Table 12-1). Microscopic changes at 1 or 2 days reveal calcification of necrotic cardiac muscle fibers (Figs. 12-9 and 12-10), and at 4 days there is macrophage invasion and early myocardial fibrosis. After 2 weeks cardiac muscle cell loss or atrophy and myocardial fibrosis are observed (Figs. 12-12 to 12-14). Histopathologic alterations of the 8-week lesions are focal cardiac muscle fiber loss or atrophy with surrounding myocardial and epicardial fibrosis. Calcified necrotic fibers have disappeared by this time. Residual morphologic damage in dog hearts after defibrillator shock is still clearly recognizable at 8 weeks but has regressed, leaving little functional effect.

ULTRASTRUCTURAL ALTERATIONS

Figs. 12-15 to 12-19 show ultrastructural changes. Two hours after shocking, major alterations in fibers with mild injury include glycogen depletion, mito-

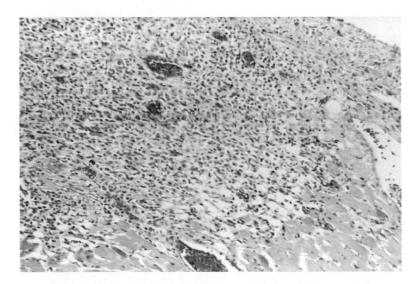

Fig. 12-12. Area of subepicardial resolving myocardial necrosis in a dog shocked ten days previously. The area of necrosis has infiltration of mononuclear leukocytes and vascular congestion. (Hematoxylin and eosin stain; magnification × 100.)

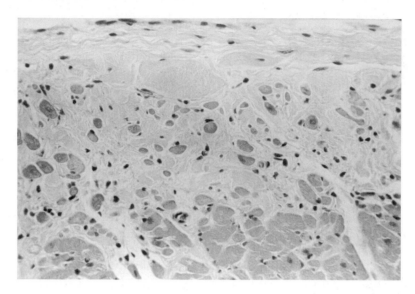

Fig. 12-13. Section of subepicardial myocardium shows fibrosis with pale eosin-ophilic collagen deposits surrounding atrophic myocytes. Left ventricle of a dog given a large single transthoracic shock (15 A/Kg body weight) eight weeks previously. (Hematoxylin and eosin stain; magnification × 400.)

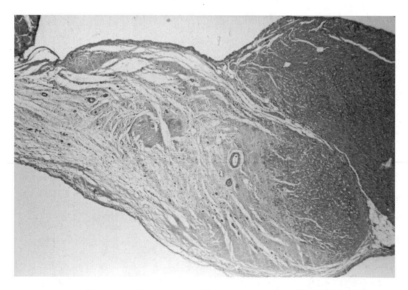

Fig. 12-14. Section of ventricular septum has myocardial fibrosis in an area of post-necrotic shock-induced damage. The dog had received multiple shocks via a right ventricular catheter electrode. (Hematoxylin and eosin stain; mag-nification × 40.)

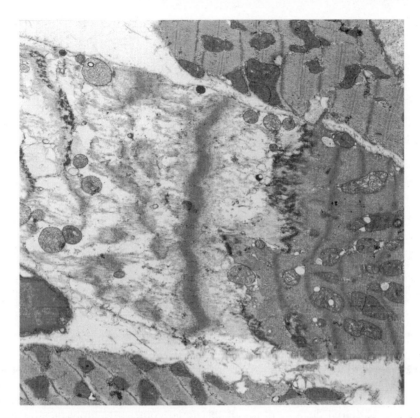

Fig. 12-15. An intercalated disk (*center*) separates the severely injured fiber (*left*) from the mildly injured fiber (*right*). In the severely injured fiber the sarcoplasm contains scattered attenuated clumps and strands of lysing fibrillar material, a dense transverse band of clumped contractile material, remnants of an intercalated disk, a few scattered mitochondria (many of which contain focal membranous thickenings), scattered tubular remnants of sarcoplasmic reticulum, and abundant lucent areas that apparently represent fluid accumulations, a few of which are membrane limited (*left center*). The sarcolemma of this fiber is composed of a persistent basal lamina and an underlying extensively disrupted plasma membrane. The mildly injured fiber segment has altered mitochondria (with decreased matrical density and disruption of cristae) and generalized loss of glycogen deposits (compared to abundant dense glycogen granules in the intact fiber on the top). The interstitium is distended by edema fluid. (Magnification × 11,000.) (From VanVleet JF et al: Acute cardiac damage in dogs given multiple transthoracic shocks with a trapezoidal waveform defibrillator, *Am J Vet Res* 38:617, 1977. With permission.)

chondrial damage, dilatation of the sarcoplasmic reticulum and T tubules, and formation of sarcoplasmic vacuoles. By 24 hours after shocking, the most prominent change in irreversibly damaged fibers is formation of hypercontraction bands and disruption of myofibrils (Figs. 12-15 and 12-16).[59] The contraction bands appear to be multiple sarcomeres laying in closely packed

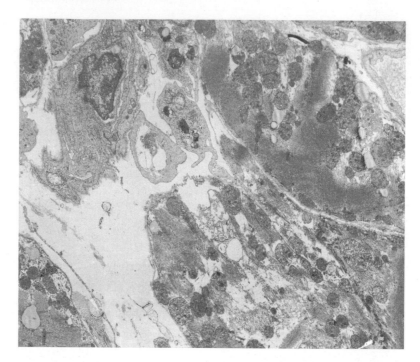

Fig. 12-16. Right ventricular myocardium 1 day after delivery of a 20 A/Kg body weight transthoracic shock. Several necrotic cardiac muscle cells and one intact fiber (*lower left*) surround a capillary. The necrotic fibers contain scattered dense clumps of disrupted contractile material and damaged mitochondria with flocculent matrical dense bodies or swelling and disruption. The interstitium contains several invading neutrophils and marked edema. The external lamina persists around necrotic fibers. (Magnification × 10,500.) (From VanVleet JF et al: Sequential ultrastructural alterations in ventricular myocardium of dogs given large, single transthoracic damped sinusoidal waveform defibrillator shocks, *Am J Vet Res* 41:493, 1980. With permission.)

stacks. These have been compared to the compressed ribs of an accordion. Often the hypercontraction pulls the sarcomeres free of their attachment to the intercalated disk. The pale intervening zones contain recognizable remnants of myofilaments, non-membrane-bound lipid droplets, and deranged mitochondria of different sizes and shapes. Some mitochondria show disrupted cristae; others contain numerous electron-dense matrical granules (Fig. 12-17). The changes of myofibrillar degeneration often stop abruptly at the intercalated disk, and apart from the sarcomere bordering the intercalated disk, which may show varying degrees of stretching and disintegration, the adjacent fibers appear relatively intact. Disruption of plasma membrane, interstitial tissue edema, scattered neutrophils, and pyknotic muscle nuclei are also seen.

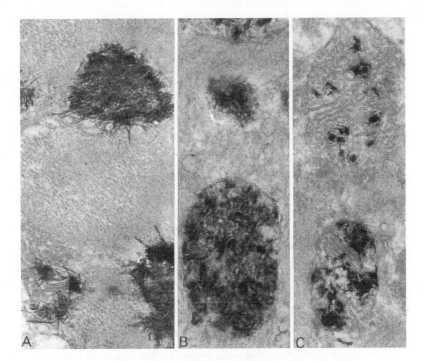

Fig. 12-17. High magnification of mitochondrial alterations in myocytes with shock-induced damage. **A**, Mineralization of mitochondria in myocyte with myofibrillar lysis. Note dark granular matrical deposits and peripheral dark interweaving spicules. (Magnification × 43,500.) **B**, Mineralized mitochondrion in necrotic myocyte has fine granular deposits in matrix and radiating "negative images" of cristae. (Magnification × 45,000.) **C**, Partially mineralized mitochondria contain focal dense granular deposits. (Magnification × 45,000.) (From VanVleet JF et al: Sequential ultrastructural alterations in ventricular myocardium of dogs given large, single transthoracic damped sinusoidal waveform defibrillator shocks, *Am J Vet Res* 41:493, 1980. With permission.)

At 2 days after shocking, necrotic myocytes have disrupted contractile material clumps. Frequently, mitochondria have matrical densities of a granular or spicular appearance indicating mineralization. The interstitium shows edema, neutrophil infiltration, and scattered fragments of sarcoplasmic debris (Fig. 12-18). Four days after shocking, numerous macrophages have infiltrated into the interstitium and within persistent "tubes" of external laminae of necrotic myocytes. At 2 and 8 weeks after shocking, the areas of myocardial necrosis have numerous active fibroblasts with prominent profiles of rough endoplasmic reticulum and deposits of collagen fibrils in the interstitium (Fig. 12-19). Scattered sublethally-injured myocytes are atrophic and have myocytolysis.

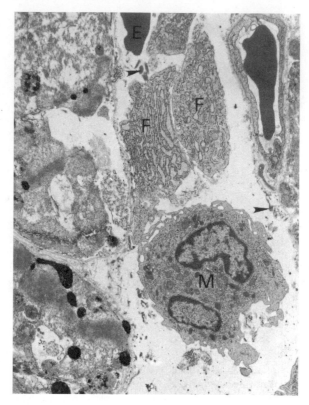

Fig. 12-18. Necrotic myocytes at 2 days postshock are separated by lucent edematous interstitium that contains a macrophage (*M*), several active fibroblasts (*F*) with distended cisternae of rough endoplasmic reticulum, an erythrocyte (*E*), and scattered dense strands of fibrin (*arrowheads*). (Magnification × 9000.) (From VanVleet JF et al: Cardiac damage in dogs with chronically implanted automatic defibrillator electrode catheters and given four episodes of multiple shocks, *Am J Vet Res* 43:909, 1982. With permission.)

CARDIAC ALTERATIONS INDUCED BY PRESENCE OF INTERNAL DEFIBRILLATORS

Recognition of shock-induced cardiac injury requires that one can confidently separate the lesions provoked by the physical presence of the defibrillator unit on the heart. Thus the reaction to the presence of epicardial electrodes, epicardial patches, and endocardial catheters must be recognized. Also it is important to be aware of the temporal changes in the body's reaction to these devices.

Van Vleet et al.[58] observed the epicardial alterations in nonshocked dogs 2 days after sham operation (thoracotomy and pericardiotomy). Grossly and microscopically, epicardial congestion, edema, and hemorrhage with overly-

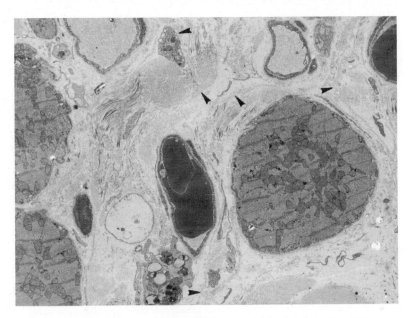

Fig. 12-19. Left ventricular myocardium from a dog euthanatized 8 weeks after receiving a 15 A/Kg transthoracic shock. An area of myocardium where several myocytes were destroyed has condensation of the interstitial tissues with prominent accumulations of collagen fibrils. Remnants of the missing cardiac muscle cells are observed as an empty tube of external lamina (*lower left*) and scattered undulating sheets of external lamina (*arrowheads*). A macrophage filled with residual bodies, probably derived from phagocytosis of sarcoplasmic debris from the necrotic myocytes, lies in the interstitium (*bottom center*). Thin, wavy cytoplasmic processes of fibroblasts are scattered in the interstitial collagen deposits. Several capillaries and intact surviving myocytes are present. (Magnification × 7000.) (From VanVleet JF et al: Sequential ultrastructural alterations in ventricular myocardium of dogs given large, single transthoracic damped sinusoidal waveform defibrillator shocks, *Am J Vet Res* 41:493, 1980. With permission.)

ing fibrin deposits were observed. The affected epicardium had neutrophilic infiltration and very occasional, necrotic myocytes were present in the subjacent myocardium.

Several studies[12,48] (as well as Van Vleet et al., unpublished observations) have described the tissue reactions to implanted, epicardial defibrillator patches. The initial alterations from surgical manipulations were similar to those described above for epicardial electrodes. Subsequently, the patches provoked proliferation of a surrounding fibrous capsule. Initially the capsule had granulation tissue and prominent fibroblastic proliferation. Weeks to months after implantation, the fibrous capsule matured into a highly collagenized outer zone with immature fibrosis and hemorrhage at the patch-cap-

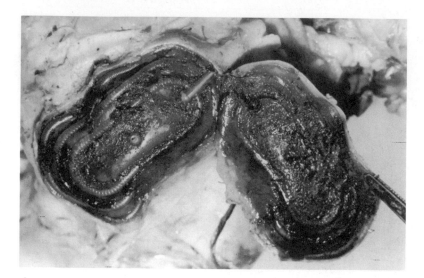

Fig. 12-20. The fibrous capsule surrounding an epicardial patch electrode has been incised to reveal dark brown deposits of blood over the inner surface. The patch was implanted in a dog 2½ years previously.

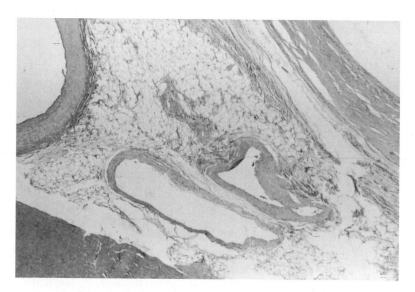

Fig. 12-21. Section of the peripatch fibrous capsule (*upper right*) that surrounded an epicardial patch electrode overlies several coronary vessels and epicardial tissue. (Hematoxylin and eosin stain; magnification × 25.)

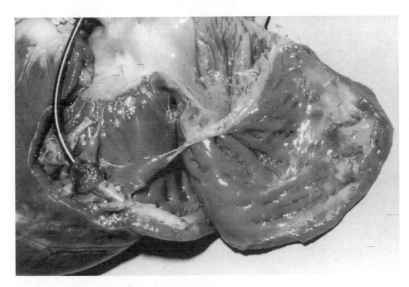

Fig. 12-22. Opened right side of the heart of a dog shows an electrode catheter implanted 26 weeks previously. The distal portion of the lead is surrounded by a thin white perilead fibrous sheath anchored to the endocardium. A reddish mass of fibrin is adhered to the edge of the sheath. The right ventricular endocardium has white thickened areas of fibrosis (*right*) from contact with the intracavitary lead.

sule interface (Figs. 12-20 and 12-21). The capsule around the patch became firmly adhered to the underlying epicardium but patency of epicardial vessels was maintained. Complications of the procedure included dislodgement of the patch and infection of the patch site.

The pathologic reactions provoked by intracavitary catheters with defibrillation electrodes have been described in human patients[12,48] and dogs.[4,55,56,57] As previously reported for endocardial pacing leads, endothelialized fibrous sheaths tend to cover the exposed intracavitary surfaces of the devices (Figs. 12-22 to 12-26). The thickness of the provoked fibrous sheath is related to the type of insulation material, with silicone rubber and polyethylene eliciting a more intense fibrotic response than polyurethane. The maturation of the fibrous sheath is similar to the events seen in the fibrous capsule surrounding epicardial patches. In dogs long-term implants had focal cartilaginous and osseous metaplasia in the sheath surrounding the lead.

Areas of the endocardium in physical contact with intracavitary leads develop fibrotic thickenings and may be adhered to the sheath surrounding the lead (Figs. 12-27 to 12-32). The thickened endocardium appears white. Small thrombi may be present at the junction of endothelialized segments of the lead and exposed segments. Occasional complications of implantation of intracavitary catheters include partial perforation of the apical, right ventricular wall and infection of the lead sheath (Fig. 12-33).

Text continues on p. 286.

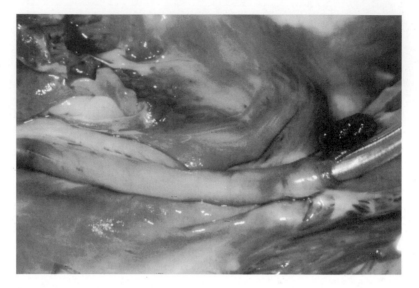

Fig. 12-23. Opened right atrium of a dog implanted with an electrode catheter 17 weeks previously has a segment of the lead surrounded by a white smooth fibrous sheath.

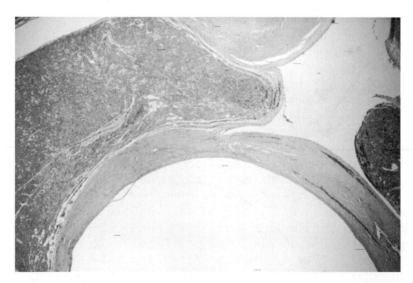

Fig. 12-24. Cross-section of perilead fibrous sheath adhered to the right ventricular endocardium. (Hematoxylin and eosin stain; magnification × 25.)

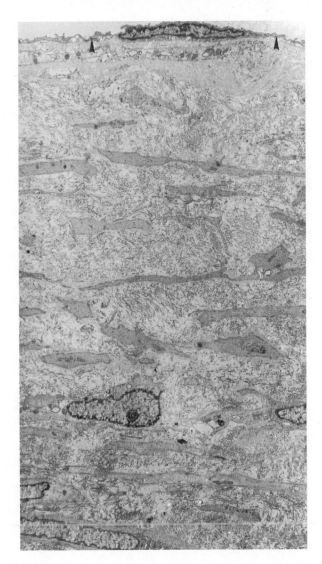

Fig. 12-25. Low-magnification electron micrograph of the outer wall of the fibrous sheath that covered a catheter implanted for 12 months in the right ventricle of a dog. The surface is covered by endothelium (*arrowheads*). The wall has myofibroblasts surrounded by abundant, pale, amorphous masses of external laminae and numerous collagen fibrils. (Magnification × 6,000.) (From VanVleet JF et al: Ultrastructural alterations in the fibrous sheath, endocardium and myocardium of dogs with chronically implanted automatic defibrillator electrode catheters and given single defibrillator shocks terminally, *Am J Vet Res* 43:909, 1982. With permission.)

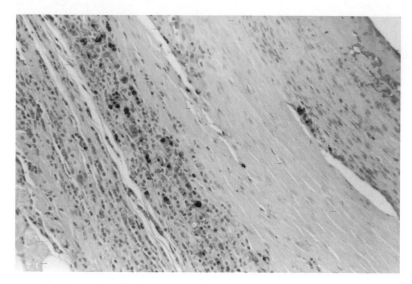

Fig. 12-26. Perilead fibrous sheath is moderately mature. Numerous fibroblasts and hemosiderin-laden macrophages are present. (Hematoxylin and eosin stain; magnification × 160.)

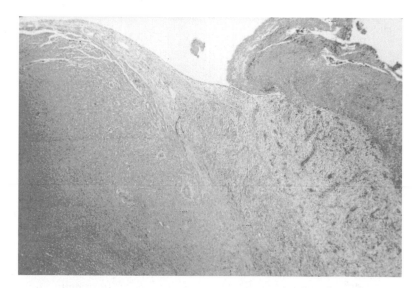

Fig. 12-27. Ventricular septum in contact with right ventricular electrode catheter has prominent endocardial thickening by a zone of granulation tissue with an overlying mass of fibrin. (Hematoxylin and eosin stain; magnification × 40.)

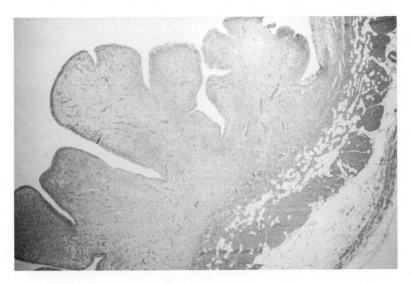

Fig. 12-28. Prominent papilliferous fibrous thickening of the right atrial endocardium at a site of contact with an electrode catheter. (Hematoxylin and eosin stain; magnification × 25.)

Fig. 12-29. Marked endocardial fibrosis of right ventricle at site of chronic contact with electrode catheter in a dog. (Hematoxylin and eosin stain; magnification × 63.)

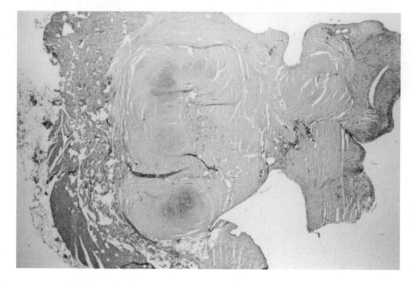

Fig. 12-30. Area of right atrial endocardial fibrosis with focal basophilic sites of carti-laginous metaplasia at contact region with electrode catheter. (Hema-toxylin and eosin stain; magnification × 25.)

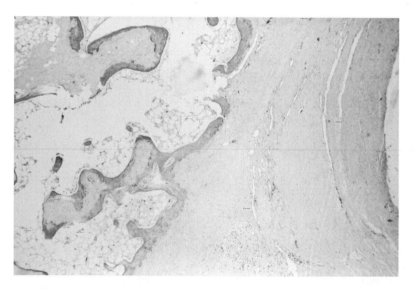

Fig. 12-31. Osseous metaplasia in the outer portion of a perilead fibrous sheath adhered to the right atrial endocardium in a dog. (Hematoxylin and eosin stain; magnification × 40.)

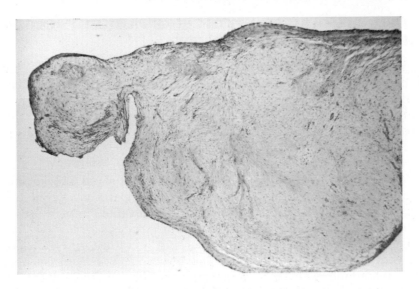

Fig. 12-32. Section of right atrioventricular valve cusp has marked thickening by myxomatous tissue. This area was in contact with a chronically implanted electrode catheter in a dog. (Hematoxylin and eosin stain; magnification × 40.)

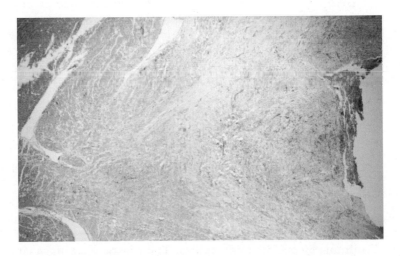

Fig. 12-33. Infected perilead fibrous sheath in a dog has extensive infiltration of inflammatory cells. (Hematoxylin and eosin stain; magnification × 25.)

PROPOSED CELLULAR AND MOLECULAR PATHOPHYSIOLOGIC MECHANISMS OF ELECTRICAL INJURY

Damage to tissues exposed to high current densities near electrodes has been attributed to thermal injury in older literature and more recently has been explained by the phenomenon of electroporation.[5,52] Electroporation, also termed electropermeabilization, is the occurrence of transiently enhanced permeability of the cellular membrane on exposure to high-intensity, pulsed electric fields.

The role of Joule heating is largely discounted as an important factor in the initiation of myocardial damage by large suprathreshold shocks. Although muscle proteins such as myosin and tropomyosin are heat labile and may undergo denaturation at 45°C or greater, these elevated temperatures are not present at sites distant from the stimulating electrodes.

Tung[54] has recently reviewed the emerging literature on electroporation. The elegant work from his laboratory has utilized microelectrodes applied to isolated individual myocytes to demonstrate onset and recovery from electrical injury. At suprathreshold shock levels, pores of 40 Å or greater in diameter have been demonstrated to develop in cell membranes in microseconds. Dependent on the extent of damage, pores may be resealed in seconds to minutes or, in the worst case, not at all. Tung[54] cites the following factors as important in the extent of electroporation damage: pulse intensity, pulse duration, number of pulses applied, time between pulses, membrane stress, and temperature. Large cells such as skeletal muscle fibers and nerve fibers are most prone to electroporation injury, but cardiac muscle cells, because of their syncytial arrangement, are also at high risk.

Tung[54] has proposed that electroporation may initiate a series of events in cardiac muscle cells, including calcium influx to produce calcium overload with subsequent hypercontraction and lethal injury. Also electroporation may result in intracellular edema and in loss of intracellular enzymes, metabolites, and electrolytes. Altered cells may become unexcitable and initiate the development of cardiac arrhythmias.

In studies of the effects of electrical injury on sheets of cultured chicken myocytes, microscopic alterations were demonstrated in sarcolemmal membranes.[16-21] Similarly cell membrane disruptions were demonstrated in isolated skeletal muscle fibers or intact skeletal muscle exposed to electrical injury.[30-31] Future research into the mechanism of shock-induced myocardial injury should provide further clarification of our current knowledge.

DAMAGE IN PROPORTION TO SHOCK STRENGTH

The extent and severity of myocardial lesions are correlated positively with shock strength, but there is considerable variability in the extent of damage between animals given identical shocks. The reason for this variability is not known. Although the damage shows many characteristics in common with ischemic necrosis, there are differentiating points. Most obvious is that the anatomic location of the defibrillator-induced damage is quite different than the location of ischemic necrosis, since the vascular pattern of the heart determines the location of ischemic damage. It is reasonable to assume that the site of damage caused by the electric shock is determined, at least in part, by the current pathway and that damage is more likely in the tissue exposed to a high current density. Measurement of current density in the heart is not easily accomplished. Models for estimating current flow have been published, and knowledge is expanding in this area. *In vitro* tissue resistivity values have been reported,[46] but they are not valid for high-current, high-voltage shocks. Most reported data are for excised tissue, usually at room temperature rather than at 37°C. Overall, the distribution of current density in the heart for defibrillation shocks is not well known.

The tissue damaged by the shock is not ischemic. Regional myocardial blood flow studies, using microspheres, scintigraphic patterns, and rate of increase of cardiac isoenzymes in plasma, show that the damaged tissue is perfused by virtually normal blood flow for many hours after application of transchest[9,26] or direct-heart shocks.[10,13]

Studies to date have often shown grossly that the border between damaged and undamaged myocardium is sharply demarcated, especially from shocks applied to the cardiac surface. Microscopically, severely damaged fibers are often immediately adjacent to normal or minimally altered fibers. This is somewhat surprising because it is difficult to explain how adjacent fibers could be exposed to vastly different current densities. Cardiac muscle fibers do have different resistivity along their longitudinal axis as compared to their transverse axis,[39] but in the area of damage one cannot invoke different resistivity of fibers to defibrillator current flow on the basis of different anatomical arrangement since the adjacent undamaged and destroyed cells are often parallel to each other. The reason for the sharp demarcation of lesions is not known. A possible mechanism might be that damage is dependent on the time in the cardiac cycle when the shock is applied. Certainly adjacent cells in a fibrillating chamber may not be in exactly the same phase of the action potential. Also Tung[54] has suggested that this may be caused by the degree of coupling between adjoining cells. Closely coupled cells may have a longer effective cell length and therefore be exposed to a greater electrical potential.

We have noted that often injured fibers are concentrated near large myocardial vessels, suggesting that columns of blood shunt the current by forming low-resistance pathways. It is difficult to compare the damaging effects of different defibrillator shocks because of the variability in damage when only one kind of shock is applied.

Babbs et al.[3] modified a classical pharmacologic technique to compare defibrillating current waveforms. In pharmacology an accepted measure of the margin of safety of a drug is the ratio of the median toxic dose (TD_{50}) and the median effective dose (ED_{50}). The ratio TD_{50}/ED_{50} (or LD_{50}/ED_{50}, where LD_{50} = median lethal dose) is known as the therapeutic index. In typical studies of the therapeutic index each subject is counted as either responding or not responding to the agent tested, according to specific criteria for effectiveness or toxicity. Then the percent of subjects responding is plotted as a function of the logarithm of the dose. ED_{50} and TD_{50} values are determined by interpolation of the plots, and the therapeutic index is calculated. The margin of safety is related to the therapeutic index and also to the slopes of the curves.

Fig. 12-34 shows curves for damped sinusoidal defibrillator shocks of 4 to 10 milliseconds duration, applied to dogs. Chest electrodes of 8 or 10 cm diameter were used. Peak voltage, peak current, and pulse duration of each

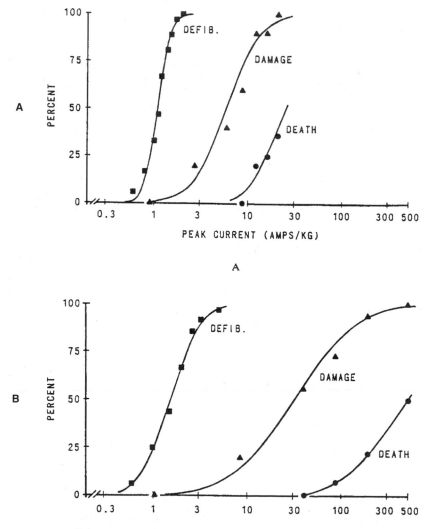

Fig. 12-34. Effectiveness, toxicity, and mortality curves for dogs given transchest damped sine wave defibrillator shocks. **A,** The current dose relationship. **B,** The energy dose relationship.

shock were recorded on a storage oscilloscope. The percent of successful defibrillation was plotted vs. the energy or current dose (Fig. 12-13); ED_{50} was then identified from these plots. The TD_{50} and LD_{50} were determined in another group of dogs that received single shocks of 0 to 25 A/kg peak current and 0 to 600 J/kg delivered energy. To determine therapeutic indices, death of an animal and/or any degree of cardiac damage found by gross or microscopic examination were considered the specific criteria analogous to drug toxicity.

Fig. 12-34 shows percent defibrillation, damage, and death as functions of shock intensity. In terms of peak current the ED_{50}, TD_{50}, and LD_{50} are 1.1, 5.8, and 24 A/kg; the therapeutic indices are $TD_{50}/ED_{50} = 5$ for damage and $LD_{50}/ED_{50} = 22$ for death. In terms of delivered energy the ED_{50}, TD_{50}, and LD_{50} are 1.5, 30, and 500 J/kg; the therapeutic indices are $TD_{50}/ED_{50} = 20$ for damage and $LD_{50}/ED_{50} = 33$ for death. Use of the technique allows comparison of defibrillation effectiveness and toxicity using different equipment and techniques even though there is considerable biological variability in the response to shock.

EFFECT OF DIVIDED DOSES OF SHOCKS

Doherty et al.[10] found that repeated, low-intensity shocks produce more PYP uptake than single, high-intensity shocks. For example, three 10 J shocks produced 20 times as much uptake as a single 30 J shock. They showed that the observation of Dahl et al.[6] was true for direct shocks; that is, a shorter interval between successive shocks increases damage. However, in the direct heart study of Doherty et al.[6] use of smaller electrodes produced the same amount of damage as larger electrodes, whereas transthoracic defibrillation damage was greater with small electrodes.

FACTORS THAT AFFECT EXTENT OF DAMAGE

There is some information in the literature that identifies certain important variables in the production of cardiac damage from a defibrillator shock. The stronger the shock, the more likely that severe myocardial damage will occur.[58,61] The smaller the defibrillation electrodes are, the more damage that is produced, presumably because small electrodes produce higher current density in the tissue.[6] Obviously a 400 J shock applied to the chest is less likely to produce damage than a 400 J shock applied directly to the heart. However, when electrodes are placed directly on the heart, lower intensity shocks are effective for defibrillation. With hand-held electrodes on the heart, the heart can be compressed and the blood, with its low resistivity, can be squeezed out so that a more homogeneous resistive load will result (because only cardiac tissue will be between the electrodes). This should minimize areas of high current density by elimination of current shunting through blood in the cardiac chambers, and one might expect more uniform current density. Paradoxically then, it may be that directly applied shocks are less likely to produce damage if near-threshold (that is, clinically effective) shock strengths are used for direct heart defibrillation. High-current density spots might naturally accompany transchest defibrillation, as a result of distribution of current in the thorax.[7,35] Of course, with ICD electrodes, the blood is not squeezed out of the fibrillating chambers.

Some waveforms produce more damage than other waveforms.[1,37] For example, the 0.2 second AC defibrillator produced more damage than the damped sine wave because of longer duration of stimulation. Application of repeated shocks causes more damage than application of a single shock. The time between repeated shocks is important because the closer together the shocks are, the more damage that will be produced.[6,10]

Several variables can be postulated in the production of myocardial damage following defibrillator shock, but their role has not been verified experimentally.

Although most damage studies have been conducted by applying shocks to nonfibrillating hearts, there are no studies in which necrosis has been related to the timing of the shock during the cardiac cycle. It is well documented that the application of shocks during the vulnerable period of the cardiac cycle (that is, the T wave) often produces ventricular fibrillation. Fibrillation production was the dominant theme of many of the early reports on deaths associated with cardioversion studies.

It is possible that myocardial cells have a range of susceptibility to damage for the same current density[33,34]; that is, some fibers may or may not become damaged by virtue of their size, shape, resting tension, or oxygen supply, for example. No study has described the application of uniform current density shocks to an area of myocardial tissue *in vivo*. Such a study should show whether cardiac muscle cells can be reproducibly damaged. Only if a uniform current density produces a uniform lesion can the variability in damage be ascribed to extracardiac factors.

The characteristic location of lesions in the dog heart appears to be somewhat related to the orientation of the electrodes. Dahl[6] reports that placement of the electrodes on the lateral chest walls results in "entry and exit" lesions on the right and left ventricular walls along an imaginary line between the two electrodes. However, they did not report lesions in the ventricular septum, which is also directly in the line between the electrodes. Other workers[60] reported that lesions are often located along the ventral cardiac surface, rather than along an "entry and exit" line. It would seem likely that these differences are the result of variation in electrode configuration. One would then expect that back-to-sternum electrode placement would produce lesions in different locations. This hypothesis has not yet been tested. However, the chest is very nonhomogeneous, and the current flow may be predominantly along low-resistivity pathways, such as columns of blood in the great vessels and heart chambers. If current is shunted by low-resistivity pathways, a change in electrode placement may not alter the lesion sites.

Metabolic state of the heart, age of the individual, blood gas and electrolyte levels, preexisting cardiac pathologic conditions, or systemic disease may play a role in defibrillator-induced damage.[14,28,29] Other possible factors in damage production include changes in resistance to electrical current flow during the respiratory cycle (resulting from the change in lung volume), variability of chest anatomy (that is, broad-chest vs. keel-chest), work load of the heart after the shock, and duration of fibrillation prior to the shock. However, these potential variables are yet to be investigated. Elevated tissue levels of catecholamines may increase the amount of myofibrillar degeneration, a common microscopic finding of several investigators. This concept is an extension of the hypothesis that catecholamines cause "myofibrillar degeneration."[42]

NONINVASIVE INDICATORS OF DAMAGE

There are three types of indirect evidence for damage: ECG changes, elevation of serum isoenzymes, and positive scintigraphic scans of the heart.

ECG CHANGES

Animal Studies

Twelve-lead ECG changes, which are often indicative of cardiac damage, include S-T segment shifts, development of Q waves, and T wave inversion. In fact, S-T segment changes may indicate either reversible or permanent changes in the heart. Q wave and T wave changes are much more likely to indicate permanent damage and usually herald necrosis. Hence, they should be more reliable indicators of cell death than S-T segment changes. There is considerable variation in ECG changes seen in different animals, but ECG changes do not always correlate well with damage.[49] Transient ECG changes frequently follow DC shocks in dogs with or without necrosis. ECG changes lasting more than 48 hours after the shock is applied or Q and T wave changes seem to be excellent indicators of necrosis. Hence, transient arrhythmias are so sensitive that they have limited specific value as indicators of necrosis. The persistent changes are not very sensitive indicators, although they are fairly specific and reliable.

Some of the reasons why many ECG changes are not reliable indicators of necrosis are as follows:

1. The changes are produced by post-shock adrenergic and cholinergic reflexes.
2. Subjects who are most seriously damaged die immediately after the shocks, and they cannot be studied for ECG changes.
3. Changes in S-T segment or Q or T waves are better indicators of lesions located on one area of the heart than of symmetrical lesions on both sides of the heart. Since defibrillator damage is often bilateral, there may be little net effect on electromotive forces of the surface ECG.

Dahl and colleagues employed precordial mapping of S-T segment shifts as an indirect measure of damage.[6] This technique may improve detection but still is insensitive to damage in some subjects.

Human Studies

Electrocardiographic changes consistent with myocardial infarction have been reported in humans following cardioversion. Resnekov and McDonald[43] found that 3% of patients show this phenomenon even when no outward symptoms of infarction are present. Furthermore, the incidence of the changes increases as shock intensity increases. Changes considered to be in this category are development of Q waves and T wave inversion. S-T segment changes may preceed Q and T wave changes, but the S-T shifts alone may reflect transient changes in electrophysiology. In humans, S-T segment changes usually persist only 20 seconds to 2 minutes after DC shocks but occasionally last longer. T wave changes usually last longer. In some cases S-T changes are associated with precordial pain and/or fever, and these findings have been ascribed to pericarditis or subepicardial myocarditis. It should be pointed out that coexistent myocardial infarction may complicate interpretation of these changes. Also CPR may traumatize the heart and produce such changes. Quantitation of injury has not yet been correlated with ECG changes, but it is reasonable to assume that they sometimes reflect permanent cardiac damage of some extent. In view of the preponderance of animal evidence showing that defibrillator damage is usually localized to epicardial and subepicardial areas, it may be that involvement of relatively small tissue mass may cause large changes in vector forces of the ECG. In any case shocks that cause ECG abnormalities should be avoided. However, this alone is not adequate reason to withhold cardioversion from a patient and, of course, is no reason to avoid shocking for ventricular fibrillation since there is no alternative therapy.

SERUM CARDIAC ISOENZYMES

Animal Studies

Early studies of serum enzyme elevation after defibrillator shocks show marked increases, mostly caused by a release of enzymes from skeletal muscle. The opportunity to determine the extent to which cardiac tissue releases enzymes after DC shock arose with the availability of enzymatic fraction tests that are more specific for cardiac tissue. Detection of these enzymes is an established procedure for indirect determination of cardiac cell death caused by ischemic injury. Ehsani et al.[11] measured total and MB fraction of serum creatine phosphokinase (CPK) in dogs following application of ten rapidly repeated, 400 J stored-energy shocks to 11 subjects. This extremely high dose of DC shock was given to assure that some dogs would show damage. All dogs had grossly elevated total CPK levels, but only six had elevated MB-CPK and myocardial necrosis at postmortem 4 days later. Each of these dogs also exhibited S-T segment elevation in the ECG recorded from the anterior chest wall. Peak total CPK elevation occurred at 6 hours, which is earlier than the typical 13 hours for dogs with myocardial infarction. The early peak is probably the result of continued perfusion of damaged cells.

Human Studies

Serum enzyme elevations have been attributed to release of enzyme from both skeletal and cardiac muscle. Early investigators attributed the rise in enzyme levels to skeletal muscle damage, but recent evidence supports the concept that small amounts of enzyme may be released from the heart.

Ehsani et al.[11] reported MB-CPK serum isoenzyme levels in 30 patients following cardioversion. Fifteen of the 30 patients had elevated total CPK activity that peaked within 4 hours. In two patients there was modest elevation of MB-CPK (cardiac origin). They concluded that the rise indicates a small lesion. Total cumulative energy in these patients was 40 to 750 J, and it was the patients receiving the highest energy who exhibited the MB-CPK rise. The authors point out that conventional cardioversion does not generally raise MB-CPK fractions, but when it does, it should not obscure diagnosis of acute myocardial infarction because the latter process raises the serum levels more than the countershock. It is not clear whether release of the MB-CPK into serum reflects reversible or irreversible changes, but it is undesirable. The potential for permanent damage cannot be ignored.

SCINTOGRAPHS

Animal Studies

DiCola et al.[9] have reported the effect in dogs of DC countershock on myocardial uptake of technetium-99 stannous pyrophosphate (PYP), which is a technique for determining the location and extent of myocardial infarction. The technique is very sensitive for detection of cardiac-cell necrosis. This study employed both the sequential myocardial imaging of the intact subject and direct cardiac tissue radioactivity in samples of myocardial tissue at postmortem examination. Shocks of 200 to 400 J were applied to dogs weighing 11 to 28 kg. Very small (4 cm diameter) electrodes were used for this study. Sometimes single shocks were applied, but usually two or three shocks were given. All dogs showed increased PYP uptake and myocardial necrosis at postmortem. The regions of heart with increased PYP uptake were the damaged areas and were predominantly epicardial in location. PYP uptake and damage increased with application of increased energy. The scintigrams were, for the most part, indistinguishable from those seen in experimental myocardial ischemia, and the abnormalities disappeared within 7 days. The right ventricular uptake of PYP was greater than uptake in the left ventricle.

Doherty et al.[10] reported that technetium-99m pyrophosphate scintigraphy is a very sensitive indicator of shock strength after direct shocks to dog hearts. There was uptake with only 10 J of energy, even though creatine kinase depletion did not occur in the heart until 30 or more Joules were applied. PYP may be too sensitive to be used as a measure of irreversible damage. Thallium-201 uptake, or regional blood flow decrease, did not occur until shock strengths were 30 J or greater and may correlate better with necrosis.

Human Studies

Werner[63] used technetium-99m pyrophosphate scintigraphy to study patients following transthoracic cardioversion, transthoracic emergency defibrillation, or direct defibrillation. They found a high incidence of positive scintigrams, ECG changes, and elevated serum MB-CPK levels. Discrete uptake of the pyrophosphate was seen only in relation to myocardial infarction or surgical damage. They also found that clinically significant scintigraphic abnormalities were not produced even when the countershock was applied directly to the epicardium.

Hence, it appears that repeated DC shocks of high intensity are potentially capable of producing positive cardiac scintigrams but that, in practice, it is unlikely that necrosis is produced. Undoubtedly, repeated use of very strong shocks would produce positive findings in some patients.

REVERSIBLE SYSTEMIC EFFECTS OF ISCHEMIA AND DEFIBRILLATION

The responses to a defibrillator shock do not always entail permanent changes or damage to the tissues and cells exposed to the shock. Indeed, the compensatory capability of the body to cope with such an event is extraordinary. In previous chapters material has been presented covering the cellular effects of defibrillator shocks, but the response of the intact organism to such shocks merits consideration. This is particularly important when evaluating the morbidity and/or mortality associated with defibrillation, as opposed to the morbidity and/or mortality associated with an episode of cardiac arrest and ischemia followed by defibrillation. The following presents a summary of reported findings. For a detailed presentation of this subject, the reader is referred to Tacker and Geddes.[50]

Of course, if the shocks are strong enough, permanent damage or death may ensue from cardiac necrosis, electromechanical dissociation, or intractable fibrillation. In contrast, low-intensity defibrillator shocks are unlikely to produce permanent damage to the subject. However, temporary changes are often seen as a result of delivery of defibrillator shocks to intact experimental animals or human subjects and include both arrhythmia production and hemodynamic alterations. As would be expected, there is no sharp demarcation between shock intensity capable of producing only transient changes and shock intensity that may produce permanent changes.

However, it is generally held that there is a relatively large safety margin between effective shock strength and damaging shock strength.[3,54]

Defibrillator shocks of progressively stronger intensity or a progressively large number of shocks of moderate intensity will produce progressively greater changes in hemodynamic function, the ECG, respiration, hematocrit, and serum corticosteroid concentrations.[50] In general, ECG changes are most often observed, and the changes seen appear in the following general order as the shocks become stronger or more numerous: ventricular fibrillation (which will be fatal if untreated) if the stimulus falls in the vulnerable period of the ventricles, atrial bradycardia followed by atrial tachycardia, premature ventricular beats, ventricular tachycardia, S-T segment elevation or depression, and conduction impairment of the A-V node or ventricular conduction system. The hemodynamic changes seen in heart rate, blood pressure, and ventricular function are not necessarily detrimental, are of relatively short duration (less than 6 minutes), and are probably in great part caused by autonomic nervous system stimulation and/or reflexes. Elevation in corticosteroid levels is probably caused by the combination of stress of the shock and direct stimulation of the nervous system.

It does appear that if an effective defibrillation shock is applied after onset of a nonperfusing arrhythmia, the predominant cause of changes in ECG and hemodynamics is the period of ischemia, rather than the shock. Consequently, the most important independent variable in the response is the duration of ischemia. Care must be taken not to attribute changes caused by the ischemia to the shock.

It must also be emphasized that in considering human clinical use of defibrillators, the complications or transient changes caused by defibrillator shocks may not be well tolerated by the diseased and compromised heart. Every attempt to minimize deleterious effects should be made.

REFERENCES

1. Anderson HN et al: An evaluation and comparison of effects of alternating and direct current electrical discharges on canine hearts, *Ann Surg* 160:251, 1964.
2. Avitall B et al: Automatic implantable cardioverter/defibrillator discharges and acute myocardial injury, *Circulation* 81:1482, 1990.
3. Babbs CF et al: Therapeutic indices for transchest defibrillator shocks: effective, damaging, and lethal electrical doses, *Am Heart J* 99:734, 1980.
4. Barker-Voelz MA et al: Pathological and physiological changes induced by a single defibrillating shock applied through a chronically implanted catheter, *J Electrocardiol* 16:167, 1983.
5. Chang DC, Reese TS: Changes in membrane structure induced by electroporation as revealed by rapid-freezing electron microscopy, *Biophys J* 58:1, 1990.
6. Dahl CF et al: Myocardial necrosis from direct current countershock—effect of paddle electrode size and time interval between discharges, *Circulation* 50:956, 1974.
7. Deale OC, Lerman BB: Intrathoracic current flow during transthoracic defibrillation in dogs, *Circ Res* 67:1405, 1990.
8. Dixon EG et al: Improved defibrillation

thresholds with large contoured epicardial electrodes and biphasic waveforms, *Circulation* 76:1176, 1987.

9. DiCola VC et al: Myocardial uptake of technetium-99M stannous pyrophosphate following direct current transthoracic countershock, *Circulation* 54:980, 1976.

10. Doherty MC et al: Cardiac damage produced by direct current countershock applied to the heart, *Am J Cardiol* 43:225, 1979.

11. Ehsani AA, Ewy GA, Sobel BE: CPK isoenzyme elevations after electrical countershock, *Am J Cardiol* 37:12, 1976.

12. Fain ES, Billingham M, Winkle RA: Internal cardiac defibrillation: histopathology and temporal stability of defibrillation energy requirements, *J Am Coll Cardiol* 9:631, 1987.

13. Gaba DM et al: Internal countershock produces myocardial damage and lactate production without myocardial ischemia in anesthetized dogs, *Anesthesiology* 66:477, 1987.

14. Gaba DM, Talner NS: Myocardial damage following transthoracic direct current countershock in newborn piglets, *Pediatr Cardiol* 2:281, 1982.

15. Harman D et al: Differences in the pathological changes in dogs' hearts after defibrillation with extrapericardial paddles and implanted defibrillator electrodes, *PACE* 14:358, 1991.

16. Jones JL, Jones RE, Balasky G: Microlesion formation in myocardial cells by high intensity electric field stimulation, *Am J Physiol* 253:H480, 1987.

17. Jones JL et al: Cellular fibrillation appearing in cultured myocardial cells after application of strong capacitor discharges, *Am J Cardiol* 39:273, 1977.

18. Jones JL et al: Ultrastructural changes produced in cultured myocardial cells by electric shock, *Fed Proc* 34:391, 1975.

19. Jones JL et al: Differentiation of myocardial cells in monolayer cell culture, *Fed Proc* 35:628, 1976.

20. Jones JL et al: Ultrastructural injury to chick myocardial cells in vitro following "electric countershock," *Circ Res* 46:387, 1980.

21. Jones JL et al: Cultured chick heart cells as a model for cardioversion trauma, *Fed Proc* 32:431, 1973.

22. Kaiser GC, Edgecomb JH, Kay JH: Ventricular fibrillation: an experimental study comparing various voltages and durations of electric shock in defibrillation of the canine heart, *J Thorac Surg* 33:537, 1957.

23. Kallock MJ et al: Catheter electrode defibrillation in dogs: threshold dependence on implant time and catheter stability, *Am Heart J* 109:821, 1985.

24. Karch SB: Resuscitation-induced myocardial necrosis. Catecholamines and defibrillation, *Am J Med Pathol* 8:3, 1987.

25. Karch SB, Billingham ME: Morphologic effects of defibrillation: a preliminary report, *Crit Care Med* 12:920, 1984.

26. Kerber R, Martins J, Gasho J: Effect of high-energy countershock on regional ventricular contractility, *Circulation* 57(suppl 2):93, 1978.

27. Kirby CK, Jensen JM, Johnson J: Defibrillation of the ventricles under hypothermic conditions, *AMA Arch Surg* 68:663, 1954.

28. Koning G, Veefkind AH, Dreschler WA: Biochemical and functional characterization of cardiac damage after experimental direct defibrillation, *Med Instrum* 12:55, 1978.

29. Koning G, Veefkind AH, Schneider H: Cardiac damage caused by direct application of defibrillator shocks to isolated Langendorff-perfused rabbit heart, *Am Heart J* 100:473, 1980.

30. Lee RC et al: Role of cell membrane rupture in the pathogenesis of electrical trauma, *J Surg Res* 44(6):709, 1988.

31. Lee RC, Kolodney MS: Electrical injury mechanisms: electrical breakdown of cell membranes, *Plast Reconstr Surg* 80:672, 1987.

32. Leeds SE, Mackay ES, Mosslin K: Production of ventricular fibrillation and defibrillation in dogs by means of accurately measured shocks across exposed heart, *Am J Physiol* 165:179, 1951.

33. Lepeschkin E et al: Local potential gradients as a unifying measure for thresholds of stimulation, standstill, tachyarrhythmia and fibrillation appearing after strong capacitor discharges, *Adv Cardiol* 21:268, 1978.

34. Lepeschkin E et al: A unifying measure for electrical myocardial stimulation and damage thresholds—comparison between in vivo and in vitro data, *Physiologist* 17:273, 1974.

35. Lerman BB, Deale OC: Relation between transcardiac and transthoracic current during defibrillation in humans, *Circ Res* 67:1420, 1990.

36. Lerman BB, et al: Myocardial injury and induction of arrhythmia by direct current shock delivered via endocardial catheters in dogs, *Circulation* 69:1006, 1984.

37. Lumb G et al: Damage in canine hearts following defibrillator shocks, *Ann Clin Lab Sci* 16:171, 1986.

38. MacLean LD, Van Tyne RA: Ventricular defibrillation, *JAMA* 175:471, 1961.

39. O'Neill RJ, Tung L: Cell-attached patch clamp study of the electropermeabilization of amphibian cardiac cells, *Biophys J* 59:1028, 1991.

40. Patel AS, Galysh FT: Experimental studies to design safe external pediatric paddles for a DC defibrillator, *IEEE Trans Biomed Eng* 19:228, 1972.

41. Pugh BR et al: Cardioversion and "false positive" technetium-99m stannous pyrophosphate myocardial scintigrams, *Circulation* 54:399, 1976.

42. Reichenbach DD, Benditt EP: Catecholamines and cardiomyopathy: the pathogenesis and potential importance of myofibrillar degeneration, *Hum Pathol* 1:125, 1970.

43. Resnekov L, McDonald L: Complications in 220 patients with cardiac dysrhythmias treated by phased direct current shock and indications for electroconversion, *Br Heart J* 29:926, 1967.

44. Resnekov L: High-energy electrical current and myocardial damage, *Med Instrum* 12:24, 1978.

45. Rivkin LM: The defibrillator and cardiac burns, *J Thorac Cardiovasc Surg* 46:755, 1963.

46. Schwan HP: Determination of biological impedance. In *Physical techniques in biological research, vol 6 (part B)*, New York, 1963, Academic Press.

47. Shephard RJ: The design of a cardiac defibrillator, *Br Heart J* 23:7, 1961.

48. Singer L et al: Pathologic findings related to the lead system and repeated defibrillations in patients with the automatic implantable cardioverter-defibrillator, *J Am Coll Cardiol* 10:382, 1987.

49. Tacker WA Jr, VanVleet JF, Geddes LA: Electrocardiographic, serum enzymic alterations associated with cardiac alterations induced in dogs by single transthoracic damped sinusoidal defibrillator shocks of various strengths, *Am Heart J* 98:185, 1979.

50. Tacker WA, Geddes LA: Physiologic response to defibrillatory shocks. In *Electrical defibrillation*, Boca Raton, Fla, 1980, CRC Press.

51. Tedeschi CG, White CW: A morphologic study of canine hearts subjected to fibrillation, electrical defibrillation and manual compression, *Circulation* 9:916, 1954.

52. Tovar O, Tung L: Electroporation of cardiac cell membranes with monophasic or biphasic rectangular pulses, *PACE* 14:1887, 1991.

53. Trouton TG et al: Metabolic changes and mitochondrial dysfunction early following transthoracic counter-shock in dogs, *PACE* 12:1827, 1989.

54. Tung L: Electrical injury to heart muscle cells. In Lee RC, Cravalho EG, Burke JF, editors: *Electrical trauma: the pathophysiology, manifestations and clinical management*, New York, Cambridge University Press (in press).

55. VanVleet JF et al: Ultrastructural alterations in the fibrous sheath, endocardium and myocardium of dogs with chronically implanted automatic defibrillator electrode catheters and given single defibrillating shocks terminally, *Am J Vet Res* 43:909, 1982.

56. VanVleet JF et al: Cardiovascular alterations induced by chronic transvenous implantation of an automatic defibrillator electrode catheter in dogs, *J Electrocardiology* 14:67, 1981.

57. VanVleet JF et al: Cardiac damage in dogs with chronically implanted automatic defibrillator electrode catheters and given four episodes of multiple shocks, *Am Heart J* 106:300, 1983.

58. VanVleet JF et al: Effect of shock strength

on survival and acute cardiac damage induced by open-thorax defibrillation of dogs, *Am J Vet Res* 39:981, 1978.

59. VanVleet JF et al: Sequential ultrastructural alterations in ventricular myocardium of dogs given large single transthoracic damped sinusoidal waveform defibrillator shocks, *Am J Vet Res* 41:493, 1980.

60. VanVleet JF et al: Acute cardiac damage in dogs given multiple transthoracic shocks with a trapezoidal waveform defibrillator, *Am J Vet Res* 38:617, 1977.

61. VanVleet JF et al: Sequential cardiac morphologic alterations induced in dogs by single transthoracic damped sinusoidal waveform defibrillator shocks, *Am J Vet Res* 39:271, 1978.

62. Warner ED, Dahl C, Ewy GA: Myocardial injury from transthoracic defibrillator countershock, *Arch Pathol* 99:55, 1975.

63. Werner JA: Personal communication.

64. Wilson CM et al: Death and damage caused by multiple direct current shocks: studies in an animal model, *Eur Heart J* 9:1257, 1988.

Chapter 13
Design of Implantable Cardioverter Defibrillators (ICDs)

W. A. Tacker

SAFETY AND EFFECTIVENESS: THE FIRST CLINICAL CHALLENGES

When the implantable defibrillator was first proposed,[7,8] considerable skepticism surrounded the concept of treating tachyarrythmias with an implantable device.[6] Engineering challenges were substantial, of course, but even the clinical value of such therapy was uncertain. Many questions were vigorously debated. What patients are suitable candidates for treatment? How will they be identified and selected? What energy is required, what waveform should be used, and what electrodes will work best for application of shocks? How will ventricular fibrillation be detected? Should ventricular tachycardia be treated? Will the device cause serious arrhythmias if it shocks a patient who is not in fibrillation? How can effectiveness be tested in a particular patient? In brief, could this technology be proven safe and effective?

It was demonstrated rather early that the device worked in animals that were fibrillated by electric stimulation of the ventricles and that a device of reasonably small size could be built if large surface area electrodes were used on the heart or pericardial surface to deliver current efficiently to a critical mass of the myocardium.[7] From this beginning many questions were addressed in experimental animals and human studies with encouraging answers. Subsequent clinical studies showed remarkable success in prevention of sudden death. Fig. 13-1 depicts a "pioneering" version of the ICD.

Of course, the current state of clinical practice is much advanced and is still changing rapidly. ICDs are now under development by many companies worldwide. The clinical aspects of ICD use are addressed in detail in Chapter 14, but many engineering design issues are of importance to the clinician and medical scientist who intends to understand the applications and limitations of ICDs. These design issues are the subject of this chapter.

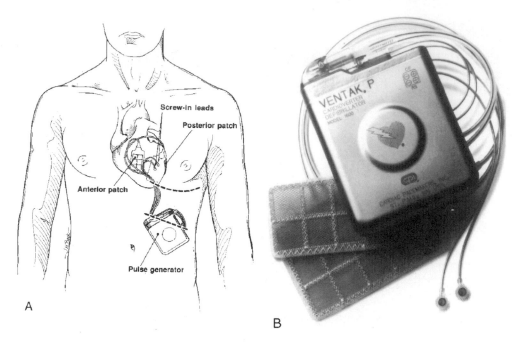

Fig. 13-1, **A** and **B.** Depiction of ICD implant, with the pulse generator in the patient's abdomen, and with two screw-in sensing leads attached to the epicardium. The two defibrillating electrodes (leads) are rectangular patches on the anterior and posterior heart surface. (Compliments of CPI, St. Paul, MN.)

SIZE: THE FIRST ENGINEERING CHALLENGE

The advent of the ICD became practical with the substantial development of new technologies in electronics and microprocessors during the past two decades. When the ICD was first envisioned, its design was theoretically possible but not very practical. Size was very important since the size bears directly on implant location, comfort, compatibility with tissues and organs in the implant location, and trade-offs between energy output and effectiveness, longevity of the device, waveform type used and electronic component selection. Several technical advances contributed to size reduction. Adequate microprocessor capability in small volume became available, as did new technologies in other components, especially batteries and capacitors.

Battery (that is, power supply) selection and use are very important for the ICD. Because of the requirement to draw a high current to charge the ICD capacitor quickly, the battery should have low internal impedance. Batteries with high internal impedance cannot deliver high current because of the internal impedance, which necessarily must be in series with the charging circuit. Batteries with low internal impedance have a disadvantage however, inasmuch as they self-discharge at a faster rate and therefore have a shorter battery life after implantation. Also the high-current, low-internal-impedance batteries are not the best for the sensing circuitry of the ICD.

Due to the need for high energy density, batteries based on lithium chemistry are used in all ICDs. Some ICDs have two batteries, one for the low-current functions and another for the high-current-capacitor charging function. However, most ICDs have only a single type of battery, and with incremental improvements in technology the trend appears to be toward a single power supply. Lithium vanadium silver pentoxide cells have favorable characteristics of high energy density, low internal impedance, and gradual voltage decline, which is advantageous for predicting end of life.[9]

Capacitor types of potential usefulness for ICDs include film capacitors and electrolytic capacitors. The former have the advantage of performing at higher voltages but the disadvantage of having lower energy density as compared to electrolytic capacitors. Both types have been used, but the trend is toward the electrolytic type as improved leads and waveforms have reduced the necessity for high voltage shocks.

Another factor in capacitor technology is the characteristic of electrolytics to perform better if they are periodically "reformed" by recharging. After a long period of nonuse, an electrolytic capacitor will charge to high voltage slowly the first time, but then will charge rapidly on subsequent uses if not much time passes between charges. For this reason capacitors may be recharged and discharged into an internal resistor periodically (either automatically or at clinical follow-up visits) to keep the capacitors well formed. Although one might expect these charging cycles to deplete batteries sooner, the cycles actually prolong battery life because the capacitors are made easier to charge by reforming.

Capacitors are the largest component in ICD pulse generators and higher energy-density capacitors would be a logical means to size reduction. Capacitor development has been slowed however because of the reluctance of vendors to develop new capacitor technology for the relatively low volume and very high reliability needs of ICD manufacturers.

Reduction in size of the pulse generator as well as improved effectiveness to defibrillate also came from several other lines of research outside the general area of circuit component size reduction. The discovery of improved ICD effectiveness using the sequential pulse waveform (two pulses with three or four electrodes to pass current through different pathways) and then using the biphasic waveform along with use of novel leads (sometimes invoking more than one current pathway) also reduced the shock strength requirements and thus the size requirements.

In addition, the development of pacing to terminate ventricular tachyarrhythmias (use of a pacemaker strength shock or bursts of these shocks) demonstrated that many of the episodes of ventricular arrhythmias could be treated with weak electrical shocks, thus reducing the battery depletion rates in a great many patients. When bursts of stimuli are used, they may be all of the same cycle length (such as 95% of the intrinsic rate) or may gradually increase in rate and then stop. Therapeutic details of burst pacing are beyond the scope of this book but it should be pointed out that the associated reduction in battery requirements provided a major engineering advantage. Of course another benefit was the elimination of pain, since the pacing pulses are of very low intensity. Because this technology had been pursued prior to the development of the ICD and was more vigorously pursued as the ICD came closer to clinical application, use of pacing strength stimuli was soon integrated into the ICD armamentarium. It was necessary however to design circuits for both the defibrillator pulse generator and the burst pacing generator that did not interact, that is, did not generate pulses in a way that caused the other one to malfunction. An example of interaction is when pulses from one generator are counted as R waves by the other generator's sensing system.

Additional size reduction/device life extension was possible, with demonstration that low-energy cardioversion shocks (stronger than pacing shocks but weaker than defibrillating shocks) from an ICD were able to cardiovert the ventricular tachycardias that often precede ventricular fibrillation.[10] The weaker cardioversion shocks deplete batteries much less than defibrillating shocks, and they are less painful. The successive use of pacing shocks first, then cardioversion strength shocks, and finally defibrillation strength shocks is referred to as ICD tiered therapy.[1]

To be sure, further reduction of size is a major issue today inasmuch as the commercially available devices are still quite large compared to pacemakers. Implantation in small adults and especially in children is problematic, and most implants require abdominal rather than thoracic wall location. However, newer-generation devices have been reduced in size, and it is anticipated that further reduction will be achieved.

WAVEFORMS

Previous chapters have included much of the relevant information on waveform characteristics, including the waveforms for ICDs. All ICD cardioverting and defibrillating waveforms are either single or multiple truncated exponential decay waveforms. These waveforms have several advantages. The truncated exponential decay waveforms are easily, accurately, and precisely controllable with solid-state switching components. Since this waveform is very amenable to solid-state switching, relays need not be included in the ICD. Such relays are large, heavy, and require substantial power to be operated. The waveforms require no inductor (needed to produce a damped sine wave) that would add considerable bulk and weight to the discharge circuit portion of the pulse generator. Also it has now been demonstrated that the shock intensity required to defibrillate can be greatly reduced by use of sequential or biphasic pulses.

PACKAGING

Development of packaging for ICDs was relatively easy due to the successes in pacemaker application and technology, which provide proven materials and technologies for implantable device reliability and longevity. Titanium cases are used for superior hermetic sealing characteristics.

ELECTRODES

Chapter 4 contains detailed information on the use, limitations, and design requirements of electrodes. A few comments about electrodes seem to be in order in this chapter however. Use of electrodes for multiple functions (such as sensing, pacing, and defibrillation) is an attractive option in theory since it reduces the number of leads required for a device and decreases some forms of complexity, and having fewer leads reduces the likelihood of some medical complications (for example, thrombosis). However multipurpose leads have practical limitations. For example, a strong ICD defibrillating shock tends to depress the myocardial response to subsequent pacing using the same electrode; large surface area defibrillating electrodes for cardioversion and defibrillation are not very efficient for pacing due to the low current density produced by the large area; and these large surface area electrodes do not provide good ECG signals for processing to analyze arrhythmias.

Materials for electrodes have been predominantly of titanium mesh for heart surface patches and of platinum-iridium for catheter-mounted ring electrodes. Platinum-iridium has lower impedance than titanium and is better for the small surface area ring electrodes on catheters. This material is biocompatible and corrosion resistant but expensive. Titanium mesh is commonly used for heart surface patch electrodes that have larger surface area and therefore lower impedance than catheter-borne ring electrodes. Insulating materials such as silicone rubber or polyurethane are used as backing for patch electrodes or for catheter surface material. Silicone rubber has been used for both heart surface patch electrodes and for catheter surfaces. Polyurethane is used on some catheters. A disadvantage of polyurethane is its degradation in the body over a period of several years. However, other characteristics such as resistance to thrombus formation are very good. Obviously circuit and lead insulation must be rated for higher voltages and currents when used for cardioversion and defibrillation than are required for pacing pulses.

SIGNAL PROCESSING AND DATA STORAGE

Other technological developments have been important to the improvement of the ICD, such as development of solid-state memory capabilities that have provided the means to record and retrieve data for analysis to improve diagnostic and therapeutic effectiveness of the ICD. Indeed it was much more difficult than originally anticipated to obtain EGM or ECG data in patients who were treated with ICDs.

Some ICDs store information only about cycle length before and after a therapeutic event. Other ICDs store a strip of EGM, which provides more information for clinical decision making as well as for improvement of device algorithms and signal processing. The trend is toward the latter approach. Storage of data facilitates therapeutic changes by reprogramming as well as improvement of algorithms for arrhythmic detection.[1]

SENSING

Electrogram (EGM) sensing of arrhythmias for therapy by the ICD has been the most successful approach to date, and even simple detection of ventricular electrograms to identify QRS or fibrillation wave components and count the rate has provided clinically acceptable reliability. Also used have been the probability density function[5] or matching of complexes with templates of previous electrogram complexes.[4] However exclusive reliance on the EGM is problematic, primarily because of difficulty in discriminating between supraventricular arrhythmias and ventricular arrhythmias, and because of the difficulty in determining whether a ventricular tachycardia is functional, that is to say, whether or not it is perfusing tissues.

Detection approaches based on EGM have evolved gradually over the past decade and are to a great extent programmable in newer-generation ICDs. Differentiation may be as simple as using a rate determination for ventricular tachycardia or ventricular fibrillation. Some minimum number of beats may be required to satisfy the diagnostic criteria, and the suddenness of onset of the tachyarrhythmia may be a diagnostic criterion. Another criterion may be stability of the cycle length, which could be of value in differentiating the irregular rate of atrial fibrillation. Another approach for ventricular fibrillation detection, which is more complex than simple rate determination, is rate determination without requirement that 100% of the EGM complexes meet the rate criterion. For example, ventricular fibrillation would be diagnosed by rate if only 75% of complexes meet the rate criterion.

Several methods have been investigated in an attempt to measure cardiac function, and in fact the earliest proposals for implantable defibrillators were based on sensing such physical parameters as blood pressure or changes in electrical impedance (as measured by intracardiac electrodes) during the cardiac cycle.[2,7] Other methods have been tried, such as detection of changes in blood temperature in the coronary sinus, which occur with each effective cardiac cycle.[3] However none of these approaches has been shown superior to EGM signal analysis alone, even when the physical sensing is used in combination with EGM analysis. Some of the problems encountered are on a physiologic basis (very low stroke volumes are hard to detect), others are on a pathophysiologic basis (blood pressure sensors become inaccurate because they are rapidly encapsulated by the body's protective mechanisms), and some are on an engineering basis (sensors have inadequate longevity after implantation).

In addition there is a fundamental issue to be resolved if new sensing modalities become available. That is whether to optimize detection systems for sensitivity (the capability to detect all rhythms that should be shocked) or for specificity (the capability to reject all rhythms that should not be shocked). Even with the current electrogram-based systems this is a difficult strategic decision and may very well be the most important factor in detection schemes. New sensors that improve only sensitivity or specificity may not be as beneficial as once envisioned due to the fundamental dilemma of whether or not to bias the ICD toward sensitivity or specificity. Of course a sensing technology that improves both would be immediately of value.

Finally there is a need for libraries of EGM signals. These could be used to develop improved detection and signal processing as well as improved algorithms. Several ECG libraries exist but are not suitable for development or testing of signals derived from electrodes on the endocardium or epicardium. Much of the data obtained for use in development is proprietary, since it is usually gathered by a company to design a specific device. Hence that database of signals is unavailable to others who wish to do signal processing development and testing. Furthermore good engineering practice requires testing with signals that are not the same signals used for development of the diagnostic hardware and software. Ideally an organization without interest in a particular company, such as a medical professional organization, would develop, evaluate, maintain, and provide a database for corporations or other organizations to use in development of arrhythmia detection systems in ICDs.

TESTING AND PHYSICIAN CONTROL

One of the advantages of the ICD as compared to transchest defibrillators is that the ICD can be custom tailored to the patient in many ways because of its prophylactic nature. This provides the opportunity at implant to test for adequate function and to set the parameters, such as burst pacing, low-energy cardioversion or high energy defibrillation sequences, energy levels, numbers of treatments of each type, and so on. Subsequent testing can also be done (using transcutaneous reprogramming of the device via radiotelemetry) to determine the patient's individual and perhaps changing needs. Use of radiofrequency communication with the ICD for reprogramming is even more important with the addition of the pacing and cardioversion modalities added to new-generation devices.

Another advantage to the testing, programming, and reprogramming capabilities provided by advanced technology is that it provides the necessary physician control for optimization of the device. Early preprogrammed ICDs with only one mode of operation were a major advance in care of the patient at high risk of sudden cardiac death but to some extent provided only a "take it or leave it" option with respect to deciding what to do in a patient with unique or difficult to control arrhythmia characteristics.

Another important development in ICDs was the introduction of devices that were not "committed." That is to say that early ICDs would monitor for a shockable arrhythmia and when such an arrhythmia was detected, the charge-discharge cycle would proceed without interruption. Newer devices have the capability to continue monitoring for reevaluation of the rhythm, and if appropriate to abort the shock delivery even after the capacitor has been charged. This has reduced the incidence of inappropriate shocks, which are painful to the patient and unnecessary, and which may even precipitate additional arrhythmias or, in theory, cause cardiac damage. Finally inclusion of multipulse pacing capability allows electrophysiologic testing without the need for repeated cardiac catheterization.[1] Uncommon but serious problems with ICDs include sensing or stimulating lead fracture, premature battery depletion, and dislodgement of catheter-mounted leads.[1]

Clinical considerations of ICD use are the subject of Chapter 14.

REFERENCES

1. Bardy et al: Clinical experiment with a tiered-therapy, multiprogrammable, anti-arrhythmia device, *Circulation* 85:1689, 1992.
2. Bourland JD et al: Automatic detection of ventricular fibrillation for an implanted defibrillator. In *Frontiers in medical signal Processing*, Midcon, 1977.
3. Hiles MC: A device to detect ventricular fibrillation using temperature. M.S. Thesis, Purdue University, 1989.
4. Langberg JJ, Griffin JC: Arrhythmia identification using the morphology of the endocardial electrogram, *Circulation* 72 (Suppl III):474, 1985.
5. Langer A et al: Considerations in the development of the automatic implantable defibrillator, *Med Instrum* 10:163, 1976.
6. Lown B, Axelrod P: Implanted standby defibrillators, *Circulation* 46:637, 1972.
7. Mirowski M et al: Standby automatic defibrillator, *Arch Int Med* 26:158, 1970.
8. Schuder JC et al: Experimental ventricular defibrillation with an automatic and completely implantable defibrillator, *Transactions of ASAIO* 16:207, 1970.
9. Visbisky M, Holmes CF: Long-term testing of defibrillator batteries, *PACE* 14:341, 1991.
10. Zipes DP, Heger JJ, Miles WM: Early experience with an implantable cardioverter, *N Engl J Med* 311:485, 1984.

Chapter 14
Clinical Use of Implantable Cardioverter-Defibrillators

Ranjan K. Thakur
Raymond Yee
George J. Klein
Gerard M. Guiraudon

The success of implantable cardioverter-defibrillators (ICDs) in terminating ventricular tachycardia (VT) and ventricular fibrillation (VF) has led to widespread acceptance and an increasing number of device implants.[133,194,201] The results of ongoing clinical trials may further expand the indications for ICD implantation by defining high-risk patients suitable for prophylactic device therapy.[11,115,153,182,215] Development of devices small enough for pectoral implantation along with transvenous leads that eliminate the need for a thoracotomy will further increase patient and physician acceptance. While it is clear that available devices have been efficacious, the technology is still evolving toward smaller devices capable of pacing, cardioversion, and defibrillation that can be implanted without a thoracotomy.* This chapter will broadly review clinical use of ICDs including indications for ICD, implantation techniques, intraoperative evaluation, complications, and follow-up, and will briefly review ongoing research that may be incorporated in future devices.

PATIENT SELECTION

Proper patient selection is paramount to the success of any therapy. Therapeutic options in patients with symptomatic ventricular arrhythmias include antiarrhythmic drugs, ablation, surgery, catheter ablation, and ICDs. The selection process involves considerations of the presenting arrhythmia and its hemodynamic stability, underlying heart disease, left ventricular function, ambient arrhythmias, and inducibility of the clinical ventricular arrhythmia.

*References 42, 138, 150, 161, 168, 218

Although there are no universally accepted guidelines, the American Heart Association, the American College of Cardiology, and the North American Society of Pacing and Electrophysiology's consensus conference have made recommendations for ICD indications based on the current literature.[33,116] NASPE's consensus conference recommendations are categorized into three classes:

Class I: ICD therapy is indicated based upon consensus.
Class II: ICD therapy is an option, but consensus does not exist.
Class III: ICD therapy is generally not justified.

NASPE's consensus conference recommendations are summarized in the accompanying box.

NASPE Recommendations for ICD Implantation

Class I
1. One or more episodes of spontaneous sustained VT or VF in a patient in whom electrophysiologic (EP) testing and/or spontaneous ventricular arrhythmias cannot be used accurately to predict efficacy of other therapies.
2. Recurrent spontaneous VT/VF despite antiarrhythmic drug therapy (EP- or Holter-guided).
3. Spontaneous VT/VF in a patient in whom antiarrhythmic drug therapy is limited by intolerance or noncompliance.
4. Persistent inducibility of ventricular arrhythmia despite drug therapy, arrhythmia surgery, or catheter ablation.

Class II
1. Syncope of undetermined etiology in a patient with inducible VT/VF and antiarrhythmic drug therapy limited by inefficacy, intolerance, or noncompliance.

Class III
1. Sustained VT/VF in the setting of acute ischemia/infarction, toxic/metabolic/electrolyte disturbance, or cause amenable to correction or reversibility.
2. Recurrent syncope of undetermined etiology in a patient without inducible sustained ventricular arrhythmias.
3. Incessant VT or VF.
4. VF secondary to atrial fibrillation in a patient with Wolff-Parkinson-White syndrome.
5. Medical, surgical, or psychiatric contraindications.

Conditions Associated with VT/VF

1. Coronary artery disease
   - (a) Previous infarction
   - (b) Aneurysm
   - (c) Ischemic cardiomyopathy
2. Cardiomyopathy:
   - (a) Dilated
     - (i) Idiopathic
     - (ii) Alcohol or toxin induced
   - (b) Hypertrophic
3. Primary electrical disease
4. Post-congenital heart disease repair
5. Cardiac tumors

INDICATIONS FOR ICDs

Sudden cardiac arrest and ventricular tachycardia comprise the major indications for ICD implantation in clinical practice. These rhythm disturbances may be manifestations of diverse etiologies (see the box above).

It has been estimated that 400,000 people experience sudden cardiac death annually in the United States and the incidence in other developed nations is comparable.[148] Approximately 20% to 30% of patients suffering out-of-hospital cardiac arrest can be successfully resuscitated in urban centers with a well organized paramedic system.[34,147,148] Cardiac arrest is usually not associated with myocardial infarction, and ventricular fibrillation is the most commonly documented cardiac rhythm.[25,34,197] Annual recurrence rate of cardiac arrest or ventricular tachycardia in out-of-hospital cardiac arrest survivors have been unacceptably high, in the range of 10% to 30% at 1 year.[8,121,122,197,211] Although implantation of the initial ICDs required that a patient survive at least two episodes of sudden death, excellent clinical results with first-generation devices established their therapeutic role in the management of sudden cardiac death survivors.* Resuscitation from out-of-hospital cardiac arrest without a reversible electrolyte, metabolic, or drug-induced disorder, in the absence of an acute myocardial infarction is now a well accepted indication for ICD therapy.

Recurrence rate of VT/VF in patients presenting with ventricular tachycardia and treated with EP-guided or Holter-guided drug therapy range from 5% to 12% at 1 to 2 years.† Hypotensive VT, recurrence of VT/VF on drug ther-

*References 1, 42, 133, 138, 150, 168, 201, 218

†References 10, 35, 71, 110, 160, 164, 180, 214

apy, or VT refractory to drug therapy by EP studies justify ICD implantation. If drug therapy is not tolerated or if drug compliance is a potential problem, an implanted device may be more acceptable to the patient and the physician.

Finally, persistent inducibility on drug therapy or inducibility after surgical or catheter ablation suggests significant risk of VT/VF recurrence that justifies device therapy.

CONTRAINDICATIONS

Contraindications to device therapy consist of reversible or correctable metabolic or electrolyte disturbance, or drug toxicity resulting in VT/VF. Risk of arrhythmia recurrence in this setting is low and does not warrant any therapy. However, it may be difficult to be certain of the triggering cause, often because of inadequate documentation.

Recurrent syncope of undetermined etiology in a patient without inducible ventricular arrhythmias and underlying structural heart disease carries a very low risk of sudden death and should not be treated with an implantable device, which would be ineffective.[93]

The risk of ventricular tachyarrhythmias in patients with the Wolff-Parkinson-White syndrome is low and is best addressed by surgical or catheter ablation.[20,63,76,104,191]

Patients with incessant VT or VF should not have an ICD implanted because such therapy does not improve survival and is associated with discomfort of repeated device discharge and early battery depletion.[220] Such patients may warrant ICD implantation if their arrhythmia frequency can be reduced by other means (drugs, surgery, or catheter ablation).

Finally, ICD implantation may not be suitable if the patient's life expectancy is diminished due to other disease, such as disseminated carcinoma, or if surgical intervention is not possible due to surgical or anesthetic contraindication, for example, in a patient with very poor left ventricular function. Implantable device therapy may not be appropriate if it is deemed that the patient may not be able to deal psychologically with the ICD or the electrical shocks.

PATIENT EVALUATION

Initial management of patients after successful resuscitation requires stabilization in an intensive-care environment. Associated myocardial infarction should be ruled out and any metabolic or electrolyte disturbances corrected. Hypokalemia is not uncommonly seen following cardiac resuscitation and may be the result of the hyperadrenergic state rather than the cause of ventricular arrhythmias.[19] Following stabilization and neurologic recovery, a thorough evaluation should be initiated (see the box).

This evaluation consists of noninvasive and invasive investigations. The first step in the evaluation is to establish the nature and severity of underlying

---

Diagnostic Evaluation of Patient with VT/VF

1. Signal averaged ECG with heart rate variability
2. 24-48 hour Holter monitoring
3. 2D-echocardiogram
4. Multi-gated nuclear angiography (MUGA)
5. Exercise stress test
6. Cardiac catheterization
7. Electrophysiologic study

---

structural heart disease. Evaluation of left ventricular function (MUGA or 2D-echo) and signal averaged ECG (with heart rate variability) are helpful for risk stratification and for identifying an underlying substrate. Two-dimensional echocardiography identifies underlying valvular disease, presence of mural thrombus, and cardiac chamber sizes. A symptom-limited exercise stress test with or without radionuclide administration is helpful in defining the presence of ischemia, provocation of arrhythmias, and the patient's physiologic heart rate response to maximal exercise. Ambulatory electrocardiographic monitoring for 24 hours or longer may be helpful in quantifying ambient ventricular arrhythmias and in defining the presence of other significant arrhythmias. These noninvasive studies are followed by complete cardiac catheterization before electrophysiologic testing in the drug-free state. Cardiac catheterization helps define the presence and extent of coronary artery disease. Based on the findings, one can decide whether it may be safe to proceed with electrophysiologic studies, which may induce hypotensive arrhythmias. In the presence of very severe coronary artery disease (e.g., critical left main disease or equivalent) revascularization may be warranted prior to electrophysiologic testing.

The results of the above investigations help define the substrate that leads to sudden cardiac death or sustained ventricular tachycardia. Integration of these investigations helps develop an individualized therapeutic approach.

TREATMENT OPTIONS

Many factors determine the selection of proper therapy for patients with life-threatening ventricular arrhythmias. These include clinical history and mode of presentation, results of noninvasive studies, electrophysiologic study results, angiographic evaluation, the patient's expectations, and the overall prognosis, especially in the presence of concomitant medical illnesses. After a thorough evaluation and careful consideration, a highly individualized therapeutic plan can be tailored based on the availability of standard and investigational devices and lead systems, experience of the electrophysiologist, and surgical expertise. Therapeutic options include drug therapy, curative surgical procedure, catheter ablation of arrhythmia substrate, and ICD therapy.

DRUGS

Pharmacologic therapies may be empiric or guided by the results of Holter monitoring or electrophysiologic testing. Empiric antiarrhythmic therapy in sudden death survivors or patients with ventricular tachycardia is fraught with a high recurrence rate.[54,139] However, empiric amiodarone therapy may have a role in patients unwilling to undergo electrophysiologic evaluation. Herre et al.[70] have reported the long-term results of empiric amiodarone therapy in 427 patients with recurrent sustained ventricular tachycardia or ventricular fibrillation. They noted the 2-year sudden death mortality to be 12% and the 2-year total mortality to be 34%.

Pharmacologic therapy can be guided by the results of Holter monitoring or electrophysiologic testing. Holter-guided therapy requires the presence of ambient arrhythmias with successful pharmacologic therapy generally defined as complete suppression of ventricular tachycardia and ≥ 90% suppression of ventricular ectopy.[21,37,214] However, as many as 30% of patients may not have adequate volume of ventricular arrhythmias to allow Holter-guided therapy.[110,180] Even patients demonstrating satisfactory response to antiarrhythmic therapy on Holter may have a cardiac arrest recurrence rate of 10% per year up to 4 years.[71,110]

Electrophysiologically guided pharmacologic therapy requires inducibility of ventricular tachycardia during the baseline drug-free study and noninducibility on drug therapy. In general, 50% to 80% of patients presenting with cardiac arrest have inducible ventricular arrhythmia during the baseline study.* Inducibility of a ventricular arrhythmia in cardiac arrest survivors depends on the underlying disease as well as the presenting arrhythmia. In general, the inducibility rate is higher in patients with underlying coronary artery disease than in patients with dilated cardiomyopathy, and is higher in patients presenting with ventricular tachycardia than in patients with ventricular fibrillation.[18,183] In the absence of inducible arrhythmia, electrophysiologically guided drug therapy is not possible, and these patients remain at risk of recurrent VT/VF.[164,186,214]

Although the majority of cardiac arrest survivors have inducible ventricular arrhythmias, appropriate antiarrhythmic therapy to render them noninducible can only be found in up to 35% of patients.[144,164,185] Patients rendered noninducible have a much better prognosis than those who remain inducible, but even with appropriate pharmacologic therapy VT/VF recurrence rate may remain as high as 10% to 15% at 2 years.[10,35,162,164,214] The Electrophysiologic Study Versus Electrocardiographic Monitoring (ESVEM) investigators recently reported more frequent and faster drug efficacy testing with repeated Holter

*References 66, 89, 164, 165, 180, 183

monitoring used in conjunction with stress testing than with repeated electrophysiology studies.[37] These two approaches to determining the appropriate pharmacologic therapy resulted in similar long-term survival, although the survival data have not yet been published. These results are very interesting and need further corroboration.

SURGERY

Surgical approaches to the management of patients surviving sudden cardiac death or VT has evolved over the last 30 years and has included revascularization alone, blind aneurysmectomy without preoperative mapping, encircling ventriculotomy, and most recently map-guided aneurysmectomy. The role of revascularization alone has been received limited attention.* Patients with coronary artery disease and cardiac arrest have a good prognosis after revascularization if they did not have an inducible arrhythmia or had VF at baseline electrophysiology study.[97,107] However, if ventricular tachycardia is inducible at baseline study, 80% remain inducible after revascularization.[97] Although revascularization may not prevent arrhythmia recurrence, it has an adjunctive role in the management of such patients by relief of ischemia to improve the underlying substrate.

Simple aneurysmectomy for cure of ventricular tachycardia was first reported in 1959.[26] Simple aneurysmectomy without electrophysiologic study and mapping, in combination with revascularization has perioperative mortality of 20% to 25% with ventricular tachycardia cure rates of only up to 40%.†

In 1978 Guiraudon et al.[61] proposed the encircling ventriculotomy procedure to isolate the arrhythmogenic tissue from normal myocardium. Cure of ventricular arrhythmias with this procedure was encouraging but was associated with increased left ventricular dysfunction and the occurrence of postoperative congestive heart failure. Modifications of this technique combining ventriculotomy with cryoablation along the border zone resulted in better hemodynamic and electrophysiologic outcome.[155]

Clinical use of invasive electrophysiologic testing in the 1970s permitted systematic evaluation of the electrophysiologic basis for recurrent ventricular tachycardia. Josephson and Harken[88] in 1979 introduced the concept of map-guided subendocardial resection. This approach required the identification of the "site of origin" of the tachycardia by preoperative catheter mapping in the electrophysiology laboratory or intraoperatively using a hand-held probe. More recently, computerized mapping systems for endocardial and epicardial mapping have been developed to simplify and speed up intraoperative mapping.[75,131,158] The tachycardia site of origin is defined as the endocardial site showing the earliest activation, usually manifested as presystolic fractionated

*References 95, 97, 104, 140, 149, 186
†References 7, 17, 55, 68, 127, 156

potentials. This is generally located in the border zone between scar tissue and the normal myocardium. The endocardium in this region is resected and postoperative electrophysiologic testing is performed 7 to 10 days later. The initial investigators reported a 9% operative mortality and postoperative tachycardia nondeductibility in 72%.[132] Other surgical centers using similar techniques have reported operative mortality of 8% to 20% and success rates of 60% to 96%.* Factors associated with operative and perioperative mortality include advanced age, severity of coronary artery disease, poor left ventricular function, absence of a resectable aneurysm, cardiopulmonary bypass time, and emergent surgery.†

Patients with a discrete aneurysm or scar due to previous myocardial infarction, preserved left ventricular function, and hemodynamically stable monomorphic ventricular tachycardia allowing adequate preoperative catheter mapping in the electrophysiology laboratory are the ideal candidates for surgical approach. The presence of more than one form of sustained ventricular tachycardia is not a contraindication but demands careful mapping of all VT morphologies. However, polymorphic ventricular tachycardia is not generally amenable to surgical cure. Patients with global left ventricular dysfunction or severe associated medical or pulmonary disease are not suitable candidates due to the high risk of perioperative mortality.

CATHETER ABLATION

Radiofrequency catheter ablation has become the preferred curative therapy for most forms of supraventricular tachycardia.[20,76,108,111] Although direct-current catheter ablation of ventricular tachycardia with underlying coronary artery disease has had some success, radiofrequency catheter ablation of ventricular tachycardia has not been studied extensively.‡

Catheter ablation for ventricular tachycardia has been directed to etiologies other than coronary artery disease with good results.[105,109,195] Recently, Morady et al.[141] have shown that radiofrequency catheter ablation of ischemic VT may be possible in a highly selected subgroup of coronary artery disease patients. However, they suggest that a reluctance to rely on catheter ablation as the only therapy for life-threatening ventricular tachycardia may relegate ablation to an adjunctive role in ischemic VT, to be used along with antiarrhythmic drugs and implantable devices. If the results from other centers with long-term follow-up are encouraging, it is possible that catheter ablation may ultimately have a more prominent role in the management of ischemic ventricular arrhythmias.

---

*References 15, 47, 67, 131, 155, 174

†References 28, 48, 49, 129, 132, 154, 155, 187

‡References 9, 13, 38, 43, 142, 143

ICD

The occurrence of ventricular tachycardia and ventricular fibrillation is an interplay between substrate and trigger with modulation by the autonomic nervous system.[27] The underlying substrate can change as the disease process evolves and may be evidenced by worsening coronary artery disease or deterioration of left ventricular function. Electrolyte imbalance and the presence of antiarrhythmic agents may also contribute to precipitating VT or VF. Given the variety of circumstances that may lead to VT/VF, the need for an effective generic therapy is evident.

The ICD is the primary therapy of choice in circumstances where antiarrhythmic therapy is unreliable or ineffective or if its efficacy cannot be assessed. The results of previously outlined evaluation help determine appropriate therapy. ICD is the primary therapy of choice in patients with hypotensive VT or VF who are not inducible during an electrophysiology study or if inducible, not suppressible with antiarrhythmic drugs. Patients with dilated cardiomyopathy or hypertrophic cardiomyopathy and hypotensive VT or VF are also appropriate candidates for ICD therapy.

ICD IMPLANTATION

Once the decision has been made to implant an ICD, the appropriate device, lead system, and surgical approach must be selected. Until recently the only FDA approved device for clinical use in the U.S. was manufactured by CPI, Inc. Therapy choices consisted of low- and high-energy shocks, and some of these devices provided back-up bradycardia pacing. In 1992 the FDA-approved release of the Medtronic PCD, a unit that offers additional tiered VT therapies (antitachycardia pacing and low-energy cardioversion) in conjunction with defibrillation, bradycardia pacing, limited stored data of events and episode data. In other countries devices manufactured by other companies are already available. Although the market-released devices and lead systems are limited at this time, several devices are available in clinical trials and it is likely that over the next few years many devices with various features of importance will become available.

SELECTION OF ICDS

Selection of the appropriate ICD requires a consideration of patient needs balanced against the myriad of device features available in current devices. For example, the patient with only ventricular fibrillation may not need a device with tiered VT therapy, and a device capable of defibrillation and back-up bradycardia pacing may be sufficient. While a complex, multifaceted device may allow flexibility in choosing initial and modifying subsequent therapy, similar results may be achievable with a less complex device. ICDs are generally described as first-, second- or third-generation based on their complexity. The first-generation devices were not programmable or were min-

---

Implantable Cardioverter/Defibrillators (ICDS)

First generation
   Nonprogrammable or minimally programmable
Second generation
   Minimal programmability and/or telemetry
   Bradycardia pacing
Third generation
   Extensive programmability and telemetry
   Bradycardia pacing
   Antitachycardia pacing

---

imally programmable, whereas the third-generation devices have multiple programmable features (see the box). Details of the FDA-approved devices and those currently in clinical trials are noted in Table 14-1.

FACILITIES AND EQUIPMENT

The ideal ICD implant center should have equipment, facilities, and personnel for patient evaluation, ICD implantation, and subsequent follow-up, as well as the ability to provide alternative and adjunctive therapies (e.g., arrhythmia surgery, catheter ablation, coronary artery bypass surgery). Support facilities for preimplant evaluation should include all noninvasive and invasive cardiac laboratories. The operating room for ICD implantation should have fluoroscopic capability so that transvenous and/or epicardial implantations can be performed.

Equipment for intraoperative testing should include a multichannel recorder, pacing system analyzer, and device implant support equipment that are usually specific to each manufacturer. Appropriate equipment and protocols for determining defibrillation efficacy, cardioversion, and tachycardia pace-termination should also be available. After implantation, critical care facilities with appropriate monitoring equipment are essential. Outpatient follow-up capability with recording and electronic analysis equipment for troubleshooting problems should be available for each specific device implanted at that center.

SURGICAL APPROACHES

The current prime determinants of the surgical approach for ICD implantation are the limited availability of lead systems and the need for concomitant surgery. Nonthoracotomy lead systems are still investigational and available

Table 14-1
Currently Available ICDs

	CPI				Intermedics Res-Q	Medtronics			Siemens Guardian	Telectronics Guardian-		Ventritex
Model	Ventak*	Ventak P	Ventak Prx	Ventak Prx II	101-01; 101-02	PCD 7216A	PCD 7217*	PCD 7219D	2120	ATP 4202/4203	4210	Cadence V-100*
Weight (gms)	235	235	234	233	220	281	200	136	210	200	200	237
Tachycardia detection algorithm	R; R+ PDF	R; R+ PDF	R,O,D,S TPM	R,O,D,S, TPM	R,O,D,S	R,O,D,S	R,O,D,S	R,O,D,S	R,O,D	R	R,O,D	R,O,D, SHR
Programmable rate threshold	Y	Y	Y	Y	Y	Y	Y	Y	Y	Y	Y	Y
Therapies												
Bradycardia pacing	N	N	Y	Y	Y	Y	Y	Y	Y	Y	Y	Y
Antitachycardia pacing	N	N	Y	Y	Y	Y	Y	Y	Y	N	Y	Y
Cardioversion												
Defibrillation												
Programmable energy	Y	Y	Y	Y	Y	Y	Y	Y	Y	Y	Y	Y
Waveform(s)	Mono	Mono	Mono	Mono/Bi	Mono/Bi	Mono/Seq/Sim	Mono/Seq/Sim	Mono/Bi/Sim	Mono	Mono	Mono	Mono/Bi
Fixed tilt or PW	Tilt	Tilt	Tilt Programmable	Tilt Programmable	PW	PW	PW	Tilt Programmable	PW	PW	PW	PW
Committed shock therapy	Y	Y	Y	Y	Y	Y	Y	Y	N	N	N	Y
Tiered VT therapy	N	N	Y	Y	Y	Y	Y	Y	Y	N	Y	Y

*FDA-approved devices in the U.S.
Mono, monophasic; Bi, biphasic; Seq, sequential; PW, pulse width; R, rate; PDF, probability density function; TPM, turning point morphology; SHR, sustained high rate; O, sudden onset; D, duration; Sim, simultaneous; S, rate stability

only to clinical investigators and investigating centers. For the remaining implanting physicians, only the epicardial patch electrodes are available. Epicardial patch electrodes have the advantage of lower defibrillation energy requirements regardless of the defibrillation waveform but require a thoracotomy for implantation.[167,190] Transvenous lead systems are easier to implant and are associated with less morbidity and mortality.[167]

Patients requiring concomitant coronary artery revascularization, valve repair or replacement, or aneurysmectomy may receive the ICD implant via a median sternotomy. However, if ICD implant alone is indicated, epicardial patch electrodes can be placed using a subxyphoid or subcostal incision, or left anterior thoractomy.[113,114,209,220] The only approved lead system at the time of this writing is the epicardial patch electrodes, although it is likely that CPI's Endotak (Fig. 14-1) and Medtronic's NTL lead systems (Fig. 14-2) will become available soon. The NTL lead system, consisting of three electrodes, is totally intravascular, whereas the Endotak lead may be implanted alone (transvenous) or in combination with a subcutaneous patch.

The original ICD lead system consisted of a superior vena cava spring electrode and a patch or apical conformal electrode.[137] Two problems became apparent with this lead system: migration of the superior vena caval electrode and the inability to defibrillate some patients.[146] This led to the use of two epicardial patch electrodes for defibrillation using monophasic waveforms.[216]

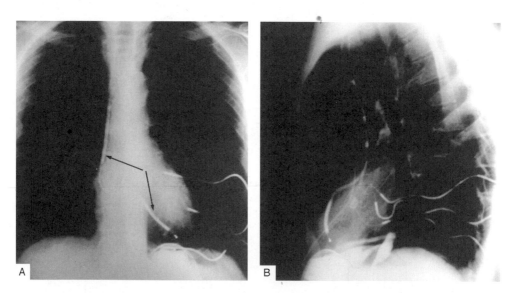

Fig. 14-1, A and **B.** PA and lateral projections of a chest x-ray demonstrating CPI's Endotak lead introduced from the left subclavian vein and a subcutaneous array lead placed over the left thorax. Arrows point to the proximal and the distal electrodes on the Endotak lead. (Courtesy of Luis M. Arisso, CPI Inc., Minneapolis, MN.)

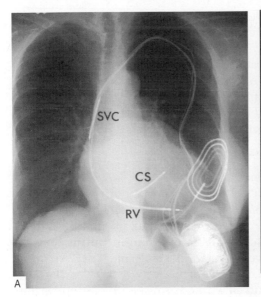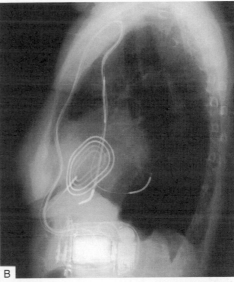

Fig. 14-2, A and **B.** PA and lateral projections of a chest x-ray demonstrating Medtronic's transvenous lead system. In this patient a subcutaneous patch electrode was also required. Transvenous electrodes are positioned in the superior vena cava (*SVC*), the coronary sinus (*CS*), and the right ventricle (*RV*). The three intravascular leads were placed via the left subclavian vein.

Subsequently, a three-patch system and sequential or simultaneous pulse defibrillation was described.[79] For either electrode system there is an inverse relationship between electrode surface area and defibrillation energy requirement.[92,202]

Epicardial patch electrodes may be placed intra- or extrapericardially. The edges of the electrodes are sutured to the parietal pericardium or directly to the epicardial surface. In patients who have had prior cardiac surgery, extrapericardial patch placement may be easier and safer. A potential disadvantage of extrapericardial patch placement is the potential rise in defibrillation energy requirement in the immediate postoperative period due to accumulation of even a modest-sized pericardial effusion.[175,193] For epicardial patch-patch defibrillation, two unipolar screw-in electrodes form a bipolar pair for pacing and sensing. Pace-sense screw-in leads are generally attached 1 to 2 cm apart and are usually on the left ventricular apex.

Transvenous defibrillation was described in an animal model well before the first human ICD implant.[134] Due to insufficient defibrillation efficacy, this approach was abandoned in favor of spring-patch and patch-patch defibrillation. Now however, transvenous defibrillation via two different lead systems has been described.[128,225] A combination of intracardiac electrode(s) and a subcutaneous patch has also been useful. A single right ventricular catheter electrode or combination of right ventricular and superior vena caval electrodes have been combined with a left chest wall subcutaneous or submuscular patch electrode or a coronary sinus electrode to direct shock current to the left ventricular myocardial mass.[2,145,225] In the transvenous lead systems the right ventricular electrode is used for rate counting.

After the electrodes are positioned and tested to ensure adequate pacing, sensing and defibrillation, a pocket is made for the ICD pulse generator. The ICD pulse generator can be placed subdiaphragmatically, or in the subcutaneous tissue, or under the rectus abdominis muscle in the left upper quadrant of the abdominal wall.[46,62]

INTRAOPERATIVE TESTING

The purpose of intraoperative testing is to ensure adequate sensing of normal rhythm as well as ventricular tachycardia and ventricular fibrillation and to ensure defibrillation efficacy with an adequate safety margin. Intraoperative testing consists of measurement of ventricular electrograms, defibrillation electrode impedance, pacing threshold, and defibrillation efficacy.

Measurement of signal amplitude and slew rate from the bipolar epicardial or endocardial rate-counting electrodes should be performed during normal rhythm using a pacing system analyzer. Ventricular pacing function should be assessed to ensure adequate pacing threshold. Intraoperative pacing threshold should be less than 1.0 to 1.5 V at 0.5 ms pulse width.

A low-energy shock (0.2 to 1 J) applied in sinus rhythm may be used to test the defibrillation pathway impedance.[118] The impedance measured with a low-energy shock has been shown to be somewhat higher than a defibrillation shock, but this technique allows a safe and simple method to ensure that all the electrodes are connected correctly and are functioning appropriately before ventricular fibrillation is induced. Defibrillation pathway impedance is dependent on the electrode system. Impedance values in humans range from 30 to 70 ohms and appear to be somewhat lower for a patch-patch electrode system than for a catheter-patch electrode system.[112,118,130,199]

Sensing during ventricular tachycardia and ventricular fibrillation can be assessed using marker channels in second- and third-generation devices. Marker channels in some devices indicate sensed and paced events, as well as detection of arrhythmia in certain zones, satisfaction of requirement for therapy, and markers to indicate that the device is charging its capacitors (Fig. 14-3). Marker channels of this kind allow rapid determination of ICD sensing function. Double counting and signal dropout are easily detected. The implanting physician should ensure that the signals satisfy or exceed the minimum requirements of the device.

Device efficacy should be tested in all cases by inducing ventricular fibrillation. If the patient has inducible ventricular tachycardia, VT termination algorithms should also be tested at some point. At some centers this is done intraoperatively at the time of implantation whereas other centers do so at a later date to minimize intraoperative testing and hypotensive episodes. Ven-

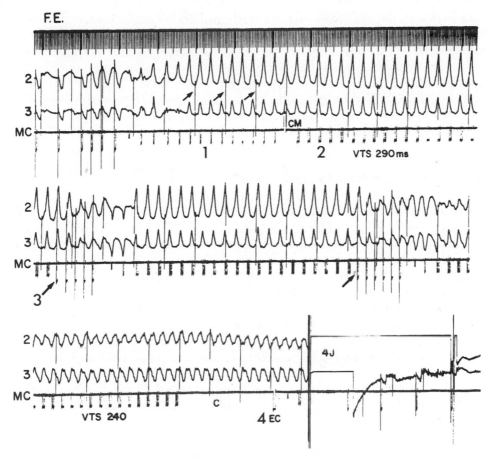

Fig. 14-3. Antitachycardia pacing (*arrow*) and low-energy cardioversion for induced ventricular tachycardia. This patient also had a unipolar atrial pacemaker (*small arrows*). The ICD marker channel (*MC*) indicates ventricular sensed beats (1), VT (2), ventricular paced beats (3), and end of capacitor charging (4) by different markers. After the capacitor is charged, a synchronous 4 J shock is delivered. Marker channels help determine if the device is functioning appropriately.

tricular fibrillation is usually induced by a brief application of alternating current or very rapid ventricular pacing pulses. Ventricular fibrillation is allowed to persist, usually for 10 seconds, after which a test shock is delivered. An unsuccessful test shock is followed by a transthoracic rescue shock of high efficacy.

Most of the defibrillation threshold protocols in use today are modifications of the original description by Bourland.[14] If the initial test shock is successful, repeat testing is performed with shocks of progressively lower energies until the test shock fails to defibrillate. If the first shock is unsuccessful, the energy is incremented until success is achieved. Defibrillation threshold is defined as the shock of least energy that successfully defibrillates the heart. At some centers implant criteria may rely on a cutoff defibrillation threshold whereas others require reliable defibrillation below a certain energy level.

The term *defibrillation threshold* implies a clear and consistent relationship between effective and ineffective shocks. However, defibrillation appears to behave in a probabilistic manner with a sigmoidal relationship between energy and defibrillation efficacy.[31] Defibrillation threshold as defined above appears to be reproducible and stable over time, and falls in the range of 62.5% to 87.5% probability of success.[31,80,163,200]

The main purpose of defibrillation threshold testing is to ensure an adequate safety margin between the threshold and the maximum output of the implanted device. The safety margin should be large enough to accommodate any future changes in defibrillation efficacy as a result of prolonged fibrillation time, progression of underlying disease, or alteration of antiarrhythmic drug therapy. The maximum acceptable defibrillation threshold above which a device should not be implanted is unknown, although most implanters would agree that inability to defibrillate consistently at the maximum output of the device constitutes a reasonable contraindication.

Intraoperative defibrillation threshold testing may require multiple VF inductions and may be time-consuming, especially if multiple variables (lead polarity, defibrillation pathway, waveform, etc.) require assessment to find an acceptable lead configuration and defibrillation threshold. However, extensive evaluation appears to be safe and well tolerated hemodynamically if clinical parameters are closely monitored.[44] An area of concern is the potential adverse neurologic effects of repeated episodes of transient hypotension induced during defibrillation trials. Using a computerized EEG technique, Singer et al. have reported that more than 6 VF episodes lasting <20 seconds each produced persistent changes on the EEG lasting up to 1 hour.[178] The clinical significance of these changes is uncertain, although similar changes during bypass surgery appear to be associated with postoperative confusional states and neurologic deficits.[106] In practice one should minimize the number of fibrillation-defibrillation trials.

PROBLEMS AND COMPLICATIONS

MORBIDITY AND MORTALITY

Morbidity and mortality following ICD implantation may be related to underlying medical illnesses, left ventricular dysfunction, and the use of concomitant cardiac surgery. Reported surgical mortality has ranged between 3% and 5.4%, although very low mortality has also been reported.* Joye et al.[90] have

---

*References 1, 50, 90, 96, 152, 204, 219, 221, 225

reported no mortality within 30 days of ICD implantation in 150 consecutive patients, whereas Winkle et al.[219] have reported 1.65% 30-day perioperative mortality in 555 patients. These excellent results may be a reflection of better patient selection, improved surgical technique, or experience and care taken by certain groups.

It has been demonstrated that left ventricular dysfunction increases surgical risk, although such patients clearly benefit from ICD therapy. Gohn et al.[51] have reported a 1.5% perioperative mortality in 137 patients with EF > 30% compared to 7.5% mortality in 134 patients with EF ≤ 30%. In a smaller group of patients Kim et al.[101] have reported 11% mortality in patients with EF < 30% and 0% in patients with EF ≥ 30%.

Concomitant surgical procedure at the time of ICD implantation may also contribute to increased mortality. Winkle et al.[221] have reported 4.6% 30-day mortality in 669 patients undergoing ICD implantation without as opposed to 3.2% mortality in 280 patients with concomitant surgery. Increased mortality with concomitant procedures have also been reported by others.[51]

Preliminary data suggest that nonthoracotomy ICD implantation may be attended by a very low 30-day surgical mortality.[45,169] Frame et al.[45] and Saksena et al.[169] have reported 0% mortality in 30 patients undergoing ICD implantation using a nonthoracotomy lead system, and the Medtronic PCD Investigators Group have reported a .3% perioperative mortality in the group with nonthoracotomy endocardial lead system as opposed to 5.5% mortality in the group receiving epicardial patch electrodes via a thoracotomy.

Overall, surgical mortality appears to be approximately 3% for ICD implantation with epicardial patch electrodes for defibrillation and may be slightly higher in patients requiring concomitant surgery. Operative mortality risk may be lower for nonthoracotomy ICD implantation since the surgical procedure is not as extensive. However, this factor may be offset by the fact that patients previously considered high risk for a thoracotomy may be offered device therapy with a transvenous lead system.

Morbidity of ICD therapy is not insignificant and the implanting center should be fully prepared to identify and address problems as they arise. Grimm et al.[57] have reported complications in 53% of 241 patients undergoing 353 device implants and followed for 24 ± 20 months. This group of patients had epicardial as well as nonthoracotomy lead systems and first-, second-, and third-generation devices were implanted. Concomitant surgery was performed in 16% of the patients. Complications were defined as any untoward effects related to the ICD implantation or function. There were no intraoperative deaths, but 30-day mortality was reported to be 3.3%. Postoperative bleeding or thrombosis occurred in 4%. Eleven percent of the patients experienced respiratory complications. ICD infection requiring removal of the device occurred in 5%. Lead migration or other complications occurred in 8%, and 22% of the patients experienced ECG-documented shocks for nonclinical arrhythmias. An operative procedure was required to correct the complication in 21% of the patients.

HIGH THRESHOLD

The incidence of defibrillation energy requirement too high to permit ICD implantation is not known, although Troup et al.[200] have reported this incidence to be approximately 0.4% for epicardial defibrillation using devices with maximum high-energy output of 35 to 40 J. The exact incidence remains elusive due to differences in DFT protocols among various implanting centers and investigators. It is evident that many parameters affect defibrillation energy requirements: lead configuration, waveform, lead polarity, antiarrhythmic drugs, etc. It may be stated that if the DFT is half of the maximum device output, adequate safety margin exists to allow for future changes in effective defibrillation energy requirements. However, the converse may not be true. This emphasizes that the decision to implant a device or to abandon the procedure intraoperatively cannot be based solely on a predetermined DFT.

Since there are multiple parameters that influence DFT, they should be considered and optimized intraoperatively if the patient's condition allows. For epicardial defibrillation, largest-size patches should be used if possible and patches should be positioned opposite each other to avoid contact between the edges of the patches, which may result in current shunting and reduced defibrillation efficacy. Cardiac tissue between the patches should be maximized and the interventricular septum should be incorporated in the defibrillation pathway. Availability of sequential monophasic pulses over two defibrillation pathways or biphasic pulse over a single pathway have been shown to decrease DFT and should be tested if clinically available. Finally, the influence of antiarrhythmic drugs should be considered and if possible drugs should be stopped or administered in lower doses. Similar principles hold true for transvenous lead systems.

The availability of biphasic, simultaneous or sequential shocks in the newer third-generation devices should allow adequate DFTs for implantation in virtually every patient deemed to require such therapy.

DEVICE-DRUG INTERACTIONS

Concomitant antiarrhythmic drug therapy is often necessary in patients with ICDs. More than half of the patients may require one or more antiarrhythmic agents.[1,206] Although the effect of most antiarrhythmic agents on defibrillation efficacy has been evaluated in animal models, human data are sparse. Drugs may increase, decrease, or have no effect on DFT (Table 14-2). Drugs of the same class may have discordant effects on defibrillation energy requirements. Therefore the effect of such therapy on defibrillation efficacy merits consideration especially in circumstances where there is inadequate safety margin. Subsequent changes in antiarrhythmic drug therapy after implantation may necessitate repeat testing of the device to ensure proper detection and termination of VT and VF since antiarrhythmic drugs may alter tachycardia rates and thereby the ability to satisfy detection criteria. Potentially, drugs may increase defibrillation energy requirements.

Table 14-2
Potential Effects of Antiarrhyhmic Drugs on Defibrillation Efficacy

Class	Increase	Decrease	No Change
IA			
Procainamide			X
Quinidine			X
IB			
Mexilitine	X		
Lidocaine	X		
IC			
Encainide	X		
ODE	X		
MODE			X
Flecainide	X		
Racainam	X		
II (β-blockers)			
Propanolol	X		X
III			
Amiodarone	X	X	X
Sotalol		X	
Bretylium			X
OTHERS			
Digoxin			X
Isoproterenol			X

Modified from Selle JC et al: Successful clinical laser ablation of ventricular tachycardia: a promising new therapeutic method, *Ann Thorac Surg* 42:380, 1986.

DEVICE-DEVICE INTERACTIONS

Interactions between bradycardia or antitachycardia pacemakers and implantable cardioverter defibrillators were a potential source of concern with first- and second-generation devices since patients may have had pacemakers (bradycardia or antitachycardia) implanted in addition to the ICD. However, with the availability of back-up bradycardia and antitachycardia pacing incorporated in the third-generation ICDs, device-device interactions of this nature are obviated unless a preexisting pacemaker is *in situ* at the time of ICD implantation. Presently only VVI pacing is available in the ICDs. If the clinical situation warrants dual chamber pacing in an ICD recepient, bipolar pacing is preferred and great care should be taken at the time of implantation to ensure that the ICD does not sense the pacing stimulus artifact.

In ICDs of a previous generation the rate-counting circuit could potentially sense the pacemaker stimulus as well as the resulting ventricular depolarization that could ultimately satisfy the detection algorithm and initiate a countershock sequence.[22,96] The pacemakers could also undersense VF and thus continue to pace. The resulting pacing stimulus artifacts could be sensed by the automatic gain control circuitry of the ICD and result in failure of the ICD to defibrillate.[103]

The only ways to avoid these problems in the past were to employ bipolar sensing electrodes and position closely spaced rate-counting electrodes oriented orthogonally and distant from the pacemaker electrode.[200] Yet another problem is the transient rise in pacing threshold following a high-energy shock. Yee et al.[223] have described an increase in ventricular pacing threshold associated with a concomitant decrease in unipolar and bipolar R wave amplitude using a catheter in which the pacing electrodes served as the common cathode for defibrillation. The transient increase in pacing threshold after a high-energy shock is surmounted in the newer devices by allowing programmability for the postshock pacing stimulus.

POSTOPERATIVE PROBLEMS

Arrhythmias

Postoperative arrhythmias may include sustained or nonsustained VT, ventricular fibrillation, sinus tachycardia, atrial fibrillation, or other supraventricular tachycardias. Any of these may satisfy detection algorithm criteria and result in device therapy delivery. Defibrillation for VT and VF is appropriate but such therapy for supraventricular tachycardias is unacceptable and should be minimized. Grimm et al.[57] have reported an incidence of 22% for ECG-documented shocks for non-VT rhythm. Gartman et al.[50] have reported new onset atrial fibrillation in 20% of patients and sustained postoperative ventricular tachycardia in 11%.

In the immediate postoperative period, while the patient is monitored in an intensive care unit or similar environment, it may be reasonable to turn the ICD off. Once postoperative supraventricular arrhythmias subside, the ICD may be turned back on. This type of approach may decrease inappropriate postoperative shocks.

Infection

The reported incidence of ICD-related infections in experienced centers vary between 2% and 9%.[203,210,218,227] Acute infections presenting within days of ICD implantation are rare. ICD system infections tend to be indolent and become apparent within the first few months after initial implant or generator replacement. Causative organisms are usually streptococci or staphylococci but other organisms including anaerobes, gram negatives, mycobacterium avium, and candida have also been reported.

The suspicion of ICD system infection should be raised by local as well as systemic signs and symptoms of infection. Since most ICD system infections involve the generator site, local symptoms such as tenderness, erythema, warmth, discoloration, drainage, and erosion provide clues to infection. Fluctuation of the ICD generator pocket occurs commonly during the first few weeks after implantation due to collection of serosanguinous fluid in the pocket. Fever, leukocytosis, and left shift of the differential count all suggest a systemic infection. Blood cultures can be very helpful if positive. The incidence of culture-negative infections is unknown. Routine computed tomography of the heart has been shown to be helpful in detecting the presence and extent of infection involving epicardial patch electrodes late after implant.[52] During the first 4 weeks after epicardial patch placement, a small amount of fluid is observed on CT images. However, accumulation of fluid around the patches after this period and distortion of the patch electrodes is suggestive of infection.[52] The use of gallium-67 imaging to detect ICD infection has been described but this technique may yield false positive results in normally healing wounds.[98]

Therapeutic strategies include (1) local debridement with irrigation and systemic antibiotic therapy, (2) pulse generator removal in addition to local measures and systemic antibiotic therapy, or (3) complete explantation of the entire system followed by systemic antibiotic therapy. Although the first two approaches have been used successfully in selected cases, the basic principle of management appears to be complete explantation of all hardware followed by systemic antibiotic therapy for several weeks.[74,98,188] Some advocate choice 1 or 2 first and complete explantation only if a full antibiotic course fails to eradicate the infection since there are serious ramifications of ICD removal. Cessation of antibiotic therapy should be followed by a period of observation during which repeated aerobic and anaerobic blood cultures should be obtained and cultures should be observed for an adequate length of time to ensure no growth. During this period of observation the patient must be free of signs of infection. At that time a new system may be reimplanted.

Because an infected ICD system can be potentially life-threatening every effort should be made to prevent infection. Basic surgical principles include keeping the operating time as short as possible, avoiding tissue trauma, keeping the number of OR personnel and equipment limited to the essential, and keeping all sterile implantable equipment in original packaging until the time of implant. Antibiotic prophylaxis has become routine practice and in some institutions the pulse generator is covered with sponges soaked with ciprofloxacin (prior to implantation) and prior to wound closure, and all operative sites are rinsed with a solution of ciprofloxacin.[177] Another issue relevant to ICD patients is the use of prophylactic antibiotics for invasive procedures that may potentially result in bacteremia. The American Heart Association does not recommend routine use of prophylactic antibiotics in these patients, although many centers prescribe them for some invasive procedures.[30]

Electromagnetic Interference

Very little clinical data are available regarding electromagnetic interference with ICDs.[3,12,170] This paucity of information is likely to become even more striking as various devices become available and are routinely implanted. The magnetic field strength required to affect device function may not be large for some devices. Schmitt et al.[170] have reported a device switched to the standby mode by magnetized screws. These observations underscore the necessity of closely monitoring these patients and their devices and scrutinizing their daily environment if phantom programming seems to have occurred. Unfortunately it is unclear as to how one should go about accomplishing this. Recently Marco et al.[126] have studied the common practice of prohibiting the pacemaker patient from using electric welding machines. They tested the work environment of 12 pacemaker patients for EMI and concluded that the effects of EMI are pacemaker- and environment-dependent. They found that most pacemaker patients could safely perform a variety of functions in several high-EMI environments previously thought to be unsafe for them. Even electric arc welding machines up to 225 A without high-frequency voltage and with the cables uncoiled were safe.

Electrocautery is the commonest preventable form of electromagnetic interference in the hospital environment. If electrocautery use is anticipated, the ICD should be turned off or inactivated.

Patient Acceptance

Patients with life-threatening arrhythmias and implanted devices are prone to anxiety and depression. Anxiety and depression have been well described in pacemaker patients and these emotions are understandably more pronounced in the ICD population.[65,159,161,206,207] Keren et al.[100] have reported anxiety and depression in ICD patients but interestingly they did not find any difference in the level of anxiety or the degree of depression between ICD patients and patients with ventricular arrhythmias treated pharmacologically. Furthermore, they did not find significant differences between ICD patients who had received a shock and those that had not. Brodsky et al.[16] reported that 59% of ICD patients feared a shock, 83% reported decreased physical activity, 52% reported decreased sexual activity, and 54% had thoughts of death. Feelings of dependency and depression occurred in 51% and 47% respectively.

While most patients may be concerned about their life-style after device implantation, many return to work and activities that they enjoyed prior to surgery. Most patients who are employed prior to ICD implantation are able to return to work.[91]

Potential ICD patients need to be prepared psychologically for the surgery and require ongoing support. These patients and their immediate family members require understandable information about the patient's disease and the recommended therapy. This is best provided by a multidisciplinary team consisting of physicians, nursing staff, social worker, psychologist, and if necessary a psychiatrist. The information should be provided in multimedia form consisting of written material (books, booklets, etc.) as well as audio and video tapes. There should be adequate discussion of the information and any individual details relevant to the particular patient should also be discussed.

Many experienced centers have organized ICD support groups for ICD patients and their families. These groups meet on a regular basis and render a social function as well as providing a forum for new information about topics of medical interest to such an audience. Members also have small group sessions mediated by a social worker or a psychologist during which they may discuss their experience and concerns. Patients and their families may find considerable comfort in knowing that their problems are not unique. Interaction between members of the support group and patients being considered for device therapy may have therapeutic benefits in relieving anxiety and stress.

Adequate psychological preparation of these patients and their families prior to device implantation cannot be overemphasized. Prior to discharge they need to be reassured that they will be followed closely and that they have constant access to a team member who is knowledgeable about their particular case.

FOLLOW-UP OF ICD PATIENTS

ROUTINE FOLLOW-UP

Regular follow-up of ICD patients is essential considering the relative novelty of this technology, the potentially life-threatening consequences of a malfunctioning device, and the reassurance felt by the patient who knows that his or her ICD is functioning optimally. Prior to discharge from the hospital, after medical therapy is optimally adjusted, the device should be tested to ensure adequate detection and termination of VF and/or VT. If the patient's clinical condition does not permit testing prior to discharge, it may be scheduled at a reasonable duration after discharge. There are no universal guidelines for the interval between ICD checks and to some extent they should be individualized depending on the patient's condition. Currently available devices have various features and not all features are present in all devices. The following is a generic outline that should apply to most third-generation devices. It includes the need to reform capacitors every 2 to 3 months.

During a particular follow-up visit the device is first interrogated to determine the programmed pacing and sensing parameters, battery status, last charge time, VT/VF detection criteria and therapies. Event counters in the device indicate occurrences of VT/VF and the effectiveness of delivered therapies. Devices may also provide R-R interval measurements or electrograms for the last detected tachycardia.

The device capacitors should then be charged to maximum output and the charge time determined. This serves two functions. First, charging the capacitors decreases the time required for recharging at a later date (formation of capacitors). Second, the charge time is one index of residual battery power and monitors battery life. At the beginning of life 6 to 10 seconds may be required to charge the capacitors to maximum output energy. As the battery ages, the charge time increases. Each device has a predetermined elective replacement index (ERI); when the ERI is exceeded, the generator should be replaced within 1 to 3 months.

Next the pacing and sensing function of the device should be evaluated using the marker channels if available. One should ensure that double sensing of a wide QRS complex, T-waves, or afterpotential does not occur.

During each visit a brief but pertinent physical examination should be performed and a 12-lead ECG should be recorded. Chest x-ray in two views (PA and lateral) should be obtained periodically to evaluate defibrillation electrodes. Assessment of left ventricular function (2-D echocardiogram or radionuclide angiography) should be performed periodically. Exercise stress tests and ambulatory monitoring may be helpful in managing patients to determine maximal heart rate and any ambient arrhythmias.

DEVICE REPROGRAMMING

The availability of multiprogrammability in the third-generation devices allows the physician to interact with the changing clinical situation and the arrhythmic substrate to optimally tailor the device features for each individual patient. It has been shown that the advent of multiprogrammability has resulted in decreased numbers of shocks due to the successful use of anti-tachycardia pacing.[59,117] Programmable features in devices currently in clinical trials include cycle length definition of two zones of VT and cycle length criterion for VF. A combination of cycle length, sudden onset, and rate stability may be programmable for detection of VT. Therapy options for VT include antitachycardia pacing and programmable energies for cardioversion. Defibrillation waveforms may allow a choice of monophasic, biphasic, and sequential pulses. Bradycardia pacing parameters can also be defined to overcome the problem of postshock increase in pacing threshold.

RETESTING DEFIBRILLATION THRESHOLDS

In general it can be stated that changes in pharmacologic therapy that may result in increased defibrillation energy requirement or evolving changes in the substrate that bring into question the efficacy of programmed therapy should prompt careful evaluation. The most notable factor in this regard is the use of amiodarone. The effect of amiodarone on defibrillation threshold has been a controversial issue.[53,179] It has been suggested that acute intravenous administration of amiodarone results in decreased defibrillation energy requirements whereas chronic oral administration results in the opposite effect.[39,40,60,64,99] The issue of repeat defibrillation threshold testing is particularly germane in those patients who lack an adequate safety margin and subsequently require the addition of an antiarrhythmic agent that may potentially further increase the DFT. Finally, repeating DFT measurements on a routine basis is probably not necessary since defibrillation thresholds are stable over time in most patients.[208]

ICD REPLACEMENT

The generator replacement procedure for a device that has reached ERI is fairly simple. Under general anesthesia the ICD pocket is opened and the old generator is disconnected. The leads should be evaluated visually and performance characteristics should be assessed in the same manner as for the original implantation procedure. Evaluation of defibrillation efficacy should be repeated.

Gross et al.[58] have reported that 37% of patients who received an ICD did not get a shock during follow-up of more than 5 years. In such patients one may be tempted to question the initial judgment to implant a device and consider not replacing the device once it has reached ERI. However, it should be noted that the arrhythmia being treated with an ICD occurs intermittently and unpredictably, and first device discharge beyond 5 years has been reported.[41,56] Unless there is a strong reason to believe that the initial device implant was not necessary, most centers would recommend generator replacement.

DRIVING RECOMMENDATIONS FOR ICD PATIENTS

The ability to resume driving after ICD implantation is a serious concern for most ICD patients, and especially for those whose livelihood depends on it or who live in rural areas or areas without a safe and reliable public transportation system. Unfortunately there are few legal and medical guidelines to help the physician and the patient deal with this issue. Driving regulations vary from nation to nation and are a state or provincial jurisdiction in the U.S. and Canada, respectively. In the United States laws vary considerably from state to state. A recent survey of state regulations by Strickberger et al.[184] concluded that there was no legal consensus concerning driving restrictions after ICD implantation. Recently DiCarlo et al.[32] conducted a survey of 58 cardiologists implanting ICDs in three midwestern states (Indiana, Michigan, and Ohio) to determine their practices with respect to driving recommendations and compatibility with existing state laws. They found that only Michigan state laws explicitly prohibited driving after impairment or loss of consciousness until the condition causing it was corrected, cured, controlled, or spontaneously abated for more than 6 months. Indiana and Ohio state laws provided for issuance of restricted licenses that limit routes of travel for a minimum of 6 months. None of the three states were found to have any laws requiring either the physician or the patient to notify the Department of Transportation regarding any advice rendered against driving.

DiCarlo et al.[32] found that 43% of implanting physicians in their survey advised all ICD patients to abstain from driving whereas 4% never proscribed driving. The remaining 53% advised abstinence only to those patients with a history of arrhythmia-induced near-loss or loss of consciousness, or if such occurred during electrophysiology study, or during postimplant testing. In the absence of legal or medical guidelines the implanting physicians have had to exercise their best judgment. It is not known whether any implanting physicians have had legal difficulties as a result but the potential for liability exposure exists. There is an immediate need for our medical leadership to make some broad recommendations to the implanting physicians regarding this very important issue.

OTHER LEGAL ISSUES

Returning to work and driving are very important personal issues to ICD patients and their families and may result in a considerable amount of anxiety and depression. Given the concern regarding potential loss of consciousness from an arrhythmic event, it may be reasonable to prohibit patients from returning to occupations where there is a potential for injury to self or others or if the work environment may interfere with the ICD. Again the physician has to exercise judgment in this matter since there are no clear guidelines. If the patient is not able to resume his or her previous occupation, every effort should be made to ensure some form of ongoing financial support: retirement, disability benefits, or especially in the younger patients job retraining.

OVERALL RESULTS

Numerous reports have attested to the success of the ICD in preventing sudden cardiac death. However, it has been said that the impressively low sudden death rates may actually overstate the benefits of the ICD since sudden death calculations do not take into consideration operative deaths and non-sudden arrhythmia-related deaths. Kim et al.[102] have used the term "total arrhythmic death" to refer to the sum of perioperative deaths, sudden deaths, and arrhythmia-related non-sudden deaths. Therefore, the parameters of interest in assessing the survival benefit of the ICD include sudden cardiac deaths, non-sudden cardiac deaths, total arrhythmic deaths, all cardiac deaths, and total deaths. Unfortunately the data from various centers are reported in different ways, making any direct comparisons or metaanalysis difficult. However, the general theme suggests an impressive benefit of the ICD.

Sudden death rates in ICD patients are very low. Winkle et al.[218,219] initially reported a 4.4% sudden death rate at 3 years and in a larger series of 555 patients reported sudden death rates of 1.5% and 4% at 1 and 5 years respectively. In some of the other larger series, Veltri et al.[205] and Fogoros et al.[42] have reported 2 year survival of 77% and 88% respectively and sudden death rates of 4% and 3% respectively. This benefit does not appear to be related to the improvement in devices or leads over the years. Nisam et al.[151] from Cardiac Pacemakers, Inc., have recently reported patient survival in three generations of ICDs encompassing a 12-year experience and more than 25,000 patients. They reported the actuarial all-cause 1-year mortality for the

Ventak, Ventak-P, and PRx to be 7.2%, 7.1%, and 9.3% respectively. The overall all-cause mortality at 5 years is approximately 25%.

Congestive heart failure is the most common cause of death in ICD patients.[189,198,218] Survival in ICD patients is influenced by left ventricular function as measured by ejection fraction and functional class.[42,96,189,198] Even though ICD patients with poor left ventricular function do not do as well as patients with good LV function, it is clear that their outcome is significantly improved by the ICD.[161] Axtell et al.[1] examined the influence of left ventricular ejection fraction on survival of 200 ICD patients followed for a mean of 2.3 years and found sudden death rate of 4.4% in the group with EF < 30% compared to 1.5% in the group with EF > 40%. Non-sudden cardiac death rate was 7.4% in the lower EF group compared to 4.6% in the higher EF group. Using the time-to-first-shock analysis, they projected an overall 5-year survival of 11% whereas the actual survival was 60%.

Another group of patients in whom ICD therapy efficacy has been examined are the elderly. Tresch et al.[198] studied a group of 54 elderly patients aged 66 to 80 years (mean age 69.8 years) who had ICDs implanted for life-threatening ventricular arrhythmias and compared their outcome to a group of younger patients aged 18 to 65 years (mean age 52.8 years) treated similarly. All patients in each group underwent extensive evaluation, including coronary angiography and repeated EP studies. The majority of patients in each group had coronary artery disease and significant left ventricular dysfunction. The mean left ventricular ejection fraction in the younger patients was 35% and 31% in the elderly group. An ICD was implanted in all patients along with concomitant cardiac surgery in 37% of the elderly and 29% of the younger patients. They did not find a significant difference in complications from evaluation or treatment between the age groups and 2-year survival was similar, suggesting that ICD therapy is very effective and well tolerated in the elderly.

Although the ICD is highly effective in treating ventricular arrhythmias, sudden death due to bradycardia or electromechanical dissociation may not be preventable. When ECG documentation of the cardiac rhythm was available at the time of death in ICD patients, non-VT/VF rhythms were observed most commonly.[125] Electromechanical dissociation, and less commonly, bradycardia have been reported in these patients. It is possible that the newer-generation ICDs with bradycardia pacing may prevent some of these deaths but may not impact significantly on others. Deaths due to malignant ventricular arrhythmias with a normally functioning device have also been reported and may be due to a rise in defibrillation threshold due to an intercurrent event.[181]

FUTURE DIRECTIONS

The initial goal of ICD research was to develop a device suitable for human implantation. The current goals are to decrease device size and volume and improve defibrillation lead systems so that a pectoral implant obviating the need for a thoracotomy is possible. Preliminary data suggest that this too has been achieved (Fig. 14-4), but the focus of attention over the next few years will probably still center on further refinement of this approach. The areas that still remain outside of immediate grasp are improvement in capacitor and battery design to further decrease generator size.

DEFIBRILLATION LEADS

Catheter defibrillation was first described by Hopps and Bigelow[73] in 1954 and subsequently Mirowski et al.[135,136] described an electrode system consisting of a catheter and a chest wall plate electrode. The initial defibrillation electrodes used in human ICD implant consisted of a spring electrode and a conformal apical electrode. However, due to high defibrillation energy requirements in some cases and the success of epicardial defibrillation using two patch electrodes in these cases, emphasis shifted to using epicardial patch electrodes. At the present time epicardial patch electrodes are the only approved lead systems in the United States, although two transvenous lead systems are likely to be available soon. Winkle et al.[217] first evaluated a catheter electrode in patients undergoing ICD implantation and showed that

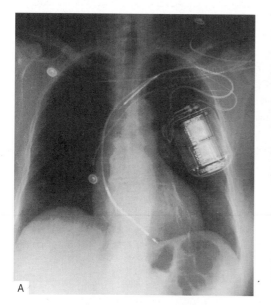
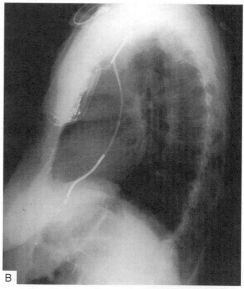

Fig. 14-4. PA and lateral projections of a chest x-ray demonstrating a device implanted in the left pectoral region. This investigational device, the Medtronic PCD Jewel (7219D), weighs 136 grams and has a volume of 83 cc. This device is capable of monophasic, biphasic, and simultaneous pulse defibrillation with a maximum energy output of 34 J.

adequate defibrillation efficacy could be demonstrated in 45% of the patients. Troup et al.[203] then implanted a similar catheter along with a submuscular left chest wall patch electrode in a patient in December, 1986, and Saksena et al.[166] reported a subsequent implant with a 5-month follow-up in 1988. The initial clinical trial of the Endotak transvenous lead with subcutaneous patch was prematurely terminated while new lead conductors were developed and tested.[36] A clinical trial using the redesigned lead began in September, 1990, and excellent clinical results have been described by various centers.[45,69,196] More recently, Yee et al.[225] described a triple electrode system consisting of leads in the right ventricle, superior vena cava, and the coronary sinus with excellent results.

Bardy et al.[5] recently described excellent results with biphasic defibrillation using a right ventricular catheter electrode as the anode and a subcutaneously placed ICD generator shell in the left infraclavicular pocket as the cathode. We prospectively compared biphasic defibrillation between two different electrode configurations and the best sequential pulse defibrillation using the lead system previously described by Yee et al.,[226] NTL-SEQ. Biphasic defibrillation pathways were (1) RV to SVC and (2) RV to shell of the pulse generator in an infraclavicular pocket, RV-CAN. Patients undergoing ICD implantation were studied. Mean DFTs and leading edge voltages were lower with the RV-CAN defibrillation pathway than with RV-SVC or the best NTL-SEQ results. In our cumulative experience in 15 patients using biphasic waveforms we have observed a mean DFT using RV-CAN of 9.7 J compared to 14.3 J using RV-SVC electrode configuration. In our experience 94% of patients with RV-CAN had DFT < 15 J, compared to 52% and 46% respectively for RV-SVC and best NTL-SEQ pathways (Fig. 14-5).

Lead systems obviating the need for a thoracotomy will be the system of choice for ICD implantation in the future, and other variables affecting defibrillation efficacy (waveform, polarity, etc.) will be optimized to preferentially use the nonthoracotomy leads when possible. However, much remains to be learned about the chronic behavior of these leads, associated complications and their management, and lead replacement.

DEFIBRILLATION WAVEFORMS

Defibrillation waveform has long been recognized to be a significant parameter affecting defibrillation efficacy. Both capacitor and noncapacitor waveforms have been used clinically, but only capacitor discharge waveforms have been used in implantable devices due to weight and volume considerations.[72,124,171] When a capacitor is charged to maximum voltage and then discharged, the voltage drops in an exponential fashion. The discharge is abruptly terminated between 4 to 8 ms later and the resultant waveform is called a monophasic truncated exponential waveform or simply a monophasic waveform. The initial ICDs provided a monophasic shock. It has been well

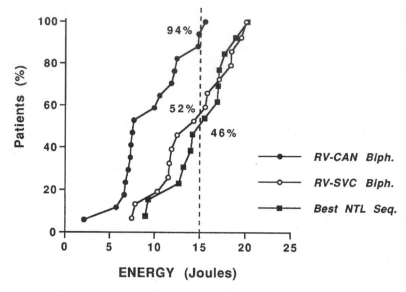

Fig. 14-5. The defibrillation efficacy curves in 15 patients undergoing evaluation for ICD implantation. Biphasic and sequential waveforms were used. *RV-Can Biph.* represents biphasic defibrillation between the RV electrode and the ICD generator can placed in a pectoral pocket. *RV-SVC Biph.* represents biphasic defibrillation between the RV electrode and an SVC electrode. Best NTL Seq. represents sequential defibrillation using the three electrodes placed in the superior vena cava, right ventricle, and the coronary sinus.

shown that biphasic shock delivered over a single pathway or sequential shocks delivered over two pathways are superior to monophasic shocks and result in lower defibrillation energy requirements.* Biphasic shocks of various durations, tilt, and interpulse separation have been examined to define the most effective waveform. The mechanism whereby biphasic shocks render more effective defibrillation is not well understood.[81,86,87]

Other efforts to improve upon the biphasic waveform have consisted of triphasic waveform and biphasic sequential waveform.[82] Triphasic waveforms are not significantly better than biphasic waveforms. Biphasic sequential waveform delivers two biphasic waves over separate pathways in a sequential manner. In a porcine model Csanadi et al.[29] showed the superiority of sequential biphasic shocks over single biphasic shocks. Yee et al.[224] compared defibrillation efficacy of biphasic, sequential and biphasic-sequential shocks

*References 23, 24, 83-85, 94

in 10 patients undergoing nonthoracotomy lead implantation. The mean defibrillation thresholds for sequential and biphasic pulse defibrillation were 20 ± 7 J and 22 ± 15 J respectively, compared to 11 ± 5 J for biphasic-sequential shocks. More recently, Johnson et al.[78] have characterized the effect of pulse separation between two sequential biphasic shocks delivered over different defibrillation pathways.

Another possible mechanism by which any of the available waveforms may be made more effective is to alter the polarity of the electrodes. Some experimental and clinical data using epicardial patches suggest a weak effect of electrode polarity on defibrillation efficacy, although the optimal electrode polarity cannot be predicted a priori.[4,157,172,212] Recently, in an animal model of nonthoracotomy defibrillation, electrode polarity has been shown to be a determinant of defibrillation efficacy for both monophasic and biphasic waveforms.[192]

For the time being it appears that a biphasic waveform is the best available for implantable devices. Devices available in the immediate future will probably provide the capability to deliver any of the three waveforms and may also allow polarity to be a programmable parameter.

TIMING OF SHOCK TO SURFACE QRS

Wiggers et al.[213] demonstrated in 1940 that electrical stimuli delivered during the vulnerable period of the cardiac cycle could induce ventricular fibrillation. To avoid this problem, transthoracic cardioversion shocks were synchronized to the R-wave of the surface ECG.[123] During the development of the ICD these observations were extrapolated to internal cardioversion with shocks being synchronized to the local ventricular electrogram.[6] However, Sharma et al.[176] have shown that the time intervals between the surface QRS onset and the local ventricular electrogram during ventricular tachycardia are quite variable.[176] In a canine preparation Jackman et al.[77] described lower cardioversion energy thresholds during the first half of the QRS interval.

Recently, Li et al.[119] reported the effect of cardioversion shock delivery at the onset of the surface QRS versus 100 msec into the QRS complex during induced ventricular tachycardia (Fig. 14-6). Minimum energy requirement and risk of VT acceleration were studied in 15 patients with inducible monomorphic ventricular tachycardia undergoing evaluation for ICD therapy. The QRS morphology was RBBB in 12 and LBBB in 3, with a mean QRS duration of 187 ± 31 ms. The interval between QRS onset and local RV endocardial electrogram was quite variable and ranged from 30 to 120 ms after onset of the earliest surface QRS complex. The VT cardioversion threshold and the risk of tachycardia acceleration were significantly lower when the shocks were delivered 100 ms from the onset than at the onset of the surface QRS. These interesting findings may find applications in future devices.

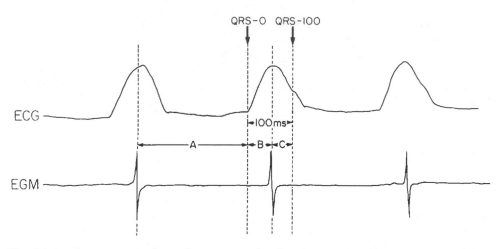

Fig. 14-6. The timing of cardioversion shocks during hemodynamically stable monomorphic ventricular tachycardia. Effect of shocks delivered at the onset of the QRS complex was compared to shocks delivered 100 ms into the QRS complex. Ventricular electrograms were used for sensing. To deliver a shock at the onset of the QRS complex, a delay value equal to the interval between the rapid upstroke or downstroke of the preceding ventricular electrogram to the QRS onset of the next beat (interval A) was introduced. To deliver a shock 100 ms into the QRS complex, the interval from the endocardial electrogram to the onset of the QRS (interval B) was measured, and an additional delay was added (interval C) such that the sum of intervals B and C was 100 ms.

OTHER PARAMETERS

Other features that would be of interest in future devices include improvements in arrhythmia discrimination with or without some form of physiological sensor, increased memory for electrogram storage, noninvasive programmed stimulation, and the ability to confirm VT/VF after capacitors have charged so as to prevent unnecessary therapy for nonsustained arrhythmias.

The incidence of unnecessary shocks for supraventricular tachycardias including atrial fibrillation is not well known. In the perioperative period these arrhythmias certainly occur and can satisfy therapy criteria resulting in a shock. The incidence of these arrhythmias on a chronic basis is not known. Improvements in tachycardia detection may diminish this undesirable event. Promising but preliminary methods include ventricular activation sequence mapping, power spectrum analysis, template correlation, and potential gradient analysis.

Atrial sensing may improve arrhythmia discrimination. Schuger et al.[173] have shown VA dissociation in 73% of sustained ventricular tachycardias and they reported that atrial sensing would have detected 100% of VT episodes. In our own experience of 66 consecutive patients undergoing evaluation for ICD therapy, ventriculoatrial conduction was present in only 23% of patients.[120] Sixty-two percent of the patients had inducible sustained monomorphic ventricular tachycardia. The shortest paced cycle length for 1:1 VA conduction was 496 ± 100 ms and was always longer than induced VT cycle length. During the induced VT none of the patients demonstrated 1:1 VA conduction and only one patient showed 2:1 VA conduction. As in Schuger's study, our findings also suggest that atrial sensing can improve VT identification.

Physiologic sensors may augment electrogram characterization of arrhythmic events. Methods of current interest include right atrial and/or right ventricular pressure and volume measurements via right-sided catheters or catheters placed in the coronary sinus.

Increased memory capacity will allow counters for arrhythmic events, therapies administered, and, most important, electrogram storage. One of the most difficult challenges in the past has been the determination of propriety of a shock when it was not preceded by hemodynamic consequences. Even tachycardia interval storage has not been a great benefit in this regard. The ability to examine electrograms associated with a therapy will greatly facilitate our understanding and thereby further improve our ability to prescribe the necessary electric therapy.

The ability to noninvasively perform programmed stimulation to induce arrhythmias and ensure therapeutic efficacy will obviate the need for additional catheter placement. This implies less discomfort for the patient and probable cost savings for the health care system.

Presently available devices are committed devices in that once the capacitor begins to charge it will deliver the shock at the end of the charging cycle. Perhaps such a strategy results in some unnecessary shocks for nonsustained arrhythmias. The magnitude of this problem is uncertain. Future devices, by confirming the persistence of arrhythmia during or immediately after the charge cycle, may be able to abort unnecessary therapies.

Undoubtedly there are many avenues for future research to improve upon the presently available technology. However, the implementation of any further refinement will probably not result in any survival advantage over what has already been achieved but may certainly improve our ability to "fine tune the electronic prescription."

EXPANDING INDICATIONS

Given the fact that 400,000 sudden cardiac deaths occur in the United States per annum with comparable incidence in other Western nations, and only a handful of patients are fortunate enough to be successfully resuscitated and even a smaller number subsequently referred for appropriate therapy, the need for identification of high-risk patients and proper prophylaxis is overwhelming. Any solutions to this problem will be costly and raise ethical and moral issues at the same time.

Several trials are currently in progress that may identify high-risk patients who may very well warrant prophylactic device therapy. The majority of studies focus on patients who have already had a myocardial infarction or are undergoing coronary artery bypass grafting. Patients with dilated cardiomyopathy and heart transplant candidates with ventricular arrhythmias are also under scrutiny. Whether ICD therapy will significantly benefit any of the high-risk groups must be examined with care. Survival benefit must be clear and the cost effectiveness of this strategy must be socioeconomically affordable before prophylaxis is widespread. If prophylaxis with ICD is realized, small devices with a limited number of advanced features and a limited number of shocks may suffice. This approach may make ICD prophylaxis economically conscionable.

REFERENCES

1. Axtell K, Tchou P, Akhtar M: Survival in patients with depressed left ventricular function treated by implantable cardioverter-defibrillator, *PACE* 14:291, 1991.

2. Bach SM Jr et al: Initial clinical experience: Endotak implantable transvenous defibrillator system, *J Am Coll Cardiol* 13:65, 1989 (abstract).

3. Barbola J et al: The automatic implantable cardioverter-defibrillator: clinical experience, complications, and follow-up in 25 patients, *Arch Intern Med* 142:70, 1988.

4. Bardy GH et al: Effect of electrode polarity on defibrillation efficacy, *Am J Cardiol* 63:433, 1989.

5. Bardy GH et al: A simplified, single lead unipolar transvenous cardioverter-defibrillator, *Circulation* 86:792, 1992 (abstract).

6. Bardy GH et al: Clinical experience with a tiered-therapy, multiprogrammable antiarrhythmia device, *Circulation* 85:1689, 1991.

7. Basta LL et al: Aneurysmectomy in treatment of ventricular and supraventricular tachyarrhythmias in patients with postinfarction and traumatic ventricular aneurysms, *Am J Cardiol* 32:693, 1973.

8. Baum RS, Alvarez HA, Cobb LA: Survival after resuscitation from out-of-hospital ventricular fibrillation, *Circulation* 50:1231, 1974.

9. Belhassen B et al: Transcatheter electrical shock ablation of ventricular tachycardia, *J Am Coll Cardiol* 7:1347, 1986.

10. Benditt BG et al: Prevention of recurrent sudden cardiac arrest: role of provocative electropharmacologic testing, *J Am Coll Cardiol* 2:418, 1983.

11. Bigger JT: Prophylactic use of implantable cardioverter defibrillators: medical, technical, economic considerations, *PACE* 14:376, 1991.

12. Bonnet CA, Elson JJ, Fogoros RN: Accidental deactivation of the automatic implantable cardioverter defibrillator, *PACE* 13:546, 1990 (abstract).

13. Borggrefe M et al: Catheter ablation of ventricular tachycardia using defibrillator pulses: electrophysiological findings and long-term results, *Eur Heart J* 10:591, 1989.

14. Bourland JD et al: Comparative efficacy of damped sine wave and square wave current for transchest defibrillation in animals, *Med Instrum* 12:42, 1978.

15. Brodman R et al: Results of electrophysiologically guided operations for drug-resistant recurrent ventricular tachycardia and ventricular fibrillation due to coronary artery disease, *J Thorac Cardiovasc Surg* 87:431, 1984.

16. Brodsky AM et al: Psychosocial adaptation of the automatic implantable cardioverter defibrillator, *Circulation* 78:155, 1988 (abstract).

17. Buda AJ, Stinson EB, Harrison DC: Surgery for life-threatening ventricular tachyarrhythmias, *Am J Cardiol* 44:1171, 1979.

18. Buxton AE et al: Role of triple extrastimuli during electrophysiologic study

of patients with documented sustained ventricular tachyarrhythmias, *Circulation* 69:532, 1984.

19. Buylaert WA et al: Serum electrolyte disturbances in the post-resuscitation period, *Resuscitation* 17:189, 1989.

20. Calkins H et al: Diagnosis and cure of the Wolff-Parkinson-White syndrome or paroxysmal supraventricular tachycardias during a single electrophysiologic test, *N Engl J Med* 324:1612, 1991.

21. The Cardiac Arrhythmia Suppression Trial (CAST) Investigators. SPECIAL REPORT. Preliminary report: effect of encainide and flecainide on mortality in a randomized trial arrhythmia suppression after myocardial infarction, *N Engl J Med* 321:406, 1989.

22. Chapman PD, Troup PJ: The automatic implantable cardioverter defibrillator: evaluating inappropriate shocks, *J Am Coll Cardiol* 7:1075, 1986.

23. Chapman PD et al: Comparative efficacy of monophasic and biphasic truncated exponential shocks for nonthoracotomy internal defibrillation in dogs, *J Am Coll Cardiol* 12:739, 1988.

24. Chapman PD et al: Comparison of monophasic with single and dual capacitor biphasic waveforms for nonthoracotomy canine internal defibrillation, *J Am Coll Cardiol* 14:242, 1989.

25. Cobb LA, Werner JA, Trobaugh GB: Sudden cardiac death: a decade's experience with out-of-hospital resuscitation, *Modern Concepts Cardiovasc Dis* 49:31, 1980.

26. Couch OA: Cardiac aneurysm with ventricular tachycardia and subsequent excision of aneurysm, *Circulation* 20:251, 1959.

27. Coumel P: The management of clinical arrhythmias. An overview on invasive versus non-invasive electrophysiology, *Eur Heart J* 8:92, 1987.

28. Cox JL, Gallagher JJ, Ungerleider RM: Encircling endocardial ventriculotomy for refractory ischemic ventricular tachycardia. IV. Clinical indications, surgical technique, mechanisms of action and results, *J Thorac Cardiovasc Surg* 83:865, 1982.

29. Csanadi Z et al: Comparison of single-biphasic versus sequential-biphasic shocks on defibrillation threshold in pigs, *PACE* 16:915, 1993 (abstract).

30. Dajani AS et al: Prevention of bacterial endocarditis: recommendations by the American Heart Association, *JAMA* 264:2919, 1990.

31. Davy J et al: The relationship between successful defibrillation and delivered energy in open-chest dogs: reappraisal of the "defibrillation threshold" concept, *Am Heart J* 113:77, 1987.

32. DiCarlo LA et al: Driving restrictions advised by midwestern cardiologists implanting cardioverter defibrillators: present practices, criteria utilized, and compatibility with existing state laws, *PACE* 15:1131, 1992.

33. Dreifus LS et al: Guidelines for implantation of cardiac pacemakers and antiarrhythmia devices. A report of the American College of Cardiology/American Heart Association Task Force on assessment of diagnostic and therapeutic cardiovascular procedures (Committee on Pacemaker Implantation), *J Am Coll Cardiol* 18:1, 1991.

34. Eisenberg MS, Hallstrom A, Bergner L: Long-term survival after out-of-hospital cardiac arrest, *N Engl J Med* 306:1340, 1982.

35. Eldar M, Sauve MJ, Scheinman MM: Electrophysiologic testing in the follow-up of patients with aborted sudden death, *J Am Coll Cardiol* 10:291, 1987.

36. Endotak lead system clinical investigation. First Annual Report. IDE # G870174. Cardiac Pacemakers, Inc. January 31, 1989.

37. The ESVEM Investigators: Determinants of predicted efficacy of antiarrhythmic drugs in the electrophysiologic study versus electrocardiographic monitoring trial, *Circulation* 87:323, 1993.

38. Evans GT, Scheinman MM, and the Executive Committee of the Percutaneous Cardiac Mapping and Ablation Registry: Catheter ablation for control of ventricular tachycardia: a report of the Percutaneous Cardiac Mapping and Ablation Registry, *PACE* 9:1391, 1986.

39. Fain ES, Lee JT, Winkle RA: Effects of acute intravenous and chronic oral amiodarone on defibrillation energy requirements, *Am Heart J* 114:8, 1987.

40. Fogoros RN: Amiodarone-induced refractoriness to cardioversion, *Ann Intern Med* 100:699, 1984.

41. Fogoros RN, Elson JJ, Bonnet CA: Actuarial incidence and pattern of occurrence of shocks following implantation of the automatic implantable cardioverter defibrillator, *PACE* 12:1465, 1989.

42. Fogoros RN et al: Efficacy of the automatic implantable cardioverter-defibrillator in prolonging survival in patients with severe underlying cardiac disease, *J Am Coll Cardiol* 16:381, 1990.

43. Fontaine G et al: Fulguration of chronic ventricular tachycardia: results of 47 consecutive cases with a follow-up ranging from 11 to 65 months. In Zipes DP, Jaliffe J, editors: *Cardiac electrophysiology: from cell to bedside*, Philadelphia, 1990, WB Saunders, pp 978-985.

44. Frame R et al: Clinical evaluation of the safety of repetitive intraoperative defibrillation threshold testing, *PACE* 15:870, 1992.

45. Frame R et al: Initial experience with transvenous implantable cardioverter defibrillator lead system: operative morbidity and mortality, *PACE* 16:149, 1993.

46. Frank G, Lowes D: Implantable cardioverter defibrillators: surgical considerations, *PACE* 15:631, 1992.

47. Gallagher JJ et al: Surgical treatment of arrhythmias, *Am J Cardiol* 61:A27, 1988.

48. Garan H et al: Perioperative and long-term results after electrophysiologically directed ventricular surgery for recurrent ventricular tachycardia, *J Am Coll Cardiol* 8:201, 1986.

49. Garan H et al: Refractory ventricular tachycardia complicating recovery from acute MI: treatment with map-guided infarctectomy, *Am Heart J* 107:571, 1984.

50. Gartman DM et al: Short-term morbidity and mortality of implantation of automatic implantable cardioverter-defibrillator, *J Thorac Cardiovasc Surg* 100:353 1990.

51. Gohn D et al: Determinants of operative mortality in implantable cardioverter defibrillator, *J Am Coll Cardiol* 17:86, 1991 (abstract).

52. Goodman LR et al: Complications of automatic implantable cardioverter-defibrillators: radiographic, CT, and echocardiographic evaluation, *Radiology* 170:447, 1989.

53. Gottlieb CD, Horowitz LN: Potential interactions between anti-arrhythmic medications and the automatic implantable cardioverter/defibrillator, *PACE* 14:898, 1991.

54. Graboys TB, Lown B, Podrid P: Long term survival of patients with malignant ventricular arrhythmias treated with antiarrhythmic drugs, *Am J Cardiol* 50:437, 1982.

55. Graham AF et al: Surgical treatment of refractory life-threatening ventricular tachycardia, *Am J Cardiol* 32:909, 1973.

56. Griffith L et al: Does an AICD generator need replacement when the battery is depleted, *PACE* 11:887, 1988.

57. Grimm W, Flores BF, Marchlinski FE: Complications of implantable cardioverter defibrillator therapy: follow-up of 241 patients, *PACE* 16:218, 1993.

58. Gross GN et al: Influence of clinical characteristics and shock occurrences on ICD patient outcome: a multicenter report, *PACE* 14:1881, 1991.

59. Gross JN et al: The antitachycardia pacing ICD: impact on patient selection and outcome, *PACE* 16:165, 1993.

60. Guarnieri T, Levine JH, Veltri EP: Success of chronic defibrillation and the role of antiarrhythmic drugs with the automatic implantable cardioverter/defibrillator, *Am J Cardiol* 60:1061, 1987.

61. Guiraudon G et al: Encircling endocardial ventriculotomy: a new surgical treatment for life-threatening ventricular tachycardias resistant to medical treatment following myocardial infarction, *Ann Thorac Surg* 26:438, 1978.

62. Guiraudon G, Klein GJ, Yee R: Left subdiaphragmatic implantation of the PCD defibrillator suppresses the problematic side-effects of bulky generators, *J Am Coll Cardiol* 19:123, 1992 (abstract).

63. Guiraudon GM, Klein GJ, Yee R: Surgery for the Wolff-Parkinson-White syndrome and supraventricular tachycardias. In Josephson ME, Wellens HJJ, editors: Tachycardias: mechanisms and management, Mount Kisco, NY, 1993, Futura.

64. Haberman RJ, Veltri EP, Mower MM: The effect of amiodarone on defibrillation threshold, *J Electrophysiol* 2:415, 1988.

65. Hackett T, Cassern N: Coping with cardiac arrest, *Adv Cardiol* 31:212, 1982.

66. Hamer A et al: Prediction of sudden death by electrophysiologic studies in high risk patients surviving acute myocardial infarction, *Am J Cardiol* 50:223, 1982.

67. Hargrove WC et al: Improved results in the operative management of ventricular tachycardia related to inferior wall infarction: importance of the annular isthmus, *J Thorac Cardiovasc Surg* 92:726, 1986.

68. Harken AH, Horowitz LN, Josephson ME: Comparison of standard aneurysmectomy with directed endocardial resection for the treatment of recurrent sustained ventricular tachycardia, *J Thorac Cardiovasc Surg* 80:527, 1980.

69. Hauser RG et al: Clinical results with nonthoracotomy ICD systems, *PACE* 16:141, 1993.

70. Herre JM et al: Long-term results of amiodarone therapy in patients with recurrent sustained ventricular tachycardia or ventricular fibrillation, *J Am Coll Cardiol* 13:442, 1989.

71. Hession MJ et al: Ethmozine therapy for complex ventricular arrhythmias, *Am J Cardiol* 60:59, 1987.

72. Hooker DR, Kouwenhoven WB, Langworthy OR: The effect of alternating currents on the heart, *Am J Physiol* 103:444, 1933.

73. Hopps JA, Bigelow WG: Electrical treatment of cardiac arrest: a cardiac stimulator-defibrillator, *Surgery* 36:833, 1954.

74. Hurst LN et al: The salvage of infected cardiac pacemaker pockets using a closed irrigation system, *PACE* 9:785, 1986.

75. Ideker RE et al: Simultaneous multichannel cardiac mapping systems, *PACE* 10:281, 1987.

76. Jackman WM et al: Catheter ablation of accessory atrioventricular pathways (Wolff-Parkinson-White syndrome) by radiofrequency current, *N Engl J Med* 324:1605, 1991.

77. Jackman WM, Zipes DP: Low-energy synchronous cardioversion of ventricular tachycardia using a catheter electrode in a canine model of subacute myocardial infarction, *Circulation* 66:187, 1982.

78. Johnson EE et al: Effect of pulse separation between two sequential biphasic shocks given over different lead configurations on ventricular defibrillation efficacy, *Circulation* 85:2267, 1992.

79. Jones D, Klein GJ, Kallok MJ: Improved internal defibrillation with twin pulse energy delivery, *Am J Cardiol* 55:821, 1985.

80. Jones DL, Fujimura O, Klein GJ: Minimum replications to estimate average threshold energy for defibrillation, *Med Instrum* 22:298, 1988.

81. Jones JL, Jones RE: Decreased defibrillator-induced dysfunction with biphasic rectangular waveforms, *Am J Physiol* 247:H792, 1984.

82. Jones JL, Jones RE: Improved safety factor for triphasic defibrillator waveforms. Circ Res 64:1172, 1989.

83. Jones DL et al: Internal cardiac defibrillation in man: pronounced improvement with sequential pulse delivery to two different lead orientations, *Circulation* 73:484, 1986.

84. Jones DL, Klein GJ, Kallok MJ: Improved internal defibrillation with twin pulse sequential energy delivery to different lead orientations in pigs, *Am J Cardiol* 55:821, 1985.

85. Jones DL et al: Internal cardiac defibrillation: single and sequential pulses and a variety of lead orientations, *PACE* 11:583, 1988.

86. Jones JL et al: Response of cultured myocardial cells to countershock-type electric field stimulation, *Am J Physiol* 235:H214, 1978.

87. Jones JL et al: Ultrastructural injury to chick myocardial cells in vitro following "electric countershock," *Circ Res* 46:387, 1980.

88. Josephson ME, Harken AH, Horowitz LN: Endocardial excision: a new surgical technique for the treatment of recurrent ventricular tachycardia, *Circulation* 60:1430, 1979.

89. Josephson ME et al: Electrophysiologic and hemodynamic studies in patients resuscitated from cardiac arrest, *Am J Cardiol* 46:948, 1980.

90. Joye JD et al: Perioperative morbidity and mortality after ICD implantation in

150 consecutive patients, *Circulation* 84:608, 1991 (abstract).

91. Kalbfleisch KR et al: Reemployment following implantation of the automatic cardioverter-defibrillator, *Am J Cardiol* 64:199, 1989.

92. Kallok MJ et al: Optimization of epicardial electrode size and implant site for reduced sequential pulse defibrillation threshold, *Med Instrum* 20:36, 1985.

93. Kapoor WN et al: A prospective evaluation and follow-up of patients with syncope, *N Engl J Med* 309:197, 1983.

94. Kavanagh KM et al: Comparison of the internal defibrillation threshold for monophasic and double and single capacitor biphasic waveforms, *J Am Coll Cardiol* 14:1343, 1989.

95. Kehoe R et al: Factors determining programmed stimulation responses and long-term arrhythmia outcome in survivors of ventricular fibrillation with ischemic heart disease, *Am Heart J* 116:355, 1988.

96. Kelly PA et al: The automatic implantable cardioverter defibrillator (AICD): efficacy, complications, and survival in patients with malignant ventricular arrhythmias, *J Am Coll Cardiol* 11:1278, 1988.

97. Kelly P et al: Surgical coronary revascularization in survivors of prehospital cardiac arrest; its effect on inducible ventricular arrhythmias and long-term survival, *J Am Coll Cardiol* 15:267, 1990.

98. Kelly PA et al: Postoperative infection with the automatic implantable cardioverter-defibrillator: clinical presentation and use of the gallium scan in diagnosis, *PACE* 11:1220, 1988.

99. Kentsch M, Kunze KP, Bleifeld W: Effect of intravenous amiodarone on ventricular fibrillation during out-of-hospital cardiac arrest, *J Am Coll Cardiol* 7:82, 1986 (abstract).

100. Keren R, Aarons D, Veltri E: Anxiety and depression in patients with life-threatening ventricular arrhythmias: impact of the implantable cardioverter-defibrillator, *PACE* 14:181, 1991.

101. Kim SG et al: The influence of left ventricular function on the outcome of patients treated with implantable defibrillators, *Circulation* 85:1304, 1992.

102. Kim SG et al: Benefits of implantable defibrillator are overestimated by sudden death rates and better represented by the total arrhythmic death rates, *J Am Coll Cardiol* 17:1587, 1991.

103. Kim SG et al: Unipolar pacemaker artifacts induce failure of the automatic implantable cardioverter/defibrillator to detect ventricular fibrillation, *Am J Cardiol* 57:880, 1986.

104. Klein GJ et al: Ventricular fibrillation in the Wolff-Parkinson-White syndrome, *N Engl J Med* 301:1080, 1979.

105. Klein LS et al: Radiofrequency catheter ablation of ventricular tachycardia in patients without structural heart disease, *Circulation* 85:1666, 1992.

106. Konstadt SN et al: The effects of normothermic hypoperfusion on processed EEG in patients, *Anesth Analg* 70:213, 1990.

107. Kron IL et al: Coronary bypass grafting in patients with ventricular fibrillation, *Ann Thorac Surg* 48:85, 1989.

108. Kuck KH et al: Radiofrequency current catheter ablation of accessory atrioventricular pathways, *Lancet* 337:1557, 1991.

109. Kuck KH et al: Successful catheter ablation of human ventricular tachycardia with radiofrequency current guided by an endocardial map of the area of slow conduction, *PACE* 14:1060, 1991.

110. Lampert S et al: Determinants of survival in patients with malignant ventricular arrhythmias associated with coronary artery disease, *Am J Cardiol* 61:791, 1988.

111. Langberg JJ et al: Catheter ablation of the atrioventricular junction with radiofrequency energy, *Circulation* 80:1527, 1989.

112. Lawrence JH et al: The characterization of human transmyocardial impedance during implantaion of the automatic internal cardioverter defibrillator, *PACE* 9:745, 1986.

113. Lawrie GM, Griffin JC, Wyndham CRC: Epicardial implantation of the automatic implantable defibrillator by left subcostal thoracotomy, *PACE* 7:1370, 1984.

114. Lawrie GM et al: High defibrillation threshold with the AICD: management with a right atrial patch electrode, *J Am Coll Cardiol* 11:209A, 1988.

115. Lehmann MH et al: Mortality in 309 patients with ischemic heart disease awaiting cardiac transplantation: implications for design of a multicenter "bridge to transplant" trial, *PACE* 14:642A, 1991.

116. Lehmann MH, Saksena S: Implantable cardioverter defibrillators in cardiovascular practice: report of the policy conference of the North American Society of Pacing and Electrophysiology, *PACE* 14:969, 1991.

117. Leitch JW et al: Reduction in defibrillator shocks with an implantable device combining antitachycardia pacing and shock therapy, *J Am Coll Cardiol* 18:145, 1991.

118. Leitch JW et al: Utility of low energy test shocks for estimation of cardiac and electrode impedance with implantable defibrillators, *PACE* 13:410, 1990.

119. Li HG et al: The effects of different shock timing during ventricular activation on the efficacy and safety of internal cardioversion for ventricular tachycardia (in press).

120. Li HG et al: Ventriculo-atrial conduction in patients with implantable cardioverter defibrillator: implications for tachycardia discrimination by dual chamber sensing (in press).

121. Liberthson PR et al: Pathophysiologic observations in prehospital ventricular fibrillation and sudden cardiac death, *Circulation* 49:790, 1974.

122. Liberthson PR et al: Pre-hospital ventricular fibrillation: prognosis and follow-up course, *N Engl J Med* 291:317, 1974.

123. Lown B: Electrical reversion of cardiac arrhythmias, *Br Heart J* 29:469, 1967.

124. Lown B et al: Comparison of alternating current with direct current electroshock across the closed chest, *Am J Cardiol* 10:223, 1962.

125. Luceri RM et al: Mechanism of death in patients with the automatic implantable cardioverter defibrillator, *PACE* 11:2015, 1988.

126. Marco D, Eisinger G, Hayes D: Testing of work environments for electromagnetic interference, *PACE* 15:2016, 1992.

127. Mason JW et al: Relative efficacy of blind left ventricular resection for the treatment of recurrent ventricular tachycardia, *Am J Cardiol* 49:241, 1982.

128. McCowan R et al: Automatic implantable cardioverter-defibrillator implantation without thoracotomy using an endocardial and submuscular patch system, *J Am Coll Cardiol* 19:490, 1992.

129. McGiffin DC et al: Relief of life-threatening ventricular tachycardia and survival after direct operations, *Circulation* 76:V93, 1987.

130. Mead RH et al: The automatic implantable defibrillator: improved defibrillation and lowered impedance using two large patch leads, *J Am Coll Cardiol* 5:454, 1985.

131. Mickleborough LL et al: A new intraoperative approach for endocardial mapping of ventricular tachycardia, *J Thorac Cardiovasc Surg* 95:271, 1988.

132. Miller JM et al: Subendocardial resection for ventricular tachycardia: predictors of surgical success, *Circulation* 70:624, 1984.

133. Mirowski M, Mower MM: The automatic implantable defibrillator: some historical notes. In Brugada P, Wellens HJJ, editors. *Cardiac arrhythmias: where do we go from here?* Mount Kisco, NY, 1987, Futura, pp 655-662.

134. Mirowski M et al: Feasibility and effectiveness of low energy catheter defibrillation in man, *Circulation* 57:79, 1973.

135. Mirowski M et al: The development of the transvenous automatic defibrillator, *Arch Int Med* 129:773, 1972.

136. Mirowski M et al: Ventricular defibrillation through a single intravascular catheter electrode system, *Clin Res* 19:228, 1971.

137. Mirowski M et al: Termination of malignant ventricular arrhythmias with an implantable automatic defibrillator in human beings, *N Engl J Med* 303:322, 1980.

138. Mirowski MM et al: Mortality in patients with implanted automatic defibrillators, *Ann Intern Med* 98:1353, 1983.

139. Moosavi AR et al: Effect of empiric antiarrhythmic therapy in resuscitated out-of-hospital cardiac arrest victims with coronary artery disease, *Am J Cardiol* 65:1192, 1990.

140. Morady F et al: Clinical features and prognosis of patients with out of hospital cardiac arrest and a normal electro-phys-

iologic study, *J Am Coll Cardiol* 4:39, 1984.

141. Morady F et al. Radiofrequency catheter ablation of ventricular tachycardia in patients with coronary artery disease, *Circulation* 87:363, 1993.

142. Morady F et al: Concealed entrainment as a guide for catheter ablation of ventricular tachycardia in patients with prior myocardial infarction, *J Am Coll Cardiol* 17:678, 1991.

143. Morady F et al: Catheter ablation of ventricular tachycardia with intracardiac shocks: results in 33 patients, *Circulation* 75:1037, 1987.

144. Morady F et al: Electrophysiologic testing in management of survivors with out of hospital cardiac arrest, *Am J Cardiol* 51:85, 1983.

145. Moser S et al: Non-thoracotomy implantable defibrillator system, *PACE* 11:887, 1988 (abstract).

146. Mower MM et al: Automatic implantable cardioverter defibrillator structural characteristics, *PACE* 7:1331, 1984.

147. Myerburg RJ et al: Clinical electrophysiologic and hemodynamic profile of patients resuscitated from prehospital cardiac arrest, *Am J Med* 68:568, 1980.

148. Myerburg RJ, Kessler KM, Castellanos A: Sudden cardiac death: structure, function, and time-dependence of risk, *Circulation* 85 (Suppl 1):12, 1992.

149. Myerburg RJ et al: Long-term survival after prehospital cardiac arrest: analysis of outcome during an 8 year study, *Circulation* 70:538, 1984.

150. Nisam S et al: Patient survival comparison in three generations of automatic cardioverter-defibrillators: review of 12 years, 25,000 patients, *PACE* 16:174, 1993.

151. Nisam S et al: Patient survival in three generations of automatic implantable cardioverter defibrillators: review of 12 years, 25,000 patients, *PACE* 16:174, 1993.

152. Nisam S et al: AICD: standardized reporting and appropriate categorization of complications, *PACE* 11:2045, 1988.

153. Nisam S et al: Identifying patients for prophylactic automatic implantable cardioverter defibrillator therapy: status of prospective studies, *Am Heart J* 122:807, 1991.

154. Ostermeyer J et al: Direct operations for the management of life-threatening ischemic ventricular tachycardia, *J Thorac Cardiovasc Surg* 94:848, 1987.

155. Ostermeyer J et al: Surgical treatment of ventricular tachycardias. Complete versus partial encircling endocardial ventriculotomy, *J Thorac Cardiovasc Surg* 87:517, 1984.

156. Ostermyer J et al: The surgical treatment of ventricular tachycardias. Simple aneurysmectomy vs electrophysiologically guided procedures, *J Thorac Cardiovasc Surg* 84:704, 1982.

157. O'Neill PG et al: The automatic implantable cardioverter-defibrillator: effect of patch polarity on defibrillation threshold, *J Am Coll Cardiol* 17:707, 1991.

158. Parsons I, Mendler P, Downer E: On-line cardiac mapping: an analog approach using video and multiplexing techniques, *Am J Physiol* 242:H526, 1982.

159. Phibbs B, Marriott HJL: Complications of permanent transvenous pacing, *N Engl J Med* 312:1428, 1985.

160. Platia EV, Reid PR: Comparison of programmed electrical stimulation and ambulatory electrocardiographic monitoring in the management of ventricular tachycardia and ventricular fibrillation, *J Am Coll Cardiol* 4:493, 1984.

161. Pycha C et al: Psychological responses to the implantable defibrillator: preliminary observations, *Psychosomatics* 12:841, 1986.

162. Rae AP et al: Antiarrhythmic drug efficacy for ventricular tachyarrhythmias associated with coronary artery disease as assessed by electrophysiologic studies, *Am J Cardiol* 55:1494, 1985.

163. Rattes MF et al: Defibrillation with the sequential pulse technique: reproducibility with repeated shocks, *Am Heart J* 111:874, 1986.

164. Roy D et al: Clinical characteristics in long-term follow-up in 119 survivors of cardiac arrest: relation to inducibility at electrophysiologic testing, *Am J Cardiol* 53:969, 1983.

165. Ruskin JN, DiMarco JP, Garan H: Out of hospital cardiac arrest: electrophysiologic observations in selection of long-term antiarrhythmic therapy, *N Engl J Med* 303:607, 1980.

166. Saksena S, Parsonnet V: Implantation of

a cardioverter/defibrillator without thoracotomy using a triple electrode system, *JAMA* 259:69, 1988.

167. Saksena S and the PCD Investigators and Participating Institutions: Defibrillation thresholds and perioperative mortality associated with endocardial and epicardial defibrillation lead systems, *PACE* 16:202, 1993.

168. Saksena S et al: Long-term multicenter experience with a second-generation implantable pacemaker-cardioverter-defibrillator, *J Am Coll Cardiol* 19:490, 1992.

169. Saksena S et al: Complications of third-generation defibrillators using endocardial or epicardial leads: a multicenter study, *J Am Coll Cardiol* 21:170, 1993 (abstract).

170. Schmitt C et al: Implantable cardioverter defibrillator: possible hazards of electromagnetic interference, *PACE* 14:982, 1991.

171. Schuder JC, Stoeckle H, Dolan AM: Transthoracic ventricular fibrillation with square-wave stimuli: one-half cycle, one cycle, and multicycle waveforms, *Circ Res* 15:258, 1964.

172. Schuder JC et al: Is the effectiveness of cardiac ventricular defibrillation dependent upon polarity? *Med Instrum* 21:262, 1987.

173. Schuger CD et al: Atrial sensing to augment ventricular tachycardia detection by the automatic implantable cardioverter defibrillator: a utility study, *PACE* 11:1456, 1988.

174. Selle JC et al: Successful clinical laser ablation of ventricular tachycardia: a promising new therapeutic method, *Ann Thorac Surg* 42:380, 1986.

175. Shapira N et al: Trans-diaphragmatic implantation of the automatic implantable cardioverter-defibrillator, *Ann Thorac Surg* 48:371, 1989.

176. Sharma AD et al: Activation of the right ventricular apical electrogram during ventricular tachycardia: suitability for synchronizing intracavitary cardioversion, *PACE* 8:186, 1985.

177. Siclari F, Klein H, Troster J: Intraventricular migration of an ICD patch, *PACE* 13:1356, 1990.

178. Singer I et al: Is defibrillation testing safe? *PACE* 14:689, 1991 (abstract).

179. Singer I, Guarnieri T, Kupersmith J: Implanted automatic defibrillators: effects of drugs and pacemakers, *PACE* 11:2250, 1988.

180. Skale BT et al: Survivors of cardiac arrest: prevention of recurrence by drug therapy as predicted by electrophysiologic testing or electrocardiographic monitoring, *Am J Cardiol* 57:113, 1986.

181. Steinaman RT et al: Clinical findings in monitored cases of sudden cardiac deaths in patients with an automatic implantable cardioverter defibrillator, *PACE* 12:646, 1989 (abstract).

182. Stevenson L et al: Poor survival of patients with idiopathic cardiomyopathy considered too well for transplantation, *Am J Med* 83:871, 1987.

183. Stevenson WG et al: Clinical, angiographic, and electrophysiologic findings in patients with aborted sudden death as compared with patients with sustained ventricular tachycardia after myocardial infarction, *Circulation* 71:1146, 1985.

184. Strickberger SA, Cantillon CO, Friedman PL: When should patients with lethal arrhythmias resume driving? *Ann Intern Med* 115:560, 1991.

185. Swerdlow CD, Blum J, Winkle RA: Decreased incidence of drug efficacy at electrophysiologic study associated with the use of a third extrastimuli, *Am Heart J* 104:1004, 1982.

186. Swerdlow CD et al: Determinants of prognosis in ventricular tachyarrhythmia patients without induced sustained arrhythmias, *Am Heart J* 111:433, 1986.

187. Swerdlow CD et al: Results of operations for ventricular tachycardia in 105 patients, *J Thorac Cardiovasc Surg* 92:105, 1986.

188. Taylor RL et al: Infection of an implantable cardioverter-defibrillator: management without removal of the device in selected cases, *PACE* 13:1352, 1990.

189. Tchou PJ et al: Automatic implantable cardioverter defibrillators and survival of patients with left ventricular dysfunction and malignant ventricular arrhythmias, *Ann Intern Med* 109:529, 1988.

190. Thakur RK et al: Comparison of non-thoracotomy and thoracotomy defibrillation for monophasic and biphasic pulses, *PACE* 12:664, 1989 (abstract).

191. Thakur RK et al: Radiofrequency catheter ablation for Wolff-Parkinson-White syndrome, *Can Med Ass J* (in press).

192. Thakur RK et al: Electrode polarity is an important determinant of defibrillation efficacy using a nonthoracotomy lead system, *PACE* (in press).

193. Thakur RK et al: Pericardial effusion increases defibrillation energy requirement, *PACE* 16:1227, 1993.

194. Thomas AC et al: Implantable defibrillation: eight years clinical experience, *PACE* 11:2053, 1988.

195. Touboul P et al: Bundle branch reentrant tachycardia treated by electrical ablation of the right bundle branch, *J Am Coll Cardiol* 7:1404, 1986.

196. Trappe HJ et al: Initial experience with a transvenous defibrillation system, *PACE* 16:134, 1993.

197. Tresch DD, Thakur RK, Duthie E: Resuscitation of elderly sustaining out-of-hospital cardiac arrest, *Am J Cardiol* 61:1120, 1988.

198. Tresch DD et al: Comparison of efficacy of automatic implantable cardioverter defibrillator in patients older and younger than 65 years of age, *Am J Med* 90:717, 1991.

199. Troup PJ: Lead system selection: implantation and testing for automatic implantable cardioverter defibrillator, *Clin Prog Electrophysiol Pacing* 4:260, 1986.

200. Troup PJ: Implantable cardioverters and defibrillators, *Curr Prob Cardiol* 14:675, 1989.

201. Troup PJ: Lessons learned from the automatic implantable cardioverter defibrillator: past, present and future, *J Am Coll Cardiol* 11:1287, 1988 (editorial).

202. Troup PJ et al: The implanted defibrillator: relation of defibrillating lead configuration and clinical variables to defibrillation threshold, *J Am Coll Cardiol* 6:1315, 1985.

203. Troup PJ et al: Clinical features of AICD system infections, *Circulation* 78:155, 1988 (abstract).

204. Veltri EP et al: Clinical efficacy of the implantable cardioverter defibrillator: 6 year cumulative experience, *Circulation* 74:109, 1986 (abstract).

205. Veltri EP et al: Follow-up of patients with ventricular tachyarrhythmia treated with the automatic implantable cardioverter-defibrillator: programmed electrical stimulation results do not predict clinical outcome, *J Electrophysiol* 3:467, 1989.

206. Vlay SC, Fricchione GL: Psychological aspects of surviving sudden cardiac death, *Clin Cardiol* 8:237, 1985.

207. Vlay SC et al: Anxiety and anger in patients with ventricular tachyarrhythmias. Responses after automatic implantable internal cardioverter defibrillator implantation, *PACE* 12:366, 1989.

208. Wathen MS et al: Chronic defibrillation threshold for automatic implantable cardioverter defibrillator, *PACE* 15:505, 1992 (abstract).

209. Watkins L et al: Implantation of the automatic defibrillator: the subxyphoid approach, *Ann Thorac Surg* 34:515, 1982.

210. Watkins J Jr, Taylor E Jr: The surgical aspects of automatic implantable cardioverter-defibrillator implantation, *PACE* 14:953, 1991.

211. Weaver WD et al: Angiographic and prognostic indications in patients resuscitated from sudden death, *Circulation* 54:895, 1976.

212. Wetherbee JN et al: Does electrode polarity affect defibrillation efficacy? *Clin Res* 37:892, 1989 (abstract).

213. Wiggers CJ, Wegria R: Ventricular fibrillation due to single, localized induction and condenser shocks applied during the vulnerable phase of ventricular asystole, *Am J Physiol* 128:500, 1940.

214. Wilber DJ et al: Out of hospital cardiac arrest: use of electrophysiologic testing in the prediction of long-term outcome, *N Engl J Med* 318:19, 1988.

215. Wilber D et al: Electrophysiological testing and non-sustained ventricular tachycardia, *Circulation* 82:330, 1990.

216. Winkle RA et al: The automatic implantable defibrillator: local bipolar sensing to detect ventricular tachycardia and fibrillation, *Am J Cardiol* 52:265, 1983.

217. Winkle RA et al: Comparison of defibrillation efficacy in humans using a new catheter and superior vena cava spring-

left ventricular patch electrode, *J Am Coll Cardiol* 11:365, 1988.

218. Winkle RA et al: Long-term outcome with the automatic implantable cardioverter-defibrillator, *J Am Coll Cardiol* 16:1353, 1989.

219. Winkle RA et al: Ten-year experience with implantable defibrillators, *Circulation* 84:416, 1991 (abstract).

220. Winkle RA et al: Practical aspects of automatic cardioverter/defibrillator implantation, *Am Heart J* 108:1335, 1984.

221. Winkle RA, Thomas A: The automatic cardioverter defibrillator: the US experience. In Brugada P, Wellens HJJ, editors: *Cardiac arrhythmias: where do we go from here?* Mount Kisco, NY, 1987, Futura, pp 663-680.

222. Wunderly D et al: Infections in implantable cardioverter defibrillator patients, *PACE* 13:1360, 1990.

223. Yee R, Jones D, Jarvis E et al: Changes in pacing threshold and R wave amplitude after transvenous catheter countershock, *J Am Coll Cardiol* 4:543, 1984.

224. Yee R et al: Improved defibrillation efficacy by combined biphasic and sequential shock delivery, *Circulation* 84 (II):649, 1991.

225. Yee R et al: A permanent transvenous lead system for an implantable pacemaker cardioverter-defibrillator: nonthoracotomy approach to implantation, *Circulation* 85:196, 1992.

226. Zardini M et al: Improved defibrillation efficacy with a simple non-thoracotomy lead configuration, *J Am Coll Cardiol* 21:66, 1993 (abstract).

227. Zilo P et al: Fate of explanted ICD patients, *PACE* 14:286, 1991.

Chapter 15
ICDs, AEDs, and Defibrillation Technology

W. A. Tacker

Defibrillation technology holds great promise for the development of improved diagnostic and therapeutic devices and treatments, and selected areas of use will be presented in this chapter. Selection is based on the criterion of being very directly related to defibrillation. For example, the subject of how arrhythmias are generated is certainly germane to the topic of defibrillation, but this writer defers to others for presentation of that extensive and complex topic.

However, many clinical and research subjects warrant a succinct presentation to bring to the reader's attention some developments that are, or in the near future may become, clinical or investigative topics. Also it is my hope to stimulate the interest of additional investigators to address the problems and opportunities that are extant. A number of applications for defibrillators have been proposed as extensions of currently available devices or as new innovations. These include several that already have been discussed in previous chapters as well as others mentioned below.

New devices and applications will be discussed in three categories: diagnostic, therapeutic, and experimental.

DIAGNOSTIC

ICDs (implantable cardioverter defibrillators) carry the microprocessor capability to collect and store data and in some cases to make diagnostic decisions. The missing components for further exploitation of this opportunity are suitable chemical and physical sensors that have both the capability for obtaining the needed information and a long lifetime of performance when implanted in the body. Information could be periodically obtained by telemetry, as is done with present-day ICDs, or could be used in an automatic mode. The range of technologies that can be envisioned is very extensive. Some examples are as follows: sensors for cardiac functions such as output, flow, stroke volume, or ejection fraction that would separate perfusing from non-perfusing tachycardias; multiple electrode sensors intended to sense and provide input for software programs to determine the site of electrical instability and apply shocks to the most suitable choice of several implanted electrodes; and implantable electro-physiologic (E-P) diagnostic devices with defibrillators incorporated for safety.

Improved diagnostic methods for defibrillation threshold (DFT) testing are also needed and hopefully are on the horizon; that is, those that have highly reliable prediction powers, but that reduce the number of fibrillation episodes and/or shocks required, as well as the ischemia time (e.g., upper limit of vulnerability testing as discussed in Chapter 2).

Finally, in the present climate of cost control for medical care, there is need for determining which patients with putative risk for arrhythmias should get ICDs since a substantial fraction of patients who have ICDs implanted never need the device.

THERAPEUTIC

IMPLANTABLE DEVICES

The extension of defibrillation technology to newer and more diverse implantable devices is almost certain to occur. The development of ICDs with improved electrode configurations and waveforms will provide for nonthoracotomy ICD use on a widespread scale with associated improvements in morbidity and mortality. Hopefully, technology will provide improvement in the currently unsolved problem of substantial pain often being associated with ICD cardioversion or defibrillation shocks.

In addition, transvenous atrial defibrillation has been reported in animals and humans and may be found practical.[1,6] Reduction of the morbidity associated with atrial fibrillation would benefit large numbers of patients, and ICD use for atrial cardioversion may be practical.

Also likely is the appearance of implantable devices that combine features of defibrillation with other capabilities such as administration of drugs stored in implanted pumps for better control of arrhythmia and cardiovascular (C-V) disease.

NONIMPLANTABLE DEVICES

It is also likely that new and improved technology and procedures will be forthcoming in transthoracic defibrillation. Transthoracic defibrillators with new electrodes and waveforms are likely to defibrillate with higher effectiveness; lower energy, current, and voltage; fewer complications such as arrhythmias; and therefore increased safety. No commercially available devices that use the benefits of multiple and biphasic waveforms or multiple (sequential) pathways for transthoracic defibrillation are now available. However, there is theoretical reason to believe that benefits are obtainable, based on technologies of ICDs.

Wearable automatic external defibrillators (AEDs) would certainly be of value if they could be designed to achieve the reliability and safety of the ICD. Patients might wear them temporarily until an ICD could be implanted, or patients who are at only low or intermediate risk for fibrillation might wear them for short periods until the need for an ICD could be determined.

Defibrillation waveforms have been used for ablation for several years but have been displaced in great part by RF (radio-frequency) or electrosurgical-type waveform ablation. Nonetheless, the defibrillation-type waveform may prove to be of benefit for myocardial tissue ablation. The relative benefits and limitations of these two electrical waveform modalities have yet to be fully determined.

Esophageal defibrillator electrodes have been tested clinically and may prove beneficial by providing a less invasive alternative for some invasive electrophysiology laboratory procedures.[5]

An area of need already mentioned in Chapters 4 and 13 is the development of a truly multifunctional electrode for use with combination monitoring-defibrillating-pacing devices. The key issues are to provide an electrode with characteristics that optimize the effectiveness of the therapies while neither compromising monitoring capability nor causing pain in the patient who is experiencing transchest pacing.

Finally the field of ergonomics of external defibrillation provides opportunity for improvement. Because of the overwhelming importance of rapid defibrillation, minor delays (of only seconds) in shock application are a major problem. Variability in controls and electrodes, for example, frequently lead to delay in treatment. Automation, simplification, standardization, or other means to reduce time to shock application would undoubtedly reduce morbidity and mortality.

EXPERIMENTAL

Obviously all of the therapeutic and diagnostic technologies mentioned previously will require experimental development and verification. Such verification will provide opportunities for better understanding of defibrillation mechanisms, and scientific opportunities are numerous.

In addition, there are technologies that can be considered predominantly experimental since their implementation will primarily expand knowledge and understanding, rather than result in near-term clinical use; for example, use of potentiometric dyes to study the electrophysiology of the heart fibers,[3] resolution of why there is so much biologic variability for defibrillation of the heart, and development and validation of better animal models for studies of defibrillation.

Finally, an area of great promise is three-dimensional modeling of the heart and the concomitant modeling of current densities and tissue resistivities associated with and responsible for defibrillation effectiveness and safety. Development of finite element numerical analysis has provided a method for mathematical description of the anatomy of the heart. Combined with new methods such as magnetic resonance imaging (MRI) for determination of chest, heart, and other organ anatomy, it is feasible to use improved computer processing to model the distribution of defibrillation current flow through the heart and other body structures.[2] This is a very challenging task because the structures, particularly the heart, are complex and three-dimensional. Also they have mechanical and electrical properties that are "nonlinear, nonhomogeneous, anisotropic, and time dependent."[4]

Schmidt et al.[8] call out several potential benefits from dimensional field distribution of voltage current and energy. These include the following:

1. Relating lumped parameters such as tissue conductivity to electrical field distribution
2. Relating field variables such as voltages and voltage gradients to each other
3. Providing insight about underlying mechanisms
4. Being able to predict experimental or clinical findings
5. Being able to interpret results based on measurements

This group also has assessed current distribution in the dog thorax using both finite element and finite difference analysis.

The technical details of modeling defibrillation fields are beyond the scope of this book, and the reader is referred to Pilkington et al.[7] for information about high-performance computing and model development in general. The prospect of using these models for better design and use of defibrillator electrodes and waveforms is both likely and exciting. Already it is evident that intuitive views of current distribution may be very inaccurate.

However, the presently available models have not yet been validated with experimental results from *in vivo* studies, nor have the models incorporated many of the known characteristics of current flow in tissues such as the nonlinear increase in conductivity of some tissues that is produced by increased current density.[9,10] Neither do the models have resolution sufficient to include thin and/or narrow structures such as skin, pericardium, and the pericardial space, which is filled with very low resistivity fluid. The field aberrations and nonuniformities created by these features have not yet been addressed. In summary, this is an exciting but embryonic field of investigation.

REFERENCES

1. Cooper RAS et al: Marked reduction in defibrillation requirements with biphasic waveforms and a coronary sinus electrode for atrial fibrillation in sheep, *PACE* 15:530, 1992

2. Hunter J et al: An anatomical heart model with application to myocardial activation and ventricular mechanics. In Pilkington TC, editor: *High-performance computing in biomedical research*, Boca Raton, Fla, 1993, CRC Press.

3. Kinosita K et al: Electroporation of cell membrane visualized under a pulsed-laser fluorescence microscope, *Biophys J* 53: 1015, 1988.

4. McCulloch A et al: Large scale finite element analysis of the beating heart. In Pilkington TC, editor: *High-performance computing in biomedical research*, Boca Raton, Fla, 1993, CRC Press.

5. McKoewn PP et al: The aesophageal approach to defibrillation, *Am Heart J* 124:840, 1992.

6. Nathan AW et al: Internal transvenous low energy cardioversion for the treatment of cardiac arrhythmias, *Br Heart J* 52:377, 1984.

7. Pilkington TC et al: *High-performance computing in biomedical research*, Boca Raton, Fla, 1993, CRC Press.

8. Schmidt J et al: Skeletal muscle grids for assessing current distributions from defibrillation shocks. In Pilkington TC, editor: *High-performance computing in biomedical research*, Boca Raton, Fla, 1993, CRC Press.

9. Tacker WA et al: Resistivity of blood to defibrillator-strength shocks. Proceedings of the 17th Annual Meeting of AAMI, 1982.

10. Tacker WA et al: Resistivity of skeletal muscle, skin, fat, and lung to defibrillation shocks. Proceedings of the 19th Annual Meeting of AAMI, 1984.

Chapter 16
Defibrillator Standards

Francis M. Charbonnier

PURPOSE OF STANDARDS

The safety, reliability, and effectiveness of medical devices are of particular concern since malfunction or misuse of a medical device may cause serious injury or even death. Hence medical devices that are life supporting or life sustaining are carefully regulated and monitored to protect both patients and medical practitioners. In every major country there are government agencies, for example, the Food and Drug Administration (FDA) in the United States, that are responsible for the regulation of medical devices. For instance, the FDA has four major responsibilities:

1. Ensuring through premarket notification or approval that only safe and effective devices are allowed on the market.
2. Ensuring through postmarket surveillance, device tracking, and mandatory device reporting that devices in use remain safe and effective even after extended use.
3. Mandating through product recall, if necessary, that serious product defects discovered in routine use are corrected by manufacturers.
4. Ensuring through "good manufacturing practices" site inspections that manufacturers have developed and practice sound processes to control the quality of their products, both hardware and software.

The purpose of safety or performance standards is to set generally accepted minimum requirements to ensure efficacy and safety of devices. There are "horizontal" standards that define general safety or performance requirements for very broad categories of devices, for example, International Electrotechnical Commission (IEC) publications 601-1 "Safety of Medical Electrical Equipment—Part 1: General requirements," 2nd edition, 1988 (replacing the 1977 first edition). These general standards are supplemented by "vertical" standards that define modified or added requirements for specific devices, for example, IEC Publication 601-2-4 "Medical Electrical Equipment—Part 2: Particular requirements for the safety of cardiac defibrillators and cardiac defibrillator monitors," 1st edition, 1983.

STANDARDS-SETTING ORGANIZATIONS

The International Organization for Standardization (ISO) has been traditionally responsible for the development and publication of standards for every kind of product. ISO has relied on the IEC for developing standards for electrical products; standards for electromedical devices are the responsibility of the Technical Committee 62 (TC 62) of the IEC. The IEC standards will be discussed in more detail later in this chapter.

Whereas in most countries standards activity is directed by government agencies (e.g., Canadian Standards Association in Canada), a unique situation occurs in the United States where a private organization, the American National Standards Institute (ANSI), has long been active in the development of standards. ANSI serves as the "coordinator of the U.S. private sector-administered voluntary standards system." Thus in the United States standards activity occurs both in government agencies for mandatory standards (particularly the National Institute of Standards and Technology [NIST] for all products and the FDA for medical devices) and in a private sector system coordinated by ANSI for voluntary consensus standards.

ANSI relies extensively on another organization, the Association for the Advancement of Medical Instrumentation (AAMI), for the development of safety and performance standards for medical devices. AAMI is an interdisciplinary association with the active participation of physicians, medical researchers, product development or quality assurance engineers from industry, biomedical and clinical engineers, and regulatory agency engineers or managers. AAMI uses this diverse background and expertise to enhance the development of standards by committees with balanced representation of these various groups. This balanced representation serves to harmonize the concerns and perspectives of manufacturers, users, and regulators and to strive for optimum resolution of efficacy and safety issues, protecting users to the maximum while recognizing the limits of present technology. Another important distinction is that ANSI and AAMI, being private organizations, develop voluntary consensus standards. Of course, the FDA reviews these standards carefully and may in some cases elect to adopt them as mandatory standards in the United States.

THE FDA 1976 MEDICAL DEVICES AMENDMENT

The 1976 Medical Devices Amendment to the Federal Food, Drug and Cosmetic Act has extended the FDA's regulatory responsibilities to include "devices," as well as food and drugs. A device is defined as an instrument, apparatus, machine, or implant that is intended for use in the diagnosis of disease or in the cure, treatment, or prevention of disease, or that is intended to affect the structure or any functions of the body. The FDA's expanded role has created an urgent need for safety and performance standards for a very large number of medical devices and has greatly stimulated the standards activities of ANSI and AAMI. Similarly, recent preparation for the contemplated economic, financial, and political integration of the European community in 1992 (EC92) has resulted in the issuance of directives, particularly the European Council Special Directive on Active Implantable Medical Devices and the Council General Directive on Medical Devices. This has increased the responsibilities of two European organizations that oversee the development of "harmonized European standards" or European norms to facilitate verification of compliance with the European community directives. These two organizations are the Committee on European Normalization (CEN) and the Committee on European Normalization of Electrical Equipment (CENELEC), which are the European counterparts of ISO and IEC, respectively. Though CENELEC is expected to review existing IEC international standards and may adopt them, it may also make significant changes in the IEC standards; it will also, alone or in collaboration with IEC, develop a number of new medical device standards. As a result standards activity is mushrooming, the pace of standards development has greatly accelerated to meet tight European community target dates for implementation of their directives, and Europe now has a dominant influence on the development of standards for all devices.

In this chapter we will review the changes at the FDA that created a much increased need for standards; then describe the structure of the main standards organizations that have an interest in defibrillator standards, that is, AAMI, IEC, and CENELEC; review the published standards that apply to conventional defibrillators, automatic defibrillators, and automatic implantable cardioverter-defibrillators (ICDs); and mention future defibrillator standards or related documents currently in development.

FDA'S MEDICAL DEVICE CLASSIFICATION AND NEED FOR STANDARDS

Since passage by Congress of the 1976 Medical Device Amendment to the Federal Food, Drug and Cosmetic Act, the FDA has regulated and monitored all medical devices made or used in the United States by means of an expanding number of rules and regulations that implement the 1976 act and the more recent "Safe Medical Devices Act of 1990." The first task of the FDA was to organize all medical devices into three classes. For that purpose expert panels were created for every general category of medical devices, for instance, cardiovascular devices. External defibrillators and external pacemakers were included in the cardiovascular therapeutic devices subcategory. The cardiovascular devices classification panel reviewed all cardiovascular devices and classified them in 1980 into three classes:

1. Class I General Controls: A device for which general controls (standards) are sufficient to provide reasonable assurance of safety and effectiveness, or a device that is not used in supporting or sustaining life and does not present a potential unreasonable risk of illness or injury.
2. Class II Performance Standards: A device for which general standards are insufficient to provide reasonable assurance of safety and effectiveness and for which there is sufficient information to establish a performance standard to provide such assurance. Class II devices must comply with performance standards (if they exist), require premarket notification applications (510K), and are subject to postmarket surveillance.
3. Class III Premarket Approval: A device that either
   a. cannot be classified as a Class II device because insufficient information exists to establish a performance standard to provide reasonable assurance of safety and effectiveness
   b. is used in supporting or sustaining life or in preventing impairment of human health, or presents a potential unreasonable risk of illness or injury.
   Class III devices are subject to premarket approval, based on submission to the FDA of considerable technical and clinical data for each specific device, to assure safety and effectiveness.

Of approximately 140 cardiovascular devices classified, only three belong to Class I, 25 belong to Class III (including external pacers and ICDs), and the vast majority belong to Class II "for which it is therefore necessary to establish a performance standard to provide reasonable assurance of the safety and effectiveness of the device." The secretary may by regulation establish a performance standard for a Class II device. The standard shall include the following provisions to provide reasonable assurance of its safe and effective performance when necessary for that purpose:

1. Provisions respecting the construction, components, and properties of the device and its compatibility with power systems.
2. Provisions for the testing of the device by a person at the direction of the secretary to verify compliance with the standard.
3. Provisions for the measurement of the performance characteristics of the device.

The secretary shall provide for periodic evaluation of performance standards to determine if the standard should be changed to reflect new medical, scientific, or technological data. Finally, in establishing performance standards for Class II devices, the secretary shall, to the maximum extent practicable:

1. Use personnel and technical support from other federal agencies.
2. Consult with nationally or internationally recognized standard-setting entities.

3. Invite appropriate participation by informed persons representative of scientific, professional, industrial, or consumer organizations.

With its long tradition and expertise in standards development for medical devices, AAMI was particularly well qualified to respond to the FDA's needs. AAMI has greatly stepped up its standards activity, both nationally since 1978 and internationally since the mid-1980s.

The classification of conventional defibrillators became a controversial issue, mostly because of concerns about the safety of defibrillators with high-delivered energy capability or with unusual waveforms. FDA's final decision was to classify into Class II defibrillators that deliver a maximum energy of 250 to 360 J into a 50 ohm load and have a discharge current waveform reasonably similar to those used in published clinical studies that demonstrated defibrillation efficacy, particularly studies by Crampton (damped sinusoidal waveforms, including "Lown" and "Edmark") and by Anderson (truncated exponential waveforms).

The FDA classified into Class III defibrillators capable of delivering more than 360 J into a 50 ohm load or defibrillators with waveforms that are markedly different from the accepted damped sinusoidal or truncated exponential waveforms and that are not supported by published clinical studies demonstrating efficacy and safety. The FDA noted however, that while enough data existed on which to base a standard for all commercially available defibrillation waveforms, future studies may show that waveforms not included in this group may be superior for safe and effective defibrillation. This is particularly important in view of the current interest in biphasic or triphasic waveforms, which are definitely outside the waveform envelope currently specified in the AAMI standard and accepted by the FDA.

External transcutaneous pacemakers were not commercially available and had only rare investigational use in 1980; consequently, they were classified into Class III. ICDs did not exist as commercial devices in 1980 and were not classified by the original FDA panel, but are Class III devices at present. FDA device classification is very important because a Class III classification requires premarket approval for the introduction of every new device. Premarket approvals are very complex and lengthy, require costly clinical investigations to establish safety and efficacy, and hence are a considerable deterrent to the development of new and improved devices. A Class II classification is much more efficient and encourages the development of new and improved devices. However, Class II devices presuppose the establishment of performance standards acceptable to the FDA. The FDA observed in 1985 that 475 medical devices had been placed in Class II, with an estimated 600 more to follow, and that its recent experience indicated that an average of 40 staff years over a period of 38 months was needed to develop and publish a standard. AAMI's past experience is similar, though there are now greater efforts to expedite the process. IEC has required significantly more time to develop an international standard in the past but is trying to expedite its work. It will be many years before the FDA is able to develop mandatory standards for all

Class II devices. In the meantime the FDA is developing a few critical standards (for example, for apnea monitors) and relies as much as possible on existing standards developed by various organizations, particularly AAMI and IEC.

Finally, the FDA's classification decisions are not immutable, and there is a process for classification changes where supported by new information. Development of a new standard for a Class III device may help justify its reclassification into Class II. Conversely, reclassification of a device from Class III to Class II may include a stipulation that the classification change shall not take effect until the effective date of an approved performance standard for that device.

AAMI/ANSI STANDARDS

The development of safety and performance standards is a major activity for AAMI, an international organization with approximately 6000 members. If approved as a new work item by the AAMI standards board, a vertical standard for a specific medical device is developed by a technical committee. For instance, the defibrillator standards committee of AAMI has been active since 1976. With the FDA's new responsibility for medical devices in 1976, and anticipating classification of defibrillators as Class II devices, AAMI recognized that a safety and performance standard for defibrillators would protect patients and would assist the FDA in discharging its regulatory responsibilities; therefore, AAMI volunteered to develop a defibrillator standard.

The main concern of AAMI is that the standard must clearly state essential but minimum requirements for safety and efficacy, while not imposing requirements that cannot be met by existing technology. It is important to understand clearly the meaning and rationale for "minimum" requirements for safety and efficacy. It is sometimes felt that standards should mandate the highest level of performance and safety that is technically feasible. However, ultimate performance and safety may be extremely costly to achieve, and medical devices will be most beneficial if they can be widely purchased and used by hospitals or physicians often on tight budgets. Therefore, a standard should not mandate ultimate requirements but only specify the minimum requirements that still assure the necessary safety and efficacy. This is often a judgment call that requires consensus in the committee writing the standard and general public approval in the public review process. An example will illustrate the rationale. The benefits of early defibrillation are now universally recognized; hence, the defibrillator charging time should be very short—the shorter the better. But a charging time of 1 or 2 seconds to 360 J would require very heavy and expensive circuitry; hence the AAMI/ANSI defibrillator standard requires that a defibrillator must charge to maximum energy within 15 seconds, even with low mains voltage or a partially depleted battery. Of course, manufacturers are encouraged to exceed the standards requirements whenever possible, and some defibrillators on the market charge to maximum energy within 5 seconds. Technical capability increases and cost may decrease with time, and physician and public expectations of needed safety and efficacy levels generally increase with time. Hence, AAMI policy requires that all existing standards be reviewed every 5 years, generally bringing additional or increased requirements.

To achieve the proper balance between medical concerns and technical constraints, the AAMI standards committees have two chairpersons, one from industry and the other a physician or university researcher, and the committee membership of about 30 represents a balance between representatives of major manufacturers and active clinicians, with a few biomedical or clinical engineers and FDA representatives also included to contribute their expertise. The standard progresses through a series of drafts that reflect consensus in the committee. A final draft is submitted to a vote of the committee, and all negative votes or comments must be addressed and resolved by the committee. The proposed standard is then subjected to public review. All criticisms or proposed changes emanating from the public review must be addressed and answered by the committee, often resulting in additional changes to the standard. The revised standard is then reviewed and approved by the AAMI Standards Board, then by ANSI, and is published as an American National Standard.

The first published defibrillator standard was the ANSI/AAMI standard for cardiac defibrillator devices DF2-1981, approved April 15, 1982, by ANSI. Examples of issues covered in the standard include range of delivered energy, pulse waveform into various impedance loads, allowed energy loss rate and automatic disarm, timing requirements for synchronized cardioversion, maximum allowed electrical risk currents, organization of controls, and information content of operator's and service manuals.

The purpose of the requirements is to ensure the level of safety and efficacy that the committee and particularly the physician members feel is necessary and achievable. For instance, the standard specifies that delivered energy must be selectable, with at least eight different values available, the lowest being 5 J or less and the highest being at least 250 J. If a defibrillator is capable of performing synchronized cardioversion, the standard places a tight timing requirement on the cardioverting pulse relative to the R wave to ensure that the discharge is not delivered during the heart's "vulnerable period" where the discharge may induce fibrillation, even for patients with ischemia or heart disease that may extend the duration of the vulnerable period. For automatic external defibrillators, the standard is particularly concerned with the accuracy and reliability of the ventricular fibrillation (VF) detection algorithm, requiring a sensitivity greater than 90% for coarse or medium VF, a sensitivity greater than 75% for shockable ventricular tachycardia, and a specificity greater than 95% for all nonshockable rhythms.

AAMI policy requires that all standards be reviewed every 5 years and reaffirmed, revised, or withdrawn. The 1981 defibrillator standard was reviewed in 1987, and substantial changes were made. The revised standard went through the same control and approval steps as the original standard, was approved by ANSI, and was published in 1989. Though it is not an official FDA or mandatory standard in the United States, it is widely used and accepted by defibrillator manufacturers, users, and regulators.

In 1984 AAMI felt that automatic or advisory external defibrillators, capable of analyzing the ECG and recognizing VF, were achieving increasing acceptance and one could anticipate their widespread use by first responders or possibly at home. It also seemed that the technology of AEDs was still rapidly evolving so that development of a standard would be premature. In the interim AAMI published a technical information report: AAMI TIR2-1987: "Design, testing and reporting performance results of automatic external defibrillators." Subsequently, AAMI judged that a standard was now timely for AEDs. The AAMI Defibrillator Committee now has a final draft of a proposed standard: "Automatic external defibrillators and remote-control defibrillators" ready for final approval by ANSI. This will likely result in a published AAMI/ANSI standard in late 1993 or early 1994.

IEC STANDARDS

The IEC is an international organization devoted to the development of international standards for electrical products. Technical Committee 62 (TC 62) of IEC is specifically responsible for electromedical devices and in turn supervises four subcommittees:

- SC 62A is responsible for "horizontal" standards applicable to all electromedical devices, with a particular emphasis on safety rather than performance. The main general standard developed by SC 62A is IEC 601-1 (2nd edition, 1988).
- SC 62B is responsible for vertical standards for imaging medical devices (for example, CT scanners, MRIs).
- SC 62C is responsible for vertical standards for particle accelerators used in radiation therapy.
- SC 62D is responsible for vertical standards for most diagnostic, monitoring, and therapeutic devices, including defibrillators. The main defibrillator standard developed by SC 62D is IEC 601-2-4, published in 1983.

The process for development and approval of IEC standards is complex and reflects a compromise between eliciting active participation of many countries in the development of international standards and preserving the right of individual countries to modify these standards to accommodate the particular laws, requirements, or philosophy of an individual country.

Within each TC 62 subcommittee, working groups have been appointed to develop specific standards. At all levels IEC is an international organization with delegates from many countries; for instance, a recent meeting of SC 62D in Germany was attended by 35 delegates from 18 countries, with several delegates from major countries such as the United States or Germany. U.S. delegates to IEC committees and working groups are approved by ANSI.

A proposal from a national group usually forms the starting point for the development of a standard by a working group. After several successive reviews a "committee draft" is circulated for consensus position statements and comments by national groups (e.g., U.S. national responses are coordinated by AAMI for SC 62D or Health Industry Manufacturers Association [HIMA] for SC 62A, with approval from ANSI); a final draft is reached that becomes a draft international standard (DIS) submitted to a vote by all participating members of the Technical Committee and by the general ISO membership. A two-thirds majority of affirmative votes is required for final approval of an IEC standard.

A serious limitation of IEC international standards is that individual countries, even if they voted affirmatively on the IEC standard, remain free to change the standard and to adopt national standards that differ from the IEC standard and do so not infrequently. Still, the national differences are often small, and an effort is made to harmonize national standards with the IEC international standards. For instance, following publication of IEC 601-2-4 for defibrillators, the AAMI Defibrillator Committee made a serious effort during its revision of the 1981 AAMI defibrillator standard to remove conflicting requirements between the AAMI and IEC standards and succeeded in doing so in 90% of the cases in its 1989 revision. Similarly the Canadian CSA national defibrillator standard No. 601.2.4-M90, published in 1990, was essentially based on the IEC 601-2-4 defibrillator standard, with minor additions or changes inspired by the AAMI 1989 standard.

The horizontal and vertical IEC standards that apply to defibrillators are as follows:

- IEC 601-1 "Safety of Medical Electrical Equipment—Part 1: General Requirements," 2nd edition, 1988, and 1st amendment to 2nd edition, 1991. This is a general or "product family" standard that covers a broad range of medical devices and is expected to be complemented by Part 2 vertical standards for specific devices.
- IEC 601-2-4 "Medical Electrical Equipment—Part 2: Particular Requirements for the Safety of Cardiac Defibrillators and Cardiac Defibrillator Monitors," 1st edition, 1983. This is a vertical standard for defibrillators, using 601-1 as a reference.

In addition, SC 62A is working on several horizontal standards collateral to 601-1 that apply to all electromedical devices, including defibrillators. The most advanced of these is the IEC 601-1-2 "Medical Electrical Equipment—collateral standard (to 601-1) on electromagnetic compatibility requirements and tests," now an approved final standard published in February 1993.

Another horizontal standard being developed by TC 62 would require that a formal and comprehensive hazard analysis be made for both software and hardware of any new product, so that every possible hardware or software failure would be identified and its possible consequences analyzed, with particular emphasis on software critical to safety.

A recent horizontal safety standard applicable to ICDs is ISO/DIS 11318 "Implants for Surgery—Cardiac Defibrillators—DF-1: Dimensional and test requirements for a connector assembly for implantable defibrillators." The purpose of this standard is to provide interchangeability between implantable defibrillator leads and defibrillator pulse generators from different manufacturers.

The main purpose of standards is to specify requirements that manufacturers must meet in the design and manufacture of medical devices. However, several studies directed by the FDA have clearly shown that a majority of defibrillator malfunctions were caused by insufficient operator training or understanding of the instrument, by faulty operation of the instrument, by failure to test the defibrillator periodically, or by insufficient or faulty maintenance.

Hence there is a great concern that issues of operator training and instrument maintenance be properly addressed. The IEC (SC 62A) is in the final stage of developing and issuing two companion reports:

- 62A (Sec) 119 Operation of cardiac defibrillators and defibrillator monitors.
- 62A (Sec) 120 Maintenance of cardiac defibrillators and defibrillator monitors.

Similar concerns in the United States led the American Society for Testing and Materials (ASTM) to publish in 1990 two ASTM standards:

- F1254-90 Standard Practice for the Performance of Prehospital Manual Defibrillation.
- F1255-90 Standard Practice for the Performance of Prehospital Automated Defibrillation.

The FDA is also very concerned with operator training and defibrillator checkout testing and maintenance for all types of defibrillators and those for both hospital and prehospital use. The FDA has conducted studies to assess possible problems and explore corrective action and may publish guidelines for efficient operator training and skills maintenance, as well as effective maintenance programs.

At least until 1992, IEC/TC 62 and its subcommittees SC 62A and SC 62D have concentrated their efforts on developing safety standards that emphasize electrical safety issues rather than performance or efficacy requirements. As stated previously, the FDA Medical Devices Amendment of 1976 to a large extent drives the development of standards in the United States and calls for both safety and efficacy to be addressed. For example, an ANSI/AAMI standard may be harmonized with an IEC standard on all electrical safety requirements but may also cover in its scope other requirements not addressed by the IEC standard. With the advent of EC 92, efficacy and performance issues have gained increasing importance. As a result the IEC/TC 62 and its subcommittees are becoming more active in setting "functional safety" (i.e., performance and efficacy) requirements and standards.

EUROPEAN NORMS AND CENELEC

The "European Medical Devices Directive" was adopted in June 1993 by the European Council of Ministers. "Harmonized European standards" will be needed to establish compliance with the "essential requirements" of the directive relating to the safety of medical devices. CEN and CENELEC are the European counterparts of the international organizations ISO and IEC. CENELEC is expected to rely as much as possible on existing IEC international standards to verify compliance with the European directive. In fact, CENELEC has a technical committee 62 that is the counterpart of IEC/TC 62, and major IEC standards have been adopted as European norms (EN) or "harmonized European standards." For instance, IEC 601-1, 2nd edition, 1988, was adopted by CENELEC as EN 60601-1, and IEC 601-2-4, 1st edition, 1983, was adopted by CENELEC as IID395.2.4.S1 in 1988.

An important difference is that national standards bodies are not obliged to adopt IEC international standards as national standards without change. However, the integration of Europe under EC 92 mandates that harmonized European standards must be adopted without change by all European countries, so that compliance with a single set of European standards becomes a precondition for the sale of any medical device, including those that are American or Japanese manufactured, in all European countries. Hence, European standards will tend to take precedence over international or American standards when EC 92 becomes a reality.

Just as fulfillment of the FDA's obligations under the Medical Device Amendment of 1976 requires eventual development of safety and performance standards for a large number of medical devices, similarly implementation of the European Directive Concerning Medical Devices will require development by CENELEC, in collaboration with IEC, of many new safety and also performance ("functional safety") standards, and these standards will have greater force than current international standards.

DEFIBRILLATOR STANDARDS PUBLISHED OR IN DRAFT FORM

CONVENTIONAL DEFIBRILLATORS

- American National Standard ANSI/AAMI DF2-1989 (second edition, revision of ANSI/AAMI DF2-1981) safety and performance standard: "Cardiac Defibrillator Devices."
- International Standard IEC 601-2-4, 1983 "Medical Electrical Equipment,

Part 2: Particular Requirements for the Safety of Cardiac Defibrillators and Cardiac Defibrillator/Monitors."
- European Standard HD395.2.4S1, 1988. Based on IEC 601-2-4.
- Canadian National Standard CAN/CSA C22.2 No. 601.2.4-M90, 1990 "Medical Electrical Equipment, Part 2: Particular Requirements for the Safety of Cardiac Defibrillators and Cardiac Defibrillator/Monitors." Based primarily on IEC 601-24, with some additions derived from ANSI/AAMI DF2-1989.

The conventional defibrillator standards just listed have clearly had a very positive impact on the safety, quality, and performance of defibrillators presently on the market. They have also increased ease of use and reduced operator errors. Hence, the public has been well served.

AUTOMATIC EXTERNAL OR REMOTE-CONTROL DEFIBRILLATORS

The ANSI/AAMI draft standard only requires ANSI final approval and will be published late 1993 or early 1994. This safety and performance standard also covers external pacers.

AUTOMATIC IMPLANTABLE CARDIOVERTER-DEFIBRILLATORS

ISO/DIS 11318 Draft International Standard: "Implants for Surgery—Cardiac Defibrillators DF-1 Dimensional and Test Requirements for a Connector Assembly for Implantable Defibrillators."

The technology of ICDs has progressed sufficiently, and their use has increased so rapidly (approximately 30,000 ICDs implanted to date) that a safety and performance standard for ICDs would be very useful. Though proposals are being considered, there is not yet an active project for development of an ICD standard.

Index

Index